THE
GERSON
THERAPY

THE
GERSON
THERAPY

The Proven Nutritional Program
for Cancer and Other Illnesses

REVISED AND UPDATED

CHARLOTTE GERSON AND
MORTON WALKER, D.P.M.

Kensington Books
http://www.kensingtonbooks.com

Kensington Publishing Corp.
850 Third Avenue
New York, NY 10022

All Kensington titles, imprints and distributed lines are available at special quantity discounts for bulk purchases for sales promotion, premiums, fund-raising, educational or institutional use.

Special book excerpts or customized printings can also be created to fit specific needs. For details, write or phone the office of the Kensington Special Sales Manager: Kensington Publishing Corp., 850 Third Avenue, New York, NY 10022. Attn: Special Sales Department. Phone: 1-800-221-2647.

Kensington and the K logo Reg. U.S. Pat. & TM Off.

ISBN 1-57566-628-6

First Trade Printing: October 2001
Revised and Updated Trade Paperback Printing: June 2006
20 19 18 17

Printed in the United States of America

Authors' Disclaimer

The Gerson Therapy is a registered service mark (trademark) of the Gerson Institute, Post Office Box 430, Bonita, California 91908-0430.

This book has been written and published strictly for informational purposes, and in no way should be used as a substitute for advice from your own health care professional. Therefore, you must not consider educational material found here as a replacement for consultation with oncologists, cardiovascular disease specialists, endocrinologists, and other types of medical practitioners.

Most of the information in this book comes from the procedures perfected and utilized by Max Gerson, M.D., as described in the original 1958 edition of his book *A Cancer Therapy: Results of Fifty Cases*. Such procedures were developed and put into practice from findings he uncovered during a thirty-year period preceding the publication of this landmark text.

Inasmuch as Dr. Gerson's 1958 publication had focused on the reversal of cancer, another book needed to be written. That's because Dr. Gerson realized early on that the Gerson Therapy employed for curing cancer works equally well as corrective treatment for nearly all other acute and chronic degenerative diseases that have been labeled "incurable." As will be learned from reading our text, what had in the past been thought "incurable" is curable.

Derived from several sources other than the first through sixth editions of *A Cancer Therapy: Results of Fifty Cases,* our new book offers a great deal of additional information. It comes from interviews with informed health care personnel who have monitored patients' progress by their use of laboratory tests and clinical examinations. Also for our readers' education, numerous patients who have experienced either low levels of wellness, subclinical illness, or outright life-threatening disease tell their stories. All the patient case histories are true, and in most instances, unless indicated as a pseudonym, the identities of patients are given.

These patients discuss their illnesses, and the alternative/complementary medical approach they used to overcome them permanently.

Although every word published here about the Gerson Therapy is documented by case studies, this book's coauthors and publisher are providing educational material and nothing more.

If information gleaned from these pages raises questions about your own or a loved one's medical condition, you should contact the Gerson Institute directly for a list of Gerson-approved health care practitioners.

Please take the above message as a disavowal of all responsibility by the authors, publisher, the Gerson Institute, listed organizations, and product or services suppliers for any practice, procedure, diagnostic technique, nutritional supplement, food, utensil, or other item mentioned in the text. Information taken from this book and acted upon by a reader or other interested parties is carried out at that individual's personal risk.

For the best information about the Gerson Therapy, please contact the nonprofit Gerson Institute.

To Max Gerson, M.D., who,
for having developed viable therapies for the permanent remission of
cancer, was challenged by individual interests in the cancer industry
because, by application of the Gerson Therapy, these interests would be
put out of business. Today, nearly half a century later, such legitimized
interests continue to flourish at the expense of ill people around the world.

Contents

About the Authors

Charlotte Gerson, the youngest daughter of Max Gerson, M.D., whom he lovingly addressed as "Lotte," was an assistant for her father in his work on an almost continuous basis. In the first edition of his book A *Cancer Therapy: Results of Fifty Cases*, Dr. Gerson thanked her for giving help "wherever she could with great interest and understanding encouragement."

Charlotte Gerson was born in Germany and underwent her early schooling there. When her family fled from Germany to Austria as a means of escaping what became the holocaust, Lotte attended school in a suburb of Vienna. Later, upon her father's moving the Gerson family to France, which he considered safer, she studied French and continued high school under the French educational system. Dr. Gerson practiced medicine in France for only a short period under the licensure of another physician.

Next, the Gersons emigrated to England to escape domination by the French Vichy government. Lotte continued school for a short time in London, where she started to learn English. She received her high school diploma in New York City, where the Gerson family finally felt safe and could settle down. Eventually Dr. Gerson established his medical practice on Park Avenue in Manhattan and at a clinic in Nanuet, a small town located between Suffern and Nyack in upstate New York.

The young woman attended Smith College. She is literate in Spanish, which stands her in good stead since the Gerson Therapy was for close to twenty-five years primarily administered in Tijuana, Mexico, just across the border from San Diego, California.

Charlotte Gerson visits patients who are currently receiving medically supervised Gerson Therapy at the Gerson Therapy Hospital. She consults with these patients' doctors, studies their progress toward health, answers many questions from the patients and their companions, lectures on the intricacies of the Gerson Therapy, and offers everyone encouragement.

This charitable and humanitarian effort is natural for Charlotte Gerson, for she was always interested in her father's work. Even as a young woman her greatest joy involved reading medical literature. She spent much of her free time assisting Dr. Gerson by translating and writing his papers. She listened to and critiqued his lectures to health professionals and medical consumers. Often Charlotte made hospital rounds with her father and acted as one of the medical assistants at his Oakland Manor Cancer Clinic in Nanuet, New York.

In fact, to become a more valuable aide, Charlotte enrolled in and completed a formal course for medical assistants, which qualified her to help in patient nursing work at the Gerson clinic. When Dr. Gerson was absent lecturing, consulting, or on vacation, she carried out his telephoned instructions regarding the clinic's patients.

After the young woman married and became Charlotte Gerson Straus, she spent a number of years in her husband's import/export enterprise, which caused her to become familiar with many business techniques. However, the marriage eventually ended in divorce.

When Dr. Gerson died in 1959, Charlotte carried on by publicizing his last, classic book, A Cancer Therapy: Results of Fifty Cases. From public demand and the need to dispose of three thousand copies, she proceeded to lecture on the Gerson Therapy. Such lecturing, locally at first and later nationally, was what gained initial broad distribution for the Gerson title and its healing program.

As a result, Charlotte Gerson has been invited to speak on the Gerson Therapy at several hundred organizations involved with aspects of health. A few of them include:

- The Cancer Control Society—every year for twenty-five years—in two California locations, Pasadena and Los Angeles
- The National Health Federation—eighteen locations around the United States.
- The Alternative and Complementary Therapies Convention in Arlington, Virginia, put on by the clinical journal publishing house Mary Ann Liebert, Inc., of Larchmont, New York
- International Association of Cancer Victors and Friends—ten cities

- Consumer Health Organization of Canada—Toronto, Ontario, Canada
- Australian Health Groups—Sydney, Melbourne, Brisbane, and the Gold Coast
- "Fit fuers Leben" (Fit for Life)—Waldthausen Verlag, Munich and Bonn
- The Municipal Hospital—Graz, Austria
- The Gerson Support Group—London, England
- Wirral Health Clinic—Manchester, England
- Gerson Practitioners Training groups—San Diego, California, and Sedona, Arizona

Moreover, Charlotte Gerson gives numerous seminars at conventions organized by the Gerson Institute that are held periodically in many of the important cities around the United States and Canada, including Honolulu, Hawaii; and Montreal, Toronto, Ottawa, Calgary, Edmonton, Victoria, and Vancouver, Canada.

The Gerson Therapy message has been carried to people on numerous television shows, including twice on Oprah Winfrey's programs in Baltimore and Chicago, before Oprah joined her national TV network. Charlotte Gerson has appeared on Christian Broadcasting, Trinity Broadcasting, PBS, cable stations, and national radio. For example, she is interviewed frequently by Gary Null, on WBAI, by the syndicated radio columnist Dr. James Winer, and for magazine articles.

With an associate in 1977, she supervised the establishment of the first Gerson Therapy hospital in Tijuana, Mexico. Her specific goal then, as it is now, was applying and teaching the Gerson Therapy to everyone interested in surviving life-threatening diseases.

To accomplish her task, she helps to train physicians, nurses, kitchen staff, and patients, and others so that they learn the elements of nutritional treatment. Some one hundred holistic physicians in the United States and many more located around the world have been trained by Charlotte Gerson and the Gerson Institute to practice the Gerson Therapy as the health professionals' medical tool to reverse degenerative diseases.

This woman, who seems to have no shortage of energy, teaches, coaches, and trains the Mexican hospital nursing staff, the kitchen staff, the receptionists who respond to potential patients' questions, and even the hospital's passenger van drivers. For the past five years she has written most of the news articles for the bimonthly *Gerson Healing News-*

letter, and she has created many articles for publication in health magazines.

Her stamina and capacity to perform are not Charlotte Gerson's only amazing characteristics. At age seventy-nine, she looks like a much younger woman. By faithfully following the Gerson Therapy program for prevention, Charlotte never needed to wear eyeglasses or contact lenses, has all of her own teeth, exhibits absolutely no liver spots (age spots), suffers from no arthritis or osteoporosis, and shows a smooth, unblemished complexion. Because she refuses to use hair dye or any other kind of cosmetic, the hair on her head is white, her skin appears fair and alabaster, her body remains strong and well proportioned, and her mind stays acutely sharp. Charlotte Gerson gracefully grows older, but she is a true reflection of her father's medical philosophy.

Morton Walker, D.P.M., a former practicing doctor of podiatric medicine for seventeen years, has for the last thirty years worked full-time as a professional freelance medical journalist. He has had seventy-three books issued by major trade publishers, including Bantam Books, Simon & Schuster, Prentice Hall, Kensington Books, Avery, G. P. Putnam's Sons, E .P. Dutton, Macmillan, M. Evans, Keats, Arco, Devin-Adair, Hampton Roads, and more. Twelve of his book titles have become 150,000- to 2,000,000-copy best-sellers.

Dr. Walker has produced 2,250 clinical journal or magazine articles for about fifty periodicals, including monthly columns for *Health Products Business, Townsend Letter for Doctors & Patients, Healthy & Natural, Nutrition Science News, Explore Professional Journal*, a British magazine, and two Australian magazines. His works have been reprinted in eleven languages in thirty-nine countries, and the numbers continue to grow.

The result is that twenty-three medical journalism awards and medals have come his way. Dr. Walker was recognized with the 1992 Humanitarian Award from the American Cancer Control Society, which named him "the world's leading medical journalist specializing in holistic medicine."

He received the 1981 Orthomolecular Award from the American Institute of Preventive Medicine for his "outstanding achievement in orthomolecular education."

Dr. Walker was presented with the 1979 Humanitarian Award from the 1,250 physician members of the American College for Advancement in

Medicine "for informing the American public on alternative methods of healing."

And he has received two prestigious Jesse H. Neal Editorial Achievement Awards from the American Business Press, Inc., for creating the best series of magazine articles published in any audited United States magazine in both 1975 and 1976.

As a medical journalist who researches and writes exclusively in the areas of holistic medicine and alternative healing methods, Dr. Morton Walker has been highlighted by, or appeared as a guest with, Oprah Winfrey, Jay Leno, Sally Jessy Raphael, Merv Griffin, Mike Douglas, and Regis Philbin and Kathie Lee Gifford, plus several dozen other television talk show hosts—a minimum of two thousand media appearances. For example, discussing his book *The Power of Color* (Avery Publishing Group), he recently was featured on the early morning *NBC's Today* show. Avery Publishing has given him his own imprint (subdivision) with the title "A Dr. Morton Walker Health Book," and this publisher has issued twelve of his books under that imprint.

Preface

Dr. Max Gerson dedicated his life to the mastery of this scourge
of cancer and all should honor his great work.
—The Honorable United States Senator
Claude Pepper (D-Florida)

This book offers readers a documented means for reversing the pathology of nearly any illness, whether acute or chronic, when its occurrence is related to malfunctioning of the immune system or essential organs. Our reader must be warned, however, that the Gerson program is stringent and difficult to follow. Assuredly it can save the life of a terminal patient. However, the menu plan is quite work-intensive and not easily acceptable to friends and acquaintances who aren't oriented to holistic health and alternative methods of healing.

The Gerson Therapy is a natural contemporary, biological treatment, either self-administered at home or under physician supervision, which uses the body's own healing mechanisms for the elimination of debilitating ailments. It was introduced to Western industrialized nations more than sixty years ago by Max Gerson, M.D. (1881–1959). This revolutionary dietary program was so far advanced at the time of its development that no scientific rationale was available to explain why it produced reversal of chronic and infectious diseases. But because it actually cured patients with advanced tuberculosis, diabetes, migraines, heart disease, cancer, arthritis, skin disorders, and numerous other life-threatening conditions, the Gerson Therapy has long since established itself as a major contributor to the medical armamentarium.

Dr. Max Gerson treated many hundreds of patients and continued to refine his therapy until he died in 1959, at the age of seventy-eight. His most famous patient was medical missionary and philosopher Albert Schweitzer, M.D., whom he cured of adult-onset diabetes when Dr.

Schweitzer was seventy-five years old. Completely well after only six weeks of Dr. Gerson's therapy, the patient returned to Lambaréné in Gabon, French Equatorial Africa. Dr. Schweitzer ministered to many thousands of African patients, won the 1952 Nobel Peace Prize, and worked past age ninety. With diabetes eliminated from his life, Albert Schweitzer lived to be ninety-three years old.

Incidentally, Dr. Gerson successfully cured lung tuberculosis for Dr. Schweitzer's dying wife, Helene. She went on to live another twenty-eight years. And he healed a serious skin disease for Dr. Schweitzer's nineteen-year-old daughter, Rhena. Lotte Gerson and Rhena Schweitzer were friends during their teen years.

As the eulogy for his close personal friend, Dr. Albert Schweitzer wrote in sadness: "I see in Dr. Max Gerson one of the most eminent geniuses in the history of medicine. Many of his basic ideas have been adopted without having his name connected with them. He has achieved more than seemed possible under adverse conditions. He leaves a legacy which commands attention and which will assure him his due place. Those whom he cured will now attest to the truth of his ideas."

The most complete presentation of the Gerson Therapy program is currently found in Dr. Gerson's book A *Cancer Therapy: Results of Fifty Cases*, originally published by him in 1958, the year before his death. It has since been reprinted thirty-eight times with over 250,000 copies in English. These were distributed by Dr. Gerson's daughter, Charlotte (Lotte) Gerson, as well as by the Gerson Institute. Some 88,000 additional copies were printed in four other languages and dispersed around the world.

Represented by the Gerson Institute, Charlotte has carried on her father's educational work and promoted his treatment protocol for eliminating chronic diseases of all types, in particular against malignancies.[1] The book you are reading now expands upon that prior book written by Max Gerson, M.D.

MAX GERSON TESTIFIES BEFORE SENATE

During a three-day period, July 1 to 3, 1946, the United States Senate took testimony from nationally known cancer researchers relating to U.S. Senate Bill 1875, also referred to as the *Pepper-Neely anticancer proposal*. In this bill, Senators Pepper and Neely recommended the appropriation of $100 million from the U.S. government's budget for cancer researchers to find a cure for cancer once and for all.

After his two Washington, D.C.–based investigators, a physician and an attorney, reported back to Senator Claude Pepper (D-Florida) that Dr. Max Gerson did, indeed, have a successful treatment for cancer for the first time in history, the United States Senate invited a medical doctor to demonstrate his specific therapeutic approach for curing cancer. Accordingly, Dr. Gerson brought five of his cured cancer patients and the records of five more for presentation before the Pepper-Neely anticancer subcommittee of the Senate Committee on Foreign Relations of the Seventy-ninth Congress.

The impressive testimony of this anticancer specialist and his patients caused Senator Pepper to call a press conference for bringing information about the Gerson Therapy before the media. However, massive numbers of lobbyists for the immensely wealthy Pharmaceutical Manufacturers' Association (PMA), the American Medical Association (AMA), and the American Cancer Society (ACS) prevailed on reporters to ignore the Gerson press conference and attend a cocktail party instead where free food would be served and libations would be flowing. The only reporter who preferred to hear the Gerson presentation was American Broadcasting Corporation newscaster Raymond Gram Swing. During World War II, Mr. Swing had been a famous war correspondent on a par with Edward R. Murrow. He attended and took copious notes at the Senate press conference for use in his East Coast 6:00 P.M. ABC network broadcast of Wednesday, July 3, 1946. Here is what Raymond Gram Swing broadcast then throughout the United States:

> I hope I have my values right if, instead of talking tonight about the agreement reached on Trieste by the Foreign Minister in Paris, or the continuing crisis of the OPA in Washington, or President Truman's signing of the Hobbs antiracketeering bill, I talk about a remarkable hearing before a Senate Subcommittee in Washington yesterday on cancer and the need for cancer research in new fields.
>
> . . . A bill is before Congress, the Pepper-Neely bill, to appropriate a hundred million dollars for cancer research with something like the zeal and bigness with which it went for the release of atomic energy, turning the job over to the scientists with resources generous enough to solve the problem.
>
> This alone would make a good theme for a broadcast, just an example of the use a great democracy can make of its intelligence and wealth. But the subject has been made peculiarly gripping by unprecedented happenings yesterday before the subcommittee which is holding hearings on this bill, and of which Senator Pepper is chairman.

He invited a witness, a refugee scientist, now a resident of New York, Dr. Max Gerson, and Dr. Gerson placed on the stand, in quick succession, five patients. They were chosen to represent the principal prevailing types of cancer, and in each instance they showed that the Gerson treatment had had what is conservatively called "favorable effect on the course of the disease." That in itself is remarkable, but it is the more so because Dr. Gerson's treatment consists mainly of a diet which he has evolved after a lifetime of research and experimentation. To say that Dr. Gerson has been curing cancer by a dietary treatment is medically impermissible, for the reason that there must be five years without recurrence before such a statement is allowed. Dr. Gerson has cured tuberculosis and other illnesses with his diet, but in the U.S.A. he has only been working on cancer for four and a half years. . . .

Yet anything that offers even a possibility of treating successfully at least some of the four hundred thousand existing cancer cases in this country is stirring news, no matter how conservatively it is formulated. There would be no Pepper-Neely bill to appropriate a hundred million dollars for cancer research if the existing research were coping with the need.

. . . I have spoken about this carefully and abstractly, which underplays some of the shock and delight of the experience yesterday at the hearing of the Pepper Committee. It is one thing to talk about chemistry and diet and vitamins and other factors in medical science. It is another to see, as the Committee yesterday saw, a seventeen-year-old girl, who had a tumor at the base of the brain, which was inoperable, and which had paralyzed her. Yesteday, she walked without assistance to the witness chair, and told clearly about her case and her treatment.

There was a sturdy man, who had been a sergeant in the army. He had had a malignant tumor, also at the base of the brain, which had been operated on but needed deep X-ray treatment, and this he could not receive because of the danger to the brain. Yesterday he was the picture of health as he testified, and quite naturally he was proud of his remarkable recovery.

There was a woman who had had cancer of the breast which spread. Yesterday she was well, and testified with poise and confidence.

A few cases showing such improvement cannot, of themselves, affect the outlook of the medical profession. But they are attested facts and not flukes, and as such they have to be accounted for. And there are many, many more cases which could have been cited.

It would seem to be the business of medical research to leap on such facts and carry every hopeful indication to a final conclusion. . . .

So the advocates for the Pepper-Neely bill can argue that, unless we learn now how to deal successfully with cancer, many millions of persons now living in this country are condemned to die from cancer. A hundred million dollars is little more than a token payment for America to make, in order to avert such a sweep of death, and they can then point to the Gerson dietary approach as a most promising field of research. . . .

Dr. Gerson was an eminent if controversial figure in pre-Hitler Germany. He was bound to be controversial because he was challenging established practice in treating tuberculosis by diet. He has been assistant to Foerster, the great neurologist of Breslau, and for years assistant to Sauerbruch, one of the great physicians on the Continent. The Sauerbruch-Gerson diet for skin tuberculosis is well-known to European medicine, and the account of it is part of accepted medical literature. Dr. Gerson told the Pepper Committee that he had first come upon his dietary theory in trying to cure himself of migraine headaches. Later he treated others, among them a man with skin tuberculosis as well. Dr. Gerson was an acknowledged dietary authority in Weimar, Germany, and was responsible for the German army of his time being placed on dehydrated, rather than canned food.[2]

PUBLIC RESPONSE TO THE BROADCAST

Raymond Gram Swing continued with his network radio broadcast and brought in some additional news too. After he ended, the telephone switchboard lit up at the American Broadcasting Corporation in New York City. People called in from all over the nation to learn about the Gerson Therapy. But other, darker, more powerful commercial and political forces had been listening as well.

The executive directors of pharmaceutical companies producing cytotoxic agents for cancer treatment—members of the PMA—threatened to cancel all radio advertising contracts for their drugs sold over the counter, an annual loss in revenue for ABC amounting to tens of millions of dollars. Within two weeks of that fateful radio broadcast which apprised people of a potential cure for cancer, after thirty years at the same job Raymond Gram Swing was fired from his position as a newscaster for the ABC network.

You might also wish to know what happened to the Senate's 227-page Pepper-Neely anticancer bill of 1946—Document No. 89471. By efforts of the lobbyists working with four senators who were also medical doctors, the bill was defeated. Today, Document No. 89471 is stored in boxes and gathers dust in the archives of the U.S. Government Printing Office.

Meanwhile, since the Pepper-Neely bill was buried, the number of people getting cancer each year has worsened beyond what anyone could have predicted. According to Reno, Nevada, oncologist, homeopath, and internal medicine specialist W. Douglas Brodie, M.D., H.M.D., in his book *Cancer and Common Sense*, the annual incidence of cancer has increased from 402,000 in 1946 to 1.9 million in 1996.[3] Thus, during a half century since the defeat of Senator Pepper's proposed anticancer legislation, the yearly occurrence of cancer among the American populace has more than quadrupled.[4] Worse still, medical journalist and author Michael Culbert points out even more graphically that at the stroke of midnight, upon our ringing in the twenty-first century, every forty-five seconds thereafter a U.S. citizen is destined to die from cancer. That number adds up to about 1,900 Americans per day.[5]

Oncologists informed about nutrition estimate that diets filled with fruits and vegetables instead of fats and animal proteins—along with taking greater amounts of exercise, more stringent weight control, and avoidance of cigarette smoke—could reduce cancer incidence by up to 40 percent. This program would amount to nearly 4 million fewer worldwide cases of malignancies per year.

Thus, dietary and lifestyle improvements among Americans as advocated by Dr. Max Gerson more than fifty years ago would be particularly effective as the means to prevent occurrence of the four most frequently occurring life-threatening malignancies in the United States. According to the November 30, 1998, issue of *Newsweek* magazine:[6]

1. *Prostate cancer* strikes with a minimum of 184,500 cases predicted in 1999. Among American men today, 17 percent will be diagnosed with prostate cancer during their lifetimes. But improved diet, nutrition, and general lifestyle would reduce that proportion to 13.6 percent.

2. *Breast cancer* hits with a minimum of 180,300 cases estimated for 1999. Among American women today, 14 percent will be diagnosed with breast cancer during their lifetimes. But improved diet, nutrition, and general lifestyle would reduce that proportion to 7 percent.

3. *Lung cancer* happens with a minimum of 171,500 cases anticipated for 1999. Among everyone in this country today, slightly more than 7 percent will be diagnosed with lung cancer during their lifetimes. Still, improved diet, nutrition, and general lifestyle (especially eliminating exposure to tobacco smoke) would lower that proportion to just 0.35 percent.

4. *Colon/rectal cancer* shows up with a minimum of 95,600 cases expected in 1999. Among the populace of the United States, 6 percent will be diagnosed with colon and/or rectal cancers during their lifetimes. But improved diet, nutrition, and general lifestyle could reduce that proportion to 1.5 percent.

"In spite of all the advances in chemotherapy and surgery," report officials of First Circle Medical, Inc., of Minneapolis, Minnesota, a main manufacturer of antimalignancy hyperthermia equipment, "over 1,800,000 patients in North America, Europe and Japan with disseminated lung, prostate, breast [cancer] and melanoma die each year."

As you read our book, three questions you may understandably raise are:

- Why didn't the U.S. Senate over half a century ago adopt the anticancer budgetary measure that came before it?
- Wasn't the prevention of or treatment for Americans coming down with cancer vital enough?
- Why weren't anticancer experts requested to at least test the Gerson Therapy back then when senators were presented with the opportunity?

Finally, are you aware of the following additional, significant, estimated statistic? Averaging between the numbers of United States residents getting cancer in 1946 and those so victimized this year, it's likely that 39,697,000 Americans could have been prevented from contracting the scourge or saved from cancerous deaths. Application of the Gerson Therapy may have accomplished that particular worthy undertaking. It can do it even now.

CHARLOTTE GERSON
Bonita, California
MORTON WALKER, D.P.M.
Stamford, Connecticut

References for the Preface

1. Gerson, M. A *Cancer Therapy: Results of Fifty Cases*, 6th ed. Bonita, Calif.: The Gerson Institute, 1999.

2. Quoted in Dego, G. *Doctor Max: The Story of Pioneering Physician Max Gerson's Acclaimed Cancer Therapy and His Heroic Struggle to Change the*

Way We Look at Health and Healing. Barrytown, N.Y.: Station Hill Press, 1997, pp. 513–516.

3. Brodie, W. D. *Cancer and Common Sense: Combining Science and Nature to Control Cancer.* White Bear Lake, Minn.: Winning Publications, August 1997, p. 46.

4. Rugo, H.S. "Cancer." In *Current Medical Diagnosis and Treatment 1997,* 36th ed., ed. by L.M. Tierney, S.J. McPhee, and M.A. Papadakis. Stamford, Conn.: Appleton and Lange, 1997, p. 69.

5. Culbert, M. *Medical Armageddon.* San Diego, Calif.: C and C Communications, 1995.

6. Cowley, G., with Underwood, A., Springen, K., and Davis, A. "Cancer and diet: eating to beat the odds: what you need to know." *Newsweek,* November 30, 1998, pp. 60–66.

INTRODUCTION

The chief of medical oncology at the Strang Cancer Prevention Center in New York City, Mitchell Gaynor, M.D., understood a lot about cancer when he finished his cancer specialty training at Cornell Medical Center, but he admits to knowing little about diet, nutrition, and their significance for preventing and treating degenerative diseases. Cancer, a specific cluster of body cells undergoing uncontrolled cell division and multiplication, is the ultimate example of a degenerative disease in progress.

Dr. Gaynor was flabbergasted when he showed up at the prestigious Rockefeller University in 1986, for a postdoctoral fellowship in molecular biology, and found his more enlightened oncology colleagues buzzing about the cancer-inhibiting qualities of brussels sprouts, cauliflower, cabbage, and certain other cruciferous vegetables rich in the chemical called sulforaphane. Sulforaphane boosts production of the body's phase II enzymes that cart off dangerous residues of procarcinogens, those cancer-causing precursors capable of damaging cellular DNA (see chapter 3 for details).

During that 1986 period, laboratory researchers had started discovering dozens of new chemicals in common fruits and vegetables. In test tube and animal studies, these obscure compounds were exhibiting a remarkable ability to disrupt the formation of malignant and benign tumors. Today our knowledge of such phytochemicals (compounds of plant origin) is exploding. And as scientists learn more about the chemistry of plants and other edibles, they are growing increasingly hopeful about sparing people from being struck by malignancies. "We've seen the future," says Dr. Gaynor, "and the future is food."[1]

Although the significance of consuming nutritious, whole, and natural foods for health and healing was originally developed and taught by Dr. Max Gerson about sixty years ago, we have finally awakened to the truth of his teachings. It is a reality that improvements in diet, nutrition, and general lifestyle are the wave of the future for beating degenerative diseases of all types.

THE UNDERLYING NUTRITIONAL CONCEPT OF DR. MAX GERSON

Dr. Gerson's therapeutic program seeks to regenerate an ailing body and bring it back to health by flooding the sick patient with nutrients and adopting other modalities. The nutrients come from raw juices plus raw and cooked solid organic vegetarian foods generously consumed. Inasmuch as the underlying nutritional concept of Dr. Max Gerson—proven by clinical studies cited in our text—is that an oxygen deficiency in the blood contributes to degenerative diseases, his treatment invariably brings about a doubling of circulatory oxygenation.

The Gerson Therapy also stimulates metabolism, eliminates toxins, and restores sluggish waste-removal functions of a patient's liver and kidneys. Thus, by using liberal amounts of high-quality nutrition, increasing the patient's oxygen availability, reinvigorating the entire organism with a well-functioning metabolism, and improving cellular detoxification, one's suppressed immune system, imperfect physiology, muddled mind, and dysfunctional brain and other essential organs are encouraged to regenerate toward homeostasis once again.

Dr. Gerson's healing program is advantageous for overcoming nearly every pathology and far superior to cancer chemotherapy. Statistically, for instance, chemotherapy boasts an overall remission rate on average of 12 percent (7 percent for colon cancer and 1 percent for pancreatic cancer) for patients first seen at early and intermediate stages of their illnesses, but the Gerson Therapy offers remission success on average for up to 42 percent of its participating, largely terminal cancer patients.

What's more, the Gerson Therapy nutrition program works permanently, in a surer manner than all other known therapies, including cytotoxicology (chemotherapy), immunology, pharmacology, roentgenology (radiation therapy), and other usual procedures provided by conventionally practiced allopathic medicine, since the goal of the Gerson Therapy is to restore all essential organs.

SYNOPSIS OF THE GERSON THERAPY NUTRITION PROGRAM

Best represented by its dietary component, the Gerson Therapy recommends a low-fat, salt-free program of food consumption to supply the body's cells with easily assimilated nutrients for strengthening one's natural immune defenses. To prevent or correct most of the fifteen hundred known degenerative diseases, the Gerson Therapy offers an ideal way to eat. In our modern society of processed packaged foods frequently containing preservatives, additives, dyes, and sometimes outright carcinogens, all forced upon us by accompanying massive amounts of media propaganda and advertising, the Gerson Therapy admittedly presents a difficult dining program to follow. Yet if a sick person is serious about recovery, then adopting the Gerson therapeutic technique does assure the restoration of wellness.

At the core of the Gerson Therapy is its diet, which includes organically grown fresh fruits and vegetables and thirteen glasses of freshly squeezed juices daily, taken at hourly intervals. The organic fresh fruits and vegetables provide the patient with elevated levels of minerals, enzymes, beta carotene, vitamins A and C, and other antioxidants that scavenge free radicals, as well as naturally occurring phytochemicals that scientists have discovered are true preventers of chronic degenerative diseases. These foods are recommended to contain no residual pesticides and fungicides.

No meat is allowed. On the Gerson therapeutic program, all animal protein is omitted for the person who is ill during the first six to twelve weeks of treatment, and it's kept to a minimum thereafter.[2]

The diet is largely fat-free but includes some nonfat and unflavored yogurt, nonfat and unsalted pot cheese, cottage cheese, and churned buttermilk when available (otherwise use nonfat yogurt), as well as flaxseed oil. Research put forth by the seven-time Nobel prize candidate Johanna Budwig, Ph.D., of Freudenstadt-Dietersweiler, Germany, shows that the omega-3 fatty acids in flax kill human cancer cells in tissue cultures without destroying normal cells in the same culture.[3]

Before Dr. Budwig published her groundbreaking works, Dr. Gerson, first in Germany, then in Austria, and finally in the United States, was applying nutritional knowledge he had gleaned about fats and oils for his patients' illnesses. Today, the Gerson Therapy menu plan is being used by the American Cancer Society (ACS). Yes, the very same ACS which once had condemned Dr. Gerson and blacklisted his therapeutic diet. Moreover, the National Cancer Institute (NCI) and the American Heart Association (AHA) both encourage the use of a modified version of the Gerson eating program.

Believing cancer to be a systemic rather than a localized disease, as was an erroneous but popular notion among health care professionals in the 1930s and 1940s, Dr. Gerson emphasized the rebalancing of a patient's entire physiology. His writings indicate he intended that the therapy should reverse any conditions sustaining the growth of malignant cells and restore those cells dysfunctioning from other forms of pathology.

THE DETOXIFICATION COMPONENT

For the body detoxification component, Dr. Gerson employed coffee enemas, which patients self-administer several times daily. Discussed in more depth below (see chapters 12 and 13), the coffee enema enables cancer patients and all others suffering from the life-threatening metabolic illnesses to eliminate toxic breakdown products of rapidly dissolving tumor masses or from the healing reactions of formerly dysfunctional cells generated by the effects of the Gerson therapy. According to Dr. Gerson's observations, there is a risk, if coffee enemas are not applied in conjunction with the diet, juices and a few supplements, that patients may succumb, not the disease process itself, but rather as a result of the liver's inability to detoxify rapidly enough.

Caffeine taken rectally stimulates the liver activity, increases bile flow, and opens bile ducts so that the liver can excrete toxic waste more easily. Coffee enemas are excellent for preventive medicine as well as for treatment. They also bring about remarkable pain relief.[4]

As a further aid to detoxification and as part of the therapeutic component involving food supplementation, Dr. Gerson's procedures require the use of a few orally self-administered dietary supplements every day or every other day. Thyroid extract, potassium iodide, liver extract, pancreatic enzymes, and niacin (nicotonic acid or vitamin B_3) are employed.

TESTIMONY BEFORE THE UNITED STATES SENATE BY DR. MAX GERSON

In our preface, we reprinted the unmodified text broadcasted by Raymond Gram Swing in his American Broadcasting Corporation news program of Wednesday, July 3, 1946, describing the appearance earlier that same day of Max Gerson, M.D., before the Pepper-Neely subcommittee of the United States Senate's Foreign Relations Committee in Washington, D.C. Relative to this description of his dietary treatment for cancer and other degenerative illnesses, what follows are the most pertinent portions of what Dr. Gerson stated during his testimony:[5]

My office and residence is at 815 Park Avenue, New York City. I am a member of the AMA, Medical Society of New York State, and Medical Society of New York County.

The dietetic treatment, which has for many years been known as the "Gerson diet," was developed first to relieve my own severe migraine condition. Then it was successfully applied to patients with allergic conditions such as asthma, as well as diseases of the intestinal tract and the liver-pancreas apparatus. By chance a patient with lupus vulgaris (skin tuberculosis) was cured following the use of the diet. After this success the dietetic treatment was used in all other kinds of tuberculosis—bones, kidneys, eyes, lungs, and so forth. It, too, was highly favorable in many other chronic diseases, such as arthritis, heart disease, chronic sinusitis, chronic ulcers, including colitis, high blood pressure, psoriasis, sclerosis multiplex [multiple sclerosis], and so forth. The most striking results were seen in the restoration of various kinds of liver and gall bladder diseases which could not be influenced by other methods up to the present.

The great number of chronic diseases which responded to the dietetic treatment showed clearly that the human body lost part of its resistance and healing power, as it left the way of natural nutrition for generations.

The fundamental damage starts with the use of artificial fertilizer for vegetables and fruits as well as for fodder. Thus, the chemically transformed vegetarian and meat nourishment, increasing through generations, transforms the organs and functions of the human body in the wrong direction.

Another basic defect lies in the waste of excrements of the cities. Instead of returning the natural manure to the fruit-bearing soil, it is let into the rivers, killing underwater life. The natural cycle is interrupted and mankind has to suffer dearly for the violation. Life in forest and wilderness should teach us the lesson.

But we can regain the lost defense and healing power if we return as close as possible to the laws of nature as they are created. Highly concentrated for speedy reaction, they are laid down in the dietetic treatment.

The first cancer patient (bile ducts) was treated in 1928 with success. Seven favorable cases followed out of twelve and remain free of symptoms up to seven years.

My experience leads me to believe that the liver is the center of the restoration process in those patients who improve strikingly. If the liver is too far destroyed, then the treatment cannot be effective.

Aware of the imperfection of this as well as any other theory, I shall try, nevertheless, to explain the end results of the Gerson diet. It is condensed in three surpassing components:

1. The elimination of toxins and poisons and returning of the displaced "extracellular" Na (sodium)-group, connected with toxins, poisons, edema, destructive inflammation from the tissues, tumors, and organs where it does not belong, into the serum and tissues where it belongs—gall bladder with the bile ducts, connective tissue, thyroid, stomach mucosa, kidney medulla, tumors, and so forth.

2. Bringing back the lost intracellular K (potassium)-group combined with vitamins, enzymes, ferments, sugar, and so forth, into the tissues and organs where they belong: liver, muscles, heart, brain, kidney cortex, and so forth; on this basis, iodine, ineffective before, is made effective, continuously added in new amounts.

3. Restoring the differentiation, tonus, tension, oxidation, and so forth, by activated iodine, where there were before growing tumors and metastases with dedifferentiation, loss of tension, oxidation, loss of resistance, and healing power.

In 1991, two decades following President Richard M. Nixon's confident December 23, 1971, declaration of another "war on cancer" and his promise of a cure by the 1976 Bicentennial, a group of sixty noted physicians and scientists declared their disgust at the failures of the medical profession in general and oncologists in particular. They called a press conference and made the following statement: "The cancer establishment confuses the public with repeated [false] claims that we are winning the war on cancer. . . . Our ability to treat and cure most cancers has not materially improved."

Rather, the best way to correct the cancer problem is through the application of dietary improvements, nutrients, whole body detoxification, and overall nutritional therapy. Some of these aspects of degenerative disease treatment are what our next chapter introduces.

References for the Introduction

1. Cowley, G. with Underwood, A.; Springen, K.; Davis, A. "Cancer and diet: Eating to beat the odds: what you need to know." *Newsweek*, November 30, 1998, pp. 60–66.

2. Walters, R. *Options: The Alternative Cancer Therapy Book.* Garden City Park, N.Y.: Avery Publishing Group, 1992, pp. 189,190.

3. Budwig, J. *Flax Oil as a True Aid against Arthritis, Heart Infarction, Cancer and Other Diseases.* Vancouver, B.C., Canada: Apple Publishing, 1994.

4. Moss, R.W. *Cancer Therapy: The Independent Consumer's Guide to Non-Toxic Treatment and Prevention.* New York: Equinox Press, 1992, p. 189.

5. Gerson, M. Testimony during hearings on Senate Bill 1875, conducted July 1, 2, 3, 1946 by Senator Claude Pepper (D-Florida), for the Pepper-Neely Subcommittee of the Foreign Relations Committee, the 79th Congress of the U.S. Senate, July 3, 1946.

Part One

How the Gerson Therapy Works

Chapter One

HOW NUTRITION HEALS

In 1992, at the Fukushima Medical College on the island of Hokkaido in northern Japan, Professor of Medicine Yoshihiko Hoshino, M.D., Ph.D., learned that he had developed cancer of the colon. During the course of surgery to remove the malignancy, his oncological surgeon discovered that Dr. Hoshino's cancer had already metastasized to the liver. While under postoperative care, the patient was advised by his personal friend and former classmate, the same surgical oncologist, to undergo multiple courses of chemotherapy.

As it happens, the Gerson therapeutic program for reversing acute and chronic degenerative diseases such as cancer, diabetes, stroke, arthritis, and other life-threatening illnesses is quite well known and highly respected in the industrialized countries of Europe and Asia. Professor Hoshino was among a growing number of health professionals aware of Dr. Max Gerson's well-established book A *Cancer Therapy: Results of Fifty Cases* (translated into Japanese) and the medical efficacy of his treatment program.

Because of well-recognized adverse side effects and an excessive rate of failure for colon/rectal cancer (93 percent of patients die after receiving chemotherapy for such malignancy) and an even worse prognosis for liver cancer metastases (97 percent of patients succumb after receiving chemotherapy), this professor of medicine refused to take cytotoxic agents. Instead, owning the broadly disseminated Japanese translation of Dr.

Gerson's book, Dr. Hoshino followed its instructions and on his own proceeded to follow the Gerson Therapy.

Today, with a decent interval of almost nine years having elapsed since Dr. Hoshino's diagnosis, he and his oncologist have declared the patient "cured" of both colon cancer and liver metastases. Here is the letter Charlotte Gerson recently received from Professor Yoshihiko Hoshino, M.D., Ph.D.:

> As you know, I suffered from colon cancer and metastatic liver cancer in 1992 and recovered from them by use of the Gerson Therapy. I have written a book introducing Gerson Therapy to medical consumers in Japan. My book was published in August 1998 and is the first about Gerson Therapy written by a medical doctor in Japan. It has caused a big sensation among Japanese people, because using the Gerson program twelve additional cancer patients also were cured. My book not only tells of my recovery but also includes the stories of these twelve Japanese who no longer suffer from cancer.

HEALING BY A POWERFUL NUTRITIONAL THERAPY

In applying the techniques of healing, all health practitioners acknowledge a common truth: there exists just one science of human immunology, which possesses specific laws of biochemistry. In the profession of medicine, however, two opposing factions or principles of practice contend with one another. Disease-oriented orthodox medicine and patient-centered holistic medicine agree only on the current facts of biochemistry and immunology but hardly on anything else.

Disease-oriented medical practice directs its efforts to finding the generalized formulas for treating types or classes of people with similar symptoms. Classification of patients into groups or categories is indispensable for finding a treatment. In order to uncover the therapy that works best, single- or double-blind, placebo-controlled clinical trials are frequently employed. Whatever is found wrong with a patient's physiology, the allopathic (drug-using) physician attempts to correct the health problem with FDA-approved pharmaceuticals, chemotherapeutics, surgery, immunotherapy, radiation therapy, or other forms of high technology. Disease-oriented medicine is a system primarily employing drugs in an attempt to produce effects in the body that will directly oppose and so alleviate the symptoms of disease. Applying chemotherapy for cancer is the perfect example of disease-oriented medicine in practice.[1]

Patient-centered medical practice develops its healing procedures by seeking out everything that can possibly be done to optimize the health of a given unique individual. An orientation like this, also defined as "functional medicine" by health professional educator Jeffrey Bland, Ph.D., of Gig Harbor, Washington, demands decisions based on judgments by holistic physicians, chiropractors, homeopaths, naturopaths, acupuncturists, *some* nurse practitioners, nutritionists, and other types of healers. It also requires close personal participation by the patients themselves. The doctor frequently devotes as much time teaching a patient as administering treatment. Even if the patient has only subclinical symptoms, as manifested by irregular laboratory tests, an effort is made in patient-centered medicine to accomplish three specific physiological responses:

1. Harmonize the person's biochemistry.
2. Elevate the workings of a suppressed immune system.
3. Correct the malfunctioning of essential organs.

Prescribing the right homeopathic remedy is a perfect example of patient-centered medicine in practice.[2]

The Gerson Therapy is another example of how one might put to use patient-centered medicine. It is the best in self-help health care, especially for the reversal of really serious degenerative illnesses. The Gerson Therapy mostly utilizes nutrition to achieve all three components of holistic, biological, patient-oriented medicine. It is the ultimate in natural healing and a powerful antidote to the highly unnatural lifestyle that prevails in all modern industrial societies.

In the following sections of this chapter, we offer a general discussion of the pathological changes within the tissues and cells typically present in cancer. And the description of such alterations from normal physiology will offer insights into abnormalities present in some of the other degenerative diseases.

Since he first introduced it around 1926, there has been no place in the allopathic medical community for Dr. Max Gerson's powerfully healing nutritional therapy. For instance, among the four deciding votes cast by legislators to defeat the U.S. Senate's 1946 Pepper-Neely anticancer Bill No. 1875, those voting negatively were four physicians turned senators. At the time, treating people with diet to eliminate their degenerative diseases was just too excessively simple. Doing so removed a great deal of decision-making power from the medical profession; consequently, those four physicians who were U.S. senators at the time voted to kill Senator Claude Pepper's bill. So cancer patients then and later became victims of the shortsighted vote for special interests.

Dr. Gerson plodded on and continued bringing sick people who consulted him back from the brink of death. Now, with the pioneer gone these past forty years or more, his daughter and the Gerson Institute carry on with their task of educating the public.

THE GERSON THERAPY IS DE FACTO RECOGNIZED BY THE U.S. GOVERNMENT

As we alluded to in our introduction, the most revolutionary and promising field of medical research against degenerative diseases is that of chemoprevention: the use of micronutrients or macronutrients, phytochemicals, nutraceuticals, and other organic components often found in foods that can prevent, stop, or retard the process of illness. By the beginning of 1995, the National Cancer Institute was pursuing forty new or established studies in the area of nutrition that involved enzymes, fiber, fat, micronutrients, vitamins, and phytochemicals.

By 1999, the forty abstracts summarizing those same 1995 beginning investigations on cancer and nutrition had been completed and sent to the U.S. government's American Association for Cancer Research. These studies are currently providing critical information on the substances needed to be added to or eliminated from the human diet to combat cancer. You probably are not surprised that nearly all of the components of the Gerson Therapy do play leading roles among these phytochemical ingredients. By such adoption, the Gerson Therapy is, in effect, recognized as a viable treatment against cancer and most other degenerative diseases. It's a de facto recognition by the United States, but without lawful authority and literally unofficial. Still, the Gerson Therapy's components are very much in evidence and being utilized to save lives. They even form the foundation for advisories given by profit makers of the cancer industry such as the American Cancer Society, the National Cancer Institute, the Sloan-Kettering Cancer Clinic, and many pharmaceutical companies merging nutrient manufacturers into their corporate structures.

As part of our preface we stated that in the United States every year, a minimum of 1.9 million people are diagnosed with some type of malignancy (excluding skin cancer and in situ cervical cancer). And we cited holistic oncologist, internist, and homeopathic physician W. Douglas Brodie, M.D., H.M.D., of Reno, Nevada, who states that at least 700,000 Americans die from cancer annually.

Almost every health care professional and most medical consumers now know that the cause of over 70 percent of malignancies is in some way related to what we eat. Denatured food, in fact, is a main source of breast and colon/rectal cancer as well as of lung cancer in nonsmokers. Every year more medical and scientific evidence accumulates revealing that what we take in as food has tremendous influence on whether we will develop cancer and whether we can cure it once malignant disease symptoms arise.[3]

This is a tremendously exciting field of scientific inquiry that the conventional medical community is just now beginning to investigate seriously. Yet, probably half a century ahead of his time, during an active professional life spanning forty years, from 1919 in Bielefeld, Germany, to 1959 in New York City, one modest physician developed the food and nutrition answers for cancer and other degenerative diseases. Max Gerson, M.D., however, was unmercifully vilified, harassed, and persecuted in the United States by the AMA, especially its journal editor, Morris Fishbein, M.D., and his physician-politician cohorts.[4]

After a 1946 patient demonstration before a committee of the U.S. Senate that received national media attention, Dr. Gerson was attacked editorially in the pages of the *Journal of the American Medical Association* (*JAMA*). Reasons for the attack were related to prevailing domestic medical politics and the various financial policies being enforced at the time by longtime AMA politician, *JAMA* editor, and nonpracticing physician Morris Fishbein, M.D.

Why has it taken organized allopathic medicine so long to appreciate the connection between diet and cancer?

Why have oncological pioneers like Dr. Max Gerson been denigrated, been stigmatized, and had their hearts broken when they've attempted to use nutrition as a therapeutic tool?

At least for the first of these penetrating questions, the authors of this book can figure out four particular answers:

1. In the United States, advances in medical technology maintain prejudicial leads over any other means of treatment. As a nation

we have tended to focus on technology for battling cancer and other health problems. Eating vegetables as recommended by Dr. Gerson employs hardly any technology.

2. The American pharmaceutical industry rules the way medicine is allowed to be practiced not only in this country but also around the world. If a therapeutic substance or method is unpatentable—without profits to be made from a synthesized drug—it's usually ignored or opposed and suppressed. No medically oriented commercial company will be amenable to investing research time and money to promote it.

3. Admitting that there's a strong relationship between what we eat and getting cancer or some other sickness, points a self-directed finger at two groups: (a) the food processors who sell us malnourishing synthetic or otherwise unnatural packaged edibles and (b) ourselves as the source of our own illness. Although we may recognize the truth of such condemnation, it truly is a discomforting mental burden nonetheless.[5]

4. Most medical doctors have had extremely poor education in the nutritional sciences. Those physicians who currently utilize nutrition as treatment are primarily self-educated.

There has been no place for the Dr. Gersons of this world—until now. Today the medical times are changing remarkably for doctors—not only financially but also nutritionally. The more conscientious of them have found it necessary to turn to nutritional therapy almost as a last resort against cancer, arthritis, heart and blood vessel disorders, diabetes, stroke, and other disabling forms of degenerative diseases. Why? Simply because too many of their patients never get well with the applications of standard, conventionally practiced allopathic medicine and oncology. Gradually, physicians are looking at the true causes of debilitating diseases like cancer and deciding that for too long they've been treating symptoms and not the underlying sources of illness, which they didn't understand.

THE VARIOUS FORMS OF CANCEROUS GROWTHS

Of the 150 different types of cancerous growths, five major groups are conventionally recognized in oncology (the study and practice of tumor treatment). They are classified in accordance with the tissues exhibiting an abnormally wild and excessive cellular growth. The classifications listed below are taken from the book *An Alternative Medicine Definitive Guide to Cancer*, coauthored by W. John Diamond, M.D., director of the Triad Medical Center in Reno, Nevada, and cardiologist W. Lee Cowden, M.D., consultant to the Conservative Medicine Institute in Richardson, Texas, with contributor Burton Goldberg, publisher for Future Medicine Publishing, Inc.[3]

Carcinomas form in the epithelial cells that cover the skin, mouth, nose, throat, lung airways, and genitourinary and gastrointestinal tracts or that line glands such as the breast or thyroid. Solid tumors invading the lung, breast, prostate, skin, stomach, and colon/rectum are labeled carcinomas.

Sarcomas develop in the bones and soft connective and supportive tissues surrounding organs and tissues, such as cartilage, muscles, tendons, fat, and the other linings of the lungs, abdomen, heart, central nervous system, and blood vessels.

Leukemias evolve in the blood and bone marrow. Abnormal white blood cells produced in those tissues travel throughout the bloodstream damaging the spleen and other tissues. They don't form solid tumors but rather are considered blood dyscrasias (imbalances).

Lymphomas are lymph gland malignancies composed of abnormal white blood cells (lymphocytes) congregating in the neck, groin, armpits, spleen, chest center, and around the intestines as solid tumors. Two of the most prevalent lymphoma types affecting North Americans are non-Hodgkin's lymphoma and Hodgkin's disease.

Myelomas, while rare, arise in the antibody-producing plasma cells or blood-cell-producing (hemopoietic) cells of the bone marrow.

Cancer cells are essentially parasitic and immortal. They fail to develop specialized functions, develop their own blood vessel network to siphon nourishment away from the normal cells, and grow to such a state of abnormality that they kill their host. Cancer cells are not encapsulated by fiber and thus may invade nearby normal cells. If they do not invade, the cancerous growth is considered to be *localized*; if they spread to other body parts, the malignancy is labeled *metastasized*.

WHY CANCER AND OTHER BODY DEGENERATIONS ARISE

In 1958, Max Gerson, M.D., was the first physician ever to state that cancer was caused by multiple interdependent factors. He had identified several such factors during his forty-one-year career as a physician. Now, after another forty-one years, the original list offered by Dr. Gerson has expanded. Environmental polluters have been releasing into the air, soil and water myriad new cancer-causing agents (at last count over 52,000 substances), thus creating new ways to suppress people's immunity and inhibit the enzymes necessary to our life processes. Today, a minimum of forty-nine stressors exist, which contribute to acute or chronic physical, mental, and emotional deterioration (see Table 1-1 on pages 19–20).

Although Dr. Gerson was the first to identify some of these stressors, his insights have been consistently ignored by conventional oncologists. Patients coming under their care inevitably suffer as a result. Incorrect allopathic cancer treatments have been employed for almost a half century to attack tumors without correcting the underlying causes that stimulate their development.

THE MULTIPLE "HITS" OF PRECURSOR CARCINOGENS

While the potential of forty-nine (or more) cancer-causing precursors exists, if an individual avoids being "hit" by most of them it's possible that symptomatic cancer won't develop in his or her lifetime. However, since one out of three (approaching one out of two) North Americans or Europeans do currently come down with cancer, the odds are high that malignancy in some form will strike you or a loved one.

According to the *multiple-hit theory*, all cancers arise from at least two changes or "hits" to cellular genes. These double hits build up and interact over time. Eventually, a breaking point is reached (the proverbial "straw that broke the camel's back") and cancerous growth is switched on. The hits will likely come from one of the precursor carcinogens we have cited in Table 1-1.

Most critical are the number and types of carcinogenic hits, their frequency, and their intensity. Some of the carcinogen hits are cancer "initiators" while others are cancer "promoters."[4]

TABLE 1-1

Everyday Factors That Contribute to the Rise of Cancer

Taken from the medical, scientific, and environmental literature as well as from our everyday experiences, here is the coauthors' listing of forty-nine predisposing, ceaseless, contributing factors as one or more sources of cancer affecting the human body's ever-weakening enzymatic, hormonal, immunological, and other defense systems:[5]

1. Atmospheric cosmic rays and X rays
2. Sunlight's ultraviolet rays
3. Chronic electromagnetic field exposure
4. Geopathic stress
5. Sick building syndrome
6. Ionizing radiation
7. Microwave oven radiation
8. Nonionizing electromagnetic radiation from domestic appliances
9. Overhead power lines
10. Nuclear radiation
11. Pesticide/herbicide residues
12. Industrial toxins
13. Drinking or bathing in polluted water
14. Drinking or bathing in chlorinated water
15. Drinking or bathing in fluoridated water
16. Tobacco and smoking
17. Hormonal therapies
18. Immune-suppressive drugs
19. Consuming irradiated foods
20. Ingesting food additives
21. Mercury toxicity from any source
22. Toxic metal syndrome
23. Dental amalgam fillings
24. Dental root canals
25. Dental cavitations (jawbone spaces left by poor tooth extraction)
26. Dental metals of all types
27. Steady use of street drugs
28. Steady use of prescription drugs
29. Steady use of nonprescription drugs
30. Nerve interference fields
31. Diet or nutritional deficiencies
32. Consumption of synthetic "nonfoods"
33. Chronic physical or mental stress
34. Destructive negative emotions
35. Depressed thyroid action
36. Intestinal toxicity or digestive impairment
37. Parasites

TABLE 1-1 (cont.)

38. Viruses
39. Bacterial infections
40. Fungal infections
41. Blocked detoxification pathways
42. Free radical pathology
43. Cellular oxygen deficiency
44. Adverse cellular terrain
45. Oncogenes (cellular genes that change normal cells into cancer)
46. Genetic predisposition
47. Miasm (energy residues of previous illnesses)
48. Physical irritants, e.g., asbestos
49. Alcohol consumption

Any of the precursor carcinogens (often referred to by oncologists as *procarcinogens*) can be a tumor initiator or a promoter. Potentially cancerous changes begin in a damaged cell's DNA (deoxyribonucleic acid) after the second devastating procarcinogenic hit. Uncontrolled growth in a damaged cell follows in due course, progressing to an eventually noticeable malignant lesion with a mass or tumor that may invade other tissues.

In the first step toward cancer development, *initiation*, the procarcinogenic hit may produce large numbers of toxic agents, known as *free radicals*, which set up a pathological process that damages the cell's DNA when the liver sets up an enzymatic reaction known as *Phase One*. This reaction causes the procarcinogen to convert into a full-fledged carcinogen. Additionally, the liver produces *Phase Two* enzymes to cart off the dangerous residue that Phase One enzymes leave behind. The liver plays a vital role in the process of cancer formation, simultaneously initiating carcinogenesis and neutralizing it.

In the second step toward cancer formation, *promotion*, the liver's neutralization may not be up to par and a damaged cell alters its pattern of mitosis (normal cell division). It begins to divide voluminously. That is when the immune system goes to work, recognizing these cells as foreign and destroying them; if it fails, however, the damaged cell can spawn a tumorous lesion.

In the third step toward a full-blown cancer, *progression*, the tumor attempts to build itself a blood supply for sustained nourishment. Then tumorous invasion of surrounding tissues may take place. Clusters of cancer cells tend to release certain essential growth factors that promote this de-

TABLE 1-2

Health Problems Successfully Treated by the Gerson Therapy

1.	Acne	27.	Hepatitis
2.	Addictions	28.	High blood pressure
3.	AIDS	29.	Hyperactivity
4.	Allergies	30.	Hypoglycemia/hyperglycemia
5.	Anemias	31.	Immune deficiency
6.	Ankylosing spondylitis	32.	Infertility
7.	Arthritis	33.	Intestinal parasites
8.	Asthma	34.	Kidney disease
9.	Cancers and leukemias	35.	Liver cirrhosis
10.	Candidiasis	36.	Lyme disease
11.	Chemical sensitivities	37.	Lupus erythematosus
12.	Chronic fatigue syndrome	38.	Macular degeneration
13.	Constipation	39.	Migraine
14.	Crohn's disease	40.	Mononucleosis
15.	Cushing's syndrome	41.	Multiple sclerosis
16.	Depression/panic attacks	42.	Obesity
17.	Diabetes	43.	Ocular histoplasmosis
18.	Emphysema	44.	Osteomyelitis
19.	Endometriosis	45.	Osteoporosis
20.	Epilepsy	46.	Phlebitis
21.	Fibroids	47.	Premenstrual syndrome
22.	Fibromyalgia	48.	Psoriasis
23.	Genital herpes	49.	Shingles
24.	Gout	50.	Stroke
25.	Heart and artery diseases	51.	Tuberculosis
26.	Hemorrhoids	52.	Ulcerative colitis

velopment of new blood vessels, called *angiogenesis*, so that malignant invasion of surrounding tissue may then take place.[6]

THE GERSON DIETARY THERAPY FOR FIFTY-TWO ILLNESSES

Each of the factors listed in Table 1-1 that can contribute to cancer or other acute and chronic debilitating illnesses may be successfully prevented or treated with dietary intervention. Certain foods fight off cancer and other degenerative diseases or bring about their physiological reversal. Every food component incorporated into the Gerson Therapy is effective against a great variety of physical and mental pathological conditions.

To date, nearly ten thousand patients have benefited from the Gerson dietary treatment. Many of these success stories are described in the Gerson Institute's bimonthly *Gerson Healing Newsletter*. Table 1-2 shows a sample of the several hundred health problems against which the Gerson Therapy has shown verified, permanent effectiveness:

References for Chapter One

1. Baker, S.M. *Detoxification and Healing: The Key to Optimal Health.* New Canaan, Conn.: Keats Publishing, 1997, p. 157.

2. *Ibid.*, p. 158.

3. Diamond, W.J.; Cowden, W. Lee. With Goldberg, B. *An Alternative Medicine Definitive Guide to Cancer.* Tiburon, Calif.: Future Medicine Publishing, Inc., 1997, pp. 518, 519.

4. Dollinger, M.; Rosenbaum, E.H.; Cable, G. *Everyone's Guide to Cancer Therapy: How Cancer Is Diagnosed, Treated, and Managed Day to Day.* 3rd edition. Kansas City, MO.: Andrews McMeel Publishing, 1997, pp. 6, 7.

5. *Op. cit., An Alternative Medicine Definitive Guide to Cancer.*

6. Cowley, G. with Underwood, A.; Springen, K.; Davis, A. "Cancer and diet: Eating to beat the odds: what you need to know." *Newsweek*, November 30, 1998, pp. 60–66.

Chapter Two

A BRIEF BIOGRAPHY OF DR. MAX GERSON

Max Gerson was born in Wongrowitz, Germany, on October 18, 1881. He was the third child and second boy in a German-Jewish family of nine healthy children. Early on, he exhibited an inquiring mind. For instance, when Max was six and a half years old, he wondered what would happen if the fertilizers were changed in the flowerbeds of his mother's garden, and he therefore carried out experiments. The lad's crude attempts at soil alterations generally resulted in the death of her flowers so, naturally, his mother quickly stopped Max's curiosity as to changing her plants' soil nutrition.

When the young man was ready to graduate from high school (called *Gymnasium* in Germany), it was required that all students pass a written mathematics examination. Max's graduation test contained a math problem of a type that he did not remember ever having seen. Yet he proceeded to set up an equation and find an answer to this very difficult problem. His teacher had never before seen such an intricate solution and couldn't judge it to be right or wrong. For a determination, the student's paper needed to be sent to a famous mathematics professor teaching at the University of Berlin. The answer came back that Max had produced an entirely new and original solution; that here was a mathematical genius, and the young man should absolutely study mathematics.

Upon his graduation from *Gymnasium*, a family council was called, and Max's future was placed before his parents and siblings. Noting that there was no Jewish mathematics professor throughout Germany, it was agreed that, should Max study mathematics, he would never be more than a simple high school math teacher. Everyone—including the new graduate himself—agreed that he should study medicine instead.

EDUCATION OF A HEALER

Max Gerson attended the universities of Breslau, Wuerzburg, Berlin, and Freiburg for his medical studies. In 1907, he completed his internship in Hoechst, Main, and subsequently worked as an assistant to Professor Albert Frankel, M.D., in Berlin. From 1909 until the beginning of the First World War, he worked in Berlin in the Friedrichshain Hospital with Professor Kronig and Professor Borottau, and for a short period at the children's clinic with Professor Minkowsky.

As a captain in the German Army Medical Corps, Dr. Gerson was a close associate for almost half a decade of the promient neurosurgeon Ottfried Foerster, M.D. In 1928, ten years after establishing his own practice in Bielefeld in 1919, Dr. Gerson treated three hopelessly ill people suffering with cancer. One of them was dying from inoperable stomach cancer. Even surprising the diet's developer, all three recovered and went on to tell numerous other cancer patients that successful treatment was at hand. Still, because Dr. Gerson recognized that some degenerative disease patients would recover and some would not, he was careful as to whom he gave the Gerson Therapy in the next ten years.

In 1933, barely escaping from capture and imprisonment in a Nazi death camp because he was Jewish, Dr. Gerson moved his family first to Vienna, Austria, where he completed his book on tuberculosis. In 1938, he was able to emigrate with his family to New York City. He passed the New York State board examinations for medicine and opened a medical practice on Park Avenue. He continued to develop his therapy to achieve success with all types of serious health difficulties, especially cancer. The physician treated hundreds of patients given up to die after receiving surgery and radiation (chemotherapy had not yet been invented). After these years of study and research, the Gerson Therapy brought really sick people up to a 50 percent rate of recovery for even far advanced cancer cases. (After chemotherapy was introduced into oncology, Dr. Gerson's natural healing success rate in patients thus treated was reduced.)

In 1946, Dr. Gerson became the first physician to demonstrate recovered cancer patients before a United States Senate committee, which was holding hearings on a bill to find means of curing and preventing cancer under the sponsorship of Senator Claude Pepper. The American Medical Association's lobbyists who supported surgery, radiation, and chemotherapies were too well financed, however, and they caused the Senate bill's defeat by four votes. If it had passed, this Senate bill would have supported extensive research into the Gerson Therapy and could have spread this cure for cancer in 1946.

PHYSICIAN, HEAL THYSELF: GERSON'S FIRST DISCOVERIES

While he was a university student, Max Gerson was plagued by a major health problem: he suffered from exceedingly severe migraine headaches, which continued throughout his undergraduate years.

By the time Max was a medical resident, these headaches were so disabling and frequent that he sometimes spent three days a week in a darkened room, experiencing nausea, vomiting, eye sensitivity, and awful one-sided head pain which felt as though his cranium were splitting in two. He sought counsel from his medical professors only to find that they couldn't help in any way. Rather, they advised him "to learn to live with it." The young physician felt he couldn't accept such suffering and would have to find an answer for himself.

Max embarked upon a search. He read numerous books and medical papers and consulted with many authorities, but found no direction. Finally he came upon a case report in an Italian medical journal about a woman who had suffered from migraines and found relief by changing her diet. No details were given, but the idea made sense to Dr. Gerson. The severe spasms with nausea and vomiting that were affecting him, the young doctor concluded, could well be caused by some foods he was unable to digest. Now he had to discover what they were.

His first thought was that every baby can digest cow's milk; his body should be able to handle it as well. Therefore, he lived on nothing but milk for the next ten days. His migraines nevertheless showed no improvement—no change whatsoever. Then it occurred to him that animals never drink milk once they are weaned. Moreover, a human's physical structure is similar to that of vegetarian animals. This being true, Max's thinking went, people with health problems should probably live on fruit, vegetables, and grains.

He tried an all-apple diet—raw and baked apples, applesauce, apple juice, apple compote—and he became well, with no migraines. Slowly thereafter, one food following another, he added other edibles. If something eaten wasn't right for his body, it could cause him a sensitivity reaction, taking the form of migraine in as little as twenty minutes.

GERSON'S "MIGRAINE DIET"

When he experienced further sensitivity problems from consuming cooked foods, Dr. Gerson hypothesized that the culprit was not the cooking process but rather the addition of salt. Upon his eliminating salt from his diet, Max was able to eat not only cooked foods but also any kind of vegetables, potatoes, grains, and so on. He named this new program of eating, which kept him free of head pain disturbances, his "migraine diet." It was predicated on the ingestion of fresh fruits and vegetables, mostly raw but some cooked, and totally free of salt. Gerson decided that salt was the source of pathology connected with diet.

In time, patients would come to him complaining of migraines. Although there was no cure according to the textbooks, Gerson revealed that he had been suffering from migraines himself until he had developed and followed his antimigraine, saltless diet.

The young physician would then suggest that the patient try it out. Invariably, migraine patients following his eating program would return for a follow-up consultation and report that they were free of headaches as long as they didn't "cheat" on the Gerson eating program. When they began eating salt again, they would suffer a relapse.

Skin Tuberculosis Is Eliminated by the Gerson Therapy

One of Dr. Gerson's patients returned after remaining on the antimigraine diet for a short period and reported that his skin tuberculosis, known medically as lupus vulgaris, had disappeared along with his migraines. The new practitioner told his patient that lupus was an "incurable" disease and that the skin problem must have come from something else. This lupus vulgaris patient, however, possessed bacteriological studies proving his diagnosis. Thus, for the first time in the history of medicine, Dr. Gerson saw skin tuberculosis healing from treatment.

In light of the patient's diagnostic reports, the young doctor could hardly believe his eyes, but he soon became convinced that his migraine diet was helpful in the treatment of tubercular skin disease. He asked the patient if he knew others suffering from the same problem. Yes, the patient replied, and he sent Dr. Gerson some of his tubercular friends from the hospital where he had been confined. After some weeks elapsed, these tuberculosis patients also recovered on Dr. Gerson's antimigraine eating plan.

News of Dr. Gerson's success with lupus vulgaris came to the attention of Professor Ferdinand Sauerbruch, M.D., the world-famous lung tuberculosis specialist who practiced in Munich. After conducting long discussions on dietary concepts with Dr. Gerson, Prof. Sauerbruch decided to set up a clinical trial using the Gerson Therapy. During an extended period, the professor treated 450 "incurable" skin tuberculosis patients using Dr. Gerson's method. Of these subjects, 446 recovered fully; Dr. Sauerbruch was deeply impressed. The renowned lung specialist reports on this successful Gerson dietary trial and its positive results in his autobiography, *Master Surgeon*.

Dr. Gerson was not satisfied to let the situation rest there. He reasoned that if lupus vulgaris could be healed with diet, why not other forms of tuberculosis, such as lung, kidney, or bone TB? He started to treat such cases and found that they too responded to the dietary therapy and were cured.

One of the lung TB cases was Albert Schweitzer's wife, Helene, who had contracted tuberculosis at an early age in the tropics and was in terminal condition when she was brought to see Dr. Gerson by her husband. Mrs. Schweitzer recovered from her disease completely and went on to live well into her eighties.

During the course of treating these various migraine and tuberculosis cases, Dr. Gerson found that many of the patients had been suffering from other problems, too: high blood pressure, asthma, allergies, kidney damage, arthritis, residual stroke, hardening of the arteries, and more. These acute or chronic degenerations also disappeared. Unquestionably, the Gerson Therapy worked toward correcting almost any degenerating illness.

Thus, Dr. Gerson recognized that he was no longer treating a disease; he was helping the body to heal itself of nearly all dysfunctions. Of course, this meant that he was no longer treating symptoms but the patient's underlying problem; he was taking a completely different direction from the usual approach of orthodox medicine: the suppression of symptoms.

Sodium/Potassium Balance as a Metabolic Healing Procedure

In the course of his work with tuberculosis patients, Dr. Gerson realized that one of the basic problems of disease was the loss of potassium from tissue cells and the penetration of sodium into the cells (known in medicine as *tissue damage syndrome* or TDS). The cell, in attempting to maintain its integrity, binds the toxic sodium material with water. Such a circumstance for the sick patient is recognized as *edematous fluid retention*.

Six years after Dr. Gerson's death, a medical textbook coauthored by Malcolm Dixon and Edwin C. Webb titled *Enzymes* (Academic Press, 1964) gave further evidence of the problems caused by sodium penetration. The book confirmed Dr. Gerson's initial findings. These two authors studied how the body builds enzymes, and they reported that, in most cases, potassium behaves like a catalyst (an activating substance) in the formation of enzymes. Sodium, on the other hand, usually acts as an inhibitor, or blocking substance. Thus, with the penetration of sodium into the cell, and therefore into tissues, enzyme function is inhibited and the normal tissue activity becomes disturbed or at worst, blocked.

While a minimum of sodium is needed by the body for normal function, this inorganic substance is also considered to be an *extracellular* mineral, since it must remain outside of body cells in their fluids. Potassium is the *intracellular* mineral, since it is needed for metabolism within body cells. When the extracellular/intracellular balance is disturbed, health problems start from damage to the cells. In normal vegetarian nutrition, plant material of all kinds contains quite adequate amounts of sodium to satisfy our needs. The problem is that, in the course of canning, bottling, preserving, freezing, and all other forms of food processing, as well as during the usual procedure of cooking, potassium is depleted and salt (sodium chloride) is invariably added to foods. Additions like these constitute an excess. The body is normally able to excrete excess sodium through the kidneys and feces, but when it becomes overwhelmed daily, year after year, with huge amounts of excess sodium, there comes a point when the body's ability to excrete this excess is reduced or lost. Now a person's many enzyme systems, his or her immune system, and eventually the liver, are damaged. The result is symptoms of illness and the creation of disease dysfunction.

As we observed earlier, the first thing Dr. Gerson did was to eliminate all added salt (sodium) from his own and his patients' diet. He then added to the patients' salt-free vegetarian diet a freshly pressed glass of organic vegetable juice taken hourly, thirteen times a day. Additionally, the doctor examined his patients' urine and found that during the first week on this treatment they often excreted from 6 to 8 grams of sodium in a day even on a sodium-free diet!

Following this salt-free program, the participating patients' ankles and legs lost their swelling (edema) and became normal once again; moreover, overabundant abdominal fluid (ascites) decreased as well. The patients ridding themselves of so much burdensome fluid invariably excreted a great deal of urine. Restoring the body's sodium/potassium tissue balance for his patients became one of Dr. Gerson's key metabolic healing procedures. (Please see chapter 10 on the Gerson saltless diet for more detailed information about the human body's sodium/potassium balance.)

OUTSIDE STRESSORS AND DISEASE

Dr. Gerson discovered that more difficulties with illness develop as well from outside stressors, before the body's defenses break down. For example, foods are raised in soil containing artificial fertilizers providing only the three particular minerals: nitrogen, phosphorus, and potassium (symbolized by the initials N, P, and K). But normal plants require something like fifty-two different chemicals for good health and strong growth. Artificially fertilized soil, as is employed in truck farming, brings nutritional deficiency to the plants growing on it. People, too, require these fifty-two minerals to be present in foods. When they are not contained in the soil and thus not in our foods, we become deficient in the same way that our plants are lacking.

Furthermore, plants, just like people, experience deficiency diseases and lose their defenses. Then, fungal or viral diseases and insects move in to destroy such weak and deficient plants, and farmers are forced to spray them with fungicides, herbicides, and pesticides to avoid losing their crops. Thus, in agriculture worldwide, deficient and toxic commercially raised foods cause peoples' bodies to become deficient, weakened, toxic, and finally diseased.

With this basic understanding as taught by Dr. Gerson, we may be able to see how health breaks down. And this description of soil and plants does not include additional damage we inflict on ourselves with cigarettes, alcohol, antibiotics, sleeping pills, pesticides, fungicides, herbicides, over-the-counter and doctor-prescribed drugs, and much more (see chapter 1). It becomes clear that, in order to reverse disease and restore health, we need to detoxify and intensively flood the body with live, fresh, active nutrients.

THE USE OF COFFEE ENEMAS FOR WASTE REMOVAL

Dr. Gerson further found that the cellular systems and body tissues also excreted waste products accumulated over many years from the taking in of poor air, bad water, food additives, viruses, germs, and other toxic items. In order not to overload the liver, which filters these poisons out of the blood, he found a way to open the bile ducts and help the liver to release the body's accumulated poisons by means of his renowned coffee enemas.

He discovered that, without such a waste-removing method, the liver was unable to handle the toxic load escaping from all dysfunctional cells and could be poisoned. In terminally ill cancer patients, Dr. Gerson observed their toxicities to be so severe that he decided to apply such coffee enemas as frequently as every four hours. The enemas worked as a primary means of detoxification (for more information on coffee enemas, see chapter 12).

And his patients reported a welcome additional benefit: pain relief quickly occurred for them as their livers released cellular toxins. Therefore, another big advantage of following the Gerson Therapy's sodium-free, high-potassium detoxifying diet was that Dr. Gerson could discontinue prescribing painkilling drugs almost at once!

High blood pressure, too, usually came down in about five days, along with discontinuation of blood pressure medication. Today, we see that the patient's immune system starts to function and, in some cases, a healing fever develops. Fever can help to destroy tumor tissue and should not be suppressed unless it goes way out of range (i.e., above 104.5°F).

With all its defenses restored, the body is again capable of destroying tumor tissue, breaking it down and excreting it. The most aggressive kinds of malignancies—melanomas, ovarian cancers, small-cell lung cancers, agressive lymphomas—retreat the most rapidly. One can almost watch them melt away. Other, less aggressive tumors grow more slowly and retreat less rapidly: the adenocarcinomas (breast cancer, prostate cancer, bone metastases, etc.) disappear slowly but steadily. At the same time, the fat-free diet, high in enzymes, also helps to dissolve atherosclerotic plaque and clear arteries, so that circulation of the blood improves, as does respiration. Now we can understand why the whole body heals; whether we are seeing patients with arthritis, emphysema, colitis, multiple sclerosis, high blood pressure, heart disease, diabetes, or any other of the multitude of acute or chronic degenerative diseases, the patients undergo healing.

VEGETABLE JUICE TO ENHANCE THE ENEMAS

Dr. Gerson found that the basic problem underlying all chronic disease is twofold: deficiency and toxicity. He clearly needed to address both these problems in order to heal his patients. The deficiency was overcome by the tremendous amount of nutrients available in the multiple vegetable juices, given every hour, made from organically grown produce.

Drinking such juices also helped to flush out the kidneys; but they caused the sick patients' tissues to release accumulated toxins into the bloodstream. These toxins were filtered out by the liver, but so much poison was burdening their livers with toxicity. Dr. Gerson realized that if he did not help the body to remove these poisons rapidly, the liver became seriously damaged and such released poisons could even cause liver coma. The coffee enemas, given in the early stages as frequently as every four hours, relieved the liver and even, in most cases, relieved pain.

As the patient continues to recover, the body dissolves tumor tissue. Toxins from this dead tissue are released into the bloodstream. At this time, it is important to increase the coffee enemas. It often takes two to three months before the number of coffee enemas can be reduced to three or four daily.

For over ten years now, coffee enemas have been more intensively studied. For instance, Peter Lechner, M.D., of the Second Surgical Division of the Landeskrankenhaus in Graz, Austria, became interested in the Gerson Therapy. He applied it to many of his outpatients and made some scientific studies on how the coffee enemas work. Dr. Lechner writes in his clinical report, "Coffee enemas have a definite effect on the colon which can be observed with an endoscope. Moreover, Wattenberg and coworkers were able to prove in 1981 that the palmitic acid found in coffee promotes the activity of the enzyme, gluthathione s-transferase, and other ligands by manifold times above the norm. It is this enzymatic group which is responsible primarily for the conjugation of free electrophile radicals which the gall bladder will then release."

In patients with addictions (to nicotine in cigarettes, heroin, morphine, cocaine, etc.) the frequent vegetable juices quickly help to overcome cravings, while the coffee enemas help to clear away any withdrawal symptoms.

Total healing for almost any degenerative condition is not complete until the patient's liver and essential organ functions are all restored to full normal activity. In most patients, healing like this takes at least two years on the full Gerson therapeutic program, including the ingestion of thirteen glasses of freshly made juices a day, organically grown vegetarian foods, regular (but slowly decreasing) coffee enemas, and the taking of potassium as well as digestive enzyme supplements.

One recent patient, MB of Canton, California, suffered from widely metastasized melanoma, had cataracts, and was unable to watch TV or read with or without glasses. Besides these difficulties, MB was suffering from advanced osteoarthritis "in all her joints," she said. Also the woman was obese and suffered from high blood pressure and diabetes.

MB's life was saved on the Gerson Therapy, supervised by her physician. When the melanoma was gone, so were this patient's other problems: she could read and watch TV, had good energy, and today at age eighty-four is "working circles" around other family members. Even her hearing has improved to the point where the family believes that "she hears more than she is supposed to." MB no longer requires insulin to control her diabetes.

Nutritional Supplements to Treat Multiple Health Problems

Dr. Gerson helped his patients' damaged body functions by adding certain digestive enzymes, plus thyroid and iodine, to activate the immune system against multiple health problems. Furthermore, because his patients were so seriously depleted, he added potassium to an already high-potassium diet. He also supported the patients' livers with liver powder capsules and liver injections and helped patients produce adequate red blood cells with extra vitamin B_{12}.

It is important to note that with the full application of the Gerson

Therapy, all the body systems are restored to full function. Dr. Gerson's healing program is a total metabolic approach, not a single treatment for a specific symptom of a disease.

Many patients have multiple problems of illness associated with their main life-threatening disability—cancer as well as diabetes, heart disease, high blood pressure, arthritis, atherosclerosis with leg cramps, macular degeneration, cataracts, and so on. When the body truly heals, all of these types of health troubles involving overall physiological degeneration disappear, not just a single disease entity. With true healing, one cannot heal selectively—all medical difficulties improve steadily and finally go away permanently.

Charlotte Gerson cites the case of a patient who was suffering from prostate cancer as well as regular kidney colics, high blood pressure, and three herniated disks resulting in severe pain and atrophy of the thigh muscle in his left leg. After two years on the Gerson Therapy, the man got rid of all these problems. His prostate was clear; he had no more kidney colics; without taking any drugs, his elevated blood pressure lowered to normal and stayed there; and the damaged vertebral disks had re-formed, thus allowing his thigh muscles also to improve. He had been on total disability due to his many health problems, but this patient returned to completely normal activity.

Following the Gerson Therapy described over fifty years ago, people become well in the same way in modern times.

One patient, Mrs. GF, was told that her arteries were 90 percent clogged and that she needed immediate coronary artery bypass surgery, or she would not see the weekend! She refused to undergo the operation and traveled instead to the Gerson Therapy hospital in Tijuana, Mexico. GF was in a very dangerous situation, needing oxygen even to sleep, and was barely able to walk across the room without assistance. But she followed the Gerson Therapy faithfully both under hospital staff supervision and on her own after returning home.

Upon reexamining her two years later, the same doctor found that GF's arteries were 100 percent clear and she was able to function normally. He claimed that some kind of medical miracle had taken place.

Why Physicians Have Failed to Tie Diet to Diseases Before Now

It has taken organized allopathic medicine too long to appreciate the connection between diet and degenerative diseases. Yet, recognizing that we have lost the war on cancer, as stated in 1986 by John C. Bailar III, Ph.D., professor of epidemiology and biostatistics at McGill University in Montreal, Canada,[1] medical doctors and their patients have now altered their thinking. Finally physicians have come to accept that diet is tied to diseases of all types.

Health professionals have had to hit upon nutritional therapy almost as a last resort against degenerative diseases, especially for cancer. Treatment using diet and nutrition is absolutely mandatory simply because too many patients never get well with the applications of standard, allopathic, conventionally practiced medicine and oncology—the disease-oriented medicine of orthodoxy. It is time to recognize diet as a powerful ally in the healing process.

Reference for Chapter Two

1. Bailar, J.C.; Smith, E.M. "Progress against cancer?" *New England Journal of Medicine.* 314:1226, 1986.

Chapter Three

THE BIOLOGICAL BASIS OF THE GERSON THERAPY

So firmly founded on scientific principles of physiology and nutrition are the therapeutic approaches developed by Max Gerson, M.D., to cancer and other chronic illnesses, they remain just as clinically valid today as in their earliest decade of establishment. One might come to believe that over a span of almost seventy years, as new medical insights and clinical protocols were uncovered, Dr. Gerson's method might have been superseded by other treatments; yet this is not the case.

The Gerson Therapy manages the body's potassium, sodium (salt), protein, and water intake. In this chapter we offer an explanation of what the Gerson biological (metabolic) concept means plus how and why it works to promote healing. There definitely is a need for animal protein restriction as the means for warding off degenerative diseases of all kinds. Required as well for reversal of cancer and other chronic diseases are potassium supplementation, acute sodium limitation, calorie restriction, protein sparing, and thyroid hormone addition. As any Gerson Therapy participant knows well, coffee enemas are featured as a way to remove circulating toxins and partial metabolites by dilating bile ducts and cleansing the liver. Dr. Gerson believed that the liver is our most important organ for maintaining the body's biochemistry for health as well as overcoming degenerative diseases, cancer in particular.

Hyperalimentation, the medication of his therapy, utilizes vegetarian foods, including raw fruit, well-cooked vegetables, salads, a special soup, oatmeal, and vegetable juices. They are the hyperalimenting medications, which have proven to be profoundly effective nutritionally, easily absorbed also by a sick body, extremely complex molecularly, and exquisite materials chemically. Ingesting them in quantity invariably restores health to an unhealthy body and prevents ill health for a well-functioning one.

Accordingly, this chapter is a preparation for utilizing the recipes of chapter 22, which describes the cooking of those specific foods for enjoying total wellness. Here we provide a full description of the biological basis for incorporating the Gerson Therapy as your personal way of life.

SUMMARIZING THE BIOLOGICAL BASIS OF THE GERSON THERAPY

Being an intensive treatment based on nutrition, designed to restore and reactivate all the body systems, the Gerson Therapy particularly strengthens one's immune system, enzyme system, and hormone system, along with correcting the functioning of all essential organs. It brings the body into homeostasis. The program's originator learned during the 1930s that in chronic degenerative diseases most of the organ systems become damaged and function poorly to the point of shutting down. He concluded that the body's innate *healing mechanism* eventually becomes inactive so that a debilitated body loses its ability to fight the attacking disease and heal.

Successful treatment for chronic illnesses requires full-bodied nutrition, specifically, a sick person must eat organic vegetarian foods, all freshly prepared. Also mandatory is the drinking of thirteen glasses of raw vegetable juices for their enzymatic effects. All foods must be free of added salt and fats, with one specific exception: flaxseed oil (high in linoleic and linolenic acids). Thus the damaged organ systems are flooded with living nutrients, easily absorbed and able to enter the deficient tissues. Required foods are high in potassium, which Dr. Gerson found to be lacking in longtime ill persons.

When active minerals and enzymes are restored to the tissues, these nutrients release the excess sodium and toxins that have accumulated during the course of years of faulty nutrition. It becomes imperative then to help the body (the liver in particular) to filter out released toxins and get rid of them. In order to achieve such a release and bring about detoxification, Dr. Gerson discovered that caffeine given rectally definitely assists the liver and its bile ducts to release their accumulated poisons into the intestinal tract for elimination.

Ozone given by rectal insufflation is also very valuable since it increases blood oxygenation, energy, and the ability of organ systems to function at higher levels. Most patients residing in a Gerson-certified health care facility also inhale air furnished by an ozone generator operating in their rooms. The machine thus provides patients with better oxygenation and overcomes antigenic odors. A similar ozone generator may be installed in the home.

Physiological Universality of the Gerson Therapy

The basic philosophy of the Gerson Therapy—hypernutrition from whole foods and detoxification—is universal for advantageous body functioning. As we have mentioned, such universality includes elimination of all toxic materials—natural and synthetic—derived from any source of additives, perfumes, cosmetics, flavorings, dyes, herbicides, fluoride, chloride, metallic poisons, pesticide residues, cleaning agents, and as much of other environmental pollutants as possible.

The Gerson Therapy has to be adjusted for particular body breakdowns with their resulting ailments and conditions, including candidiasis, diabetes, colitis, ascites in terminal cancer patients, cardiovascular disease, and high doses of chemotherapy, radiotherapy, prednisone, and other common drugs, plus a myriad of additional difficulties. Often patients suffer from infections, low-grade fevers, lack of appetite, pain, and many more complications, some of them subclinical. All of these disabilities are addressed individually and collectively during the course of administering the Gerson program. For human physiology, the Gerson Therapy is restorative and completely enhancing.

Along with the basic nutrition and detoxification, certain food supplements are also used to overcome deficiencies of vitamins, minerals, hormones, enzymes, and other physiological items. The limited number of Gerson Therapy nutritional supplements include a potassium compound, digestive enzymes, thyroid hormone, iodine (Lugol's solution), vitamin B_3 (niacin), and vitamin B_{12} (cobalamin), as well as injectable crude liver extract and/or liver powder or tablets. These "medications" are also adjusted to each patient's needs.

How the Gerson Therapy Aligns with Conventional Treatments

A few of the treatments used in conventional medicine are compatible with the Gerson Therapy, including hydrotherapy, oxygen, antibiotics, in some cases radiation, and certain surgical operations (as for gastrointestinal tract blockage or the debulking of tumors). Surprisingly, perhaps, certain other physical therapies such as deep massage, vigorous exercise, and saltwater swimming are harmful.

Chemotherapy is not encouraged at all because it is highly toxic, suppressive of the immune system, and sometimes palliative but hardly curative. Someone who undergoes chemotherapy prior to adopting Dr. Gerson's treatment starts off at a true immunological disadvantage. The Gerson Therapy in no way advocates the use of cytotoxic chemicals for killing off cancer cells because such chemicals frequently bring patients closer to more serious illness and death.

Yet numerous cancer patients pretreated with chemotherapy can still respond positively to the Gerson approach. These people include especially those suffering from ovarian cancer, lymphomas, kidney cancer, and some of the glandular malignancies, such as breast and prostate cancer. For those with pancreatic cancer, the Gerson Institute has seen a number of long-term, total recoveries with the Gerson Therapy (see chapter 21); however, we are sorry to report that poor responses are likely to result for the pancreas-cancer patient if chemotherapy was previously applied. The organ becomes just too damaged by the cytotoxicity of chemicals applied.

Long-Term Survival and Side Effects

The largest body of evidence offering proof of the Gerson Therapy's value was given in Dr. Gerson's original text, *A Cancer Therapy: Results of Fifty Cases*, first published in 1958. Even back then, almost all of his patients had been biopsied prior to starting the Gerson Therapy by different accredited medical institutions around the United States. All but two of the patients shown in this description of fifty cases were in terminal condition. They survived a minimum of five years; at least a dozen people have remained alive for forty-five years from when they first began their Gerson treatment plan.

Since the Gerson Therapy has been promoted more and reestablished during the last twenty years, numbers of documented cases of recovered patients have been assembled. You will read about three such situations in chapter 21. Admittedly, the only cancer that has been documented statistically with a retrospective analysis peer-reviewed and published in a medical journal is malignant melanoma (see chapter 6). In other cancers, the Gerson Institute records many individual recovered cases, all with prior biopsies and long-term survival, but exact figures are still not available because the Gerson Institute loses track of patients. They tend to stop communicating and go on with their lives. But now the Gerson Institute's Client Services department has created a Patient Support Network to provide a listing of fellow patients to those undertaking the treatment on their own.

There have been no untoward side effects from the use of the Gerson Therapy. Dr. Gerson's recommended fresh organic foods and juices—his medication consisting of only normal body substances and the cleansing enemas—in no way cause bodily damage. Certain patients are not treatable: those with organ transplants, patients on dialysis, and patients who have had essential organs removed. Some uninformed persons warn about dehydration or another imagined difficulty. They just don't know what they are talking about. Such people are down on what they are not up on.

In contrast, sometimes Gerson patients jokingly refer to certain "side effects" of their program—the beneficial ones. These advantageous effects include the clearing up of high blood pressure, elimination of arthritis, sight restoration in glaucoma, self-correction of herniated disks, pulmonary improvement in asthma, and many more betterments for health troubles.

Please take note of the following double fact, which may seem obvious to you after having read this book, but it's something that uninformed persons do not acknowledge:

- It is often impossible to heal a specific disease such as cancer while the body continues to suffer from diabetes, arthritis, heart disease, and most other chronic disturbances.
- We see that eventually all the other afflictions also disappear when the Gerson Therapy is utilized for healing cancer.

MANAGING POTASSIUM, SALT, AND WATER INTAKE

Around every tumor or arthritic joint, in most chronic viral conditions such as genital herpes, and in other long-standing pathologies, the patients' tissues which have lost potassium do gain sodium and swell with too much water. Today it has been established in modern medicine that this is a physiological fact.

When he studied tuberculous infections, Dr. Gerson observed the same phenomenon and recorded it in his published works. Around every tubercular cavern and cavity he saw a puffy malfunctioning sphere of adjacent tissue damaged by toxins escaping from the tuberculosis organism. Partial metabolites in the disease lesions cause difficulties because they are merely waste material that continues with destructive processes when left in place. Their presence upsets otherwise normal tissue so that it, in turn, becomes damaged.

By restricting sodium and substituting elevated amounts of potassium by providing his patients with a fresh fruit and vegetable diet, Dr. Gerson was able to bring about absorption of cellular edema. The patients' swellings disappeared by eliminating the tissue damage syndrome that surrounds not only tubercular tissue but also tumor tissue.

The Gerson Therapy, therefore, creates a physiological situation in which distressed cells slowly return to normal. What brings this about is the unspiced low-sodium, high-potassium diet required by the Gerson Therapy. It works therapeutically—nothing else known in drug-oriented allopathic, traditional Indian Ayurvedic, Central American shaman, traditional Chinese, holistic, complementary and alternative, chiropractic, naturopathic, homeopathic, or other form of medicine achieves this same beneficial effect in damaged cells. We repeat, this diet developed by Max Gerson, M.D., is a primary reason for the Gerson Therapy's efficaciousness against cancer and other chronic illnesses.

Gilbert Ning Ling, Ph.D., father of the new cellular biology that's based on "dry" physics rather than "wet" chemistry (which had previously been the foundation of modern allopathic medicine), early in the 1970s, predicted the value of a high-potassium, low-sodium nutritional intake for the obliteration of chronic disease.[1] Dr. Ling's research had evolved from Dr. Gerson's original investigations and treatments, which he had employed, first for the elimination of migraine headaches, and then for allergies, tuberculosis, and chronic diseases, and later adapted as his anticancer program.

Then another pioneering physician, the medical physicist and researcher Freeman W. Cope, M.D., Ph.D., in 1978, uncovered evidence to prove that Dr. Ling's association-induction hypothesis derived from the Gerson work was correct. Dr. Cope demonstrated that cells are poisoned by any one of a unifying set of occurrences which usually includes oxygen starvation, one or more physical traumas, and/or some type of chemical insult such as the toxic metal syndrome.[2]

No matter what is the tissue's origin of dysfunction, the same responses occur in cells throughout any part of the body: first the damaged cell loses most of its potassium, next it accepts an abundance of sodium, and finally it swells with excessive water (to dilute the sodium). This bloated cell's required life-sustaining energy in the form of adenosine triphosphate (ATP), created from the burning of sugar through oxidation, dissipates. Without ATP the cell dies. Lose enough cells and the tissue dies. Experience a dramatic drop in tissue substance and the organ dies. Lack a necessary organ and the human being dies. In his two major published works, Dr. Cope informed physiologists about this pathologic occurrence.[3,4]

About a decade ago, Dr. Cope's concept was proved to be true by the additional medical research of the respected Mexican physiologist and cardiologist Demetrio Sodi-Pallares, M.D. Then Raymond Damadian, M.D., inventor of the diagnostic device magnetic resonance imaging (MRI), confirmed that human cells behave more like ion exchange granules in a water softener than like bags of water. Prior to Dr. Damadian's theory, medicine's idea of "cells as bags of water" had been the basis on which almost all medical treatments were built (until now). But medical science is evolving.

Going back chronologically, collectively, and in summary, Dr. Damadian, Dr. Sodi-Pallares, Dr. Cope, Dr. Ling, and Dr. Gerson have brought forth a new medical foundation for why diseases become chronically degenerative and how they may be reversed. The foundation developed by these five medical scientists is that the cellular cytoplasm becomes latticed with a protein-lipid macromolecule through which an electron current flows. Energy-storing ATP is complexed with this macromolecule, polarizing and energizing it, to form many interactive, cooperative association sites which prefer potassium over sodium. Give the sick cell potassium, and it gets well. Then restrict animal protein, and it becomes even healthier.

Protein Restriction

With the aim of ridding damaged body cells of more sodium, Dr. Gerson eliminated animal protein from the patient's diet—at least for a period of six or eight weeks. He caused the condition of sodium outflooding (what he named *"Natrium Ausschuss"*) so that the detrimental mineral poured out of the body in its urine waste. That way, edema gets absorbed by the cells, tissues, and organs. In the context of Dr. Ling's modern work on biophysics, Dr. Gerson's healing procedure is absolutely correct. During studies that he conducted in Egypt, Robert Good, M.D., former director of the Sloan-Kettering Institute for Cancer Research, showed that the Gerson method of protein restriction tends to stimulate T-lymphocyte activity and cell-mediated immunity.

Bioavailable protein derives from the content of potatoes, vegetables, vegetable juices, and oatmeal. About 40 grams of protein lost each day by waste excretion is replaced through the Gerson basic vegan diet with some added dairy protein. The patient is kept in a positive nitrogen balance.

In addition to protein restriction, the Gerson diet does reduce calories (despite the patient's consuming 20 pounds of produce daily) by means of limiting fat intake. In this diet the only fats allowed are from the ongoing eating of oatmeal (1.5 percent calories in fat), flaxseed oil, and the fatty acids in some vegetables and fruits—a total of just 90 calories of fat daily.

The Gerson Therapy was perfected, therefore, to offer potassium supplementation, sodium near-elimination, calorie limitation, protein restriction, and thyroid hormone addition. Additionally, there is restructuring of all the cells' water content to produce molecular reorganization of their protoplasmic water.

The ill person's body activities are speeded along as well. It's done on purpose, for the Gerson Therapy specifically is a metabolic treatment that stimulates all body processes.

Metabolism is the sum total of all the biochemical processes going on inside the body, and metabolic therapies focus on ways to balance these chemical processes—enabling normal cells to thrive and cancer cells to become depleted and die, or revert back to normal. The therapeutic goal of metabolic therapies such as Dr. Gerson's approach is to rebuild and revitalize all of the body's life-sustaining functions, thereby helping to stop and reverse cancer or to prevent a recurrence.[5]

Metabolism consists of two fundamental phases, anabolism and catabolism. Anabolism is the constructive, building-up phase, fostering growth and order, storage of energy, and production of organic substances such as enzymes, hormones, antibodies, and cell membrane receptors. Catabolism is the destructive phase, in which matter is broken down and energy (ATP) is used. All fundamental biochemical processes are either anabolic or catabolic in nature. The Gerson Therapy stimulates both so that the body finds its required homeostatic balance.[6]

METABOLIC SPEEDUP

Dr. Gerson wanted cellular metabolism, so he turned it on with large loading dosages of the iodides, iodine, and up to 5 grains of thyroid hormone too. With their ingestion, the patient's metabolism speeds up as manifested by his or her racing pulse, perhaps over 100 beats per minute.

Thyroid hormone signals mitochondria (organelles in the cytoplasm of cells that contain genetic material and many enzymes important for cell metabolism) to multiply and increase production of ATP for more cellular energy. Iodides and iodine affect many metabolizing tissues directly in the same way.

When tumor tissue is present, it spreads pathology outward like a sphere (resembling the sun's penumbra), which is several times the tumor's volume. Within this sphere, cellular tissue works poorly because it is waterlogged, insulted, and damaged by cancerous toxins. Metabolic waste escapes from the tumor and poisons what had been normal tissue. Not functioning well at all, the tissue just sits there stewing in its own waste without any good immunity, in a state of poor blood circulation, lacking resistance, and experiencing bad drainage.

Even with the tumor removed surgically, the sphere of tissue remains waterlogged unless the cancer patient is provided a way to correct that tissue damage. With the Gerson Therapy, the sodium ring around tumors disappears within weeks, beause that's how effective Dr. Gerson's management has shown itself against the kind of tissue damage syndrome that is seen as the penumbra around tumors.

THE BIOLOGICAL BASIS FOR COFFEE ENEMAS

Capable of removing circulating toxins and partial metabolites, the coffee enema dilates bile ducts. This happens because the coffee administered by means of a cleansing enema stimulates an enzyme system in the liver known as *glutathione S-transferase* (GST) that removes a vast variety of free radicals (electrophiles) from the bloodstream.

Electrophiles are atomic particles with one or more electrons in unpaired spins which have an affinity for other electrons. They want to get involved where they should not. As charged particles, these free radicals damage membranes of cells and inflict disturbances in cellular metabolism.

Under the influence of a coffee enema the GST enzyme system increases in activity to 650 percent above normal and removes electrophiles from the bloodstream. No material other than coffee (not even coenzyme Q_{10} or oligomeric proanthocyanidine [OPC]) is known to stimulate free radical quenching in such a proportion. The free radicals are mopped up and removed by GST enzymes through the use of coffee cleansing of the lower bowel (gut).

During the time coffee is being held in the gut, all the blood in the body passes through the liver at least five times. The blood circulates through the liver every three minutes. (According to concepts espoused in Ayurvedic medicine, the liver regrows and replaces itself about every three months.) The palmitate compounds and the caffeine, theobromine, and theophylline in coffee cause dilation of the liver's blood vessels and bile ducts, relaxation of smooth muscles, stimulation of intestinal peristalsis, and elevation of bile flow.

The quart of distilled water being used as a vehicle for this internally supplied therapeutic coffee concentrate assists in these various actions too. Toxic bile is flushed out along with its bile salts to bring about effective dialysis that is advantageous.

The coffee enema removes ammonialike products, toxic-bound nitrogen, protein derivatives, polyamines, amino acids, coagulated clumps, and complexes, all of which are waste products of metabolism. Getting rid of them frees the body from becoming poisoned by its own wastes.

THE GERSON TECHNIQUE OF HYPERALIMENTATION

We have stated a number of times that for the Gerson patient, vegetarian foods, raw fruit, and vegetable juices act as the medications of choice. Collectively consuming such foods brings about hyperalimentation. And we've emphasized that such organically grown, freshly prepared natural foods are profoundly effective, extremely complex, chemically exquisite substances that heal better than anything ever invented by the mind of man. Now please accept our warning: Tamper with such nourishment at your own risk. Our advice is to avoid synthetic substances, including prescribed drugs, whenever you can do so.

Macronutrient hyperalimentation, the practice of selecting only food substances produced in nature under ideal conditions to feed the body optimal nourishment, is the method employed in the Gerson Therapy. It works to heal ill health in the body and restore it to homeostasis.

As described again, the biological basis for the Gerson Therapy is predicated on sodium restriction, potassium supplementation, protein limitation, calorie reduction through avoidance of fat, dialysis of the bloodstream for reduction of electrophiles, macronutrient hyperalimentation, salt and water management, and accelerated metabolism. This health-revitalization program has come out of the thinking of one man, Max Gerson, M.D. By studious application of his clinical work with patients, his search of the medical literature, and his strong scientific foundations, we are the beneficiaries.

References for Chapter Three

1. Ling, G.N. *In Search of the Physical Basis of Life*. New York: Plenum Press, 1984.

2. Casdorph, H.R.; Walker, M. *Toxic Metal Syndrome*. Garden City Park, N.Y.: Avery Publishing Group, 1995.

3. Cope, F.W. "Pathology of structured water and associated cations in cells (the tissue damage syndrome) and its medical treatment." *Physiological Chemistry and Physics*. 9(6):547–553, 1977.

4. Cope, F.W. "The Ling association-induction hypothesis: the high potassium, low sodium diet of the Gerson cancer therapy." *Physiological Chemistry and Physics*, 10(5):465–468, 1978.

5. Diamond, W.J.; Cowden, W.L.; Goldberg, B. *An Alternative Medicine Definitive Guide to Cancer.* Tiburon, Calif.: Future Medicine Publishing, 1997, p. 309.

6. *Ibid.*, p. 310.

Chapter Four

THE CORE OF
THE GERSON THERAPY

Residing in the county of Devon, England, for all of his fifty-eight years, Xavier Naude, an independently wealthy, refined British gentleman, has been an exponent of experiencing life in full measure, including heavy smoking. By 1992 Mr. Naude had developed emphysema, the result of his smoke inhalation, which grew steadily worse with each carton of cigarettes he consumed. Indeed, Mr. Naude burned up three packs daily.

In *pulmonary emphysema*, the air sacs (alveoli) of the lungs lose their permeability and become damaged, which reduces their surface area for the exchange of oxygen and carbon dioxide. The condition's worst and most frightening symptom is breathlessness, which may be complicated by infections. There has been no specific drug or other medical treatment, and the patient often becomes dependent on the intake of oxygen by mechanical means such as the use of oxygen mask and tank plus inhalant devices.

How emphysema develops is hardly understood at all, although it is known to be particularly common in men. While it is associated with chronic bronchitis and advancing age, inhaling cigarette smoke is the main source of this disease.

Xavier Naude started to use mechanical drug inhalants and vasodilators to help him breathe. But more and more, he found himself suffering from exhaustion. In June 1993, he learned about the healing qualities of the Gerson Therapy, and by September of that year he had traveled to San

Diego, crossed the U.S./Mexican border and enrolled as a patient at a Tijuana clinic providing the Gerson Therapy.

Prior to participating in the Gerson Therapy, even after giving up smoking, using the inhalants, and taking other medications in England, Mr. Naude felt severe pressure on his chest. He was unable to climb stairs and encountered great difficulty breathing all the time. His doctors in the United Kingdom had explained that 70 percent of his lung tissue was lost. In addition, he experienced awful leg cramps when he tried to sleep. The poor man also felt arthritic pain in his fingers so severely that he could not close them around a glass of juice.

In Mexico, all of these symptoms disappeared one after the other while he was receiving the Gerson program. Mr. Naude reported, in fact, that even after the first day of his participation in such dietary treatment approach, his leg cramps were gone. Some days later he could make a fist, an action previously impossible, but now he felt no more finger pain. And at the end of a week, the pressure on his chest eased too. By the conclusion of two weeks on the Gerson Therapy, Mr. Naude discovered that he could walk without stopping to catch his breath.

He remained at the Gerson hospital for three weeks all together, and afterward followed the therapeutic program on his own at home. He continued to thrive. For Xavier Naude, there was nothing mysterious about the Gerson Therapy. It had a clear-cut self-treatment plan, open and understandable to anyone willing to give the dietary/detoxification combination some study. Mr. Naude stated, "I am totally satisfied with the tremendous progress I've made away from the disability of emphysema."

Xavier Naude's Harley Street thoracic specialist also confirmed by written report that his patient's lung capacity had increased in a relatively short period from 30 to 50 percent. The doctor found this astonishing. No longer could emphysema be considered uncorrectable.

PATIENTS LIKE XAVIER NAUDE
ARE TYPICAL

If there's any secret connected with the Gerson Therapy, it is that Gerson patients are helped past the burden of not only cancer but nearly every other acute or chronic degenerative disease. Emphysema is but one example among dozens.

Cytotoxic poisons used in oncology merely attack tumor tissue while damaging normal cells at the same time. The Gerson Therapy does not do this. Rather, Dr. Gerson's fundamental idea, as he stated, is the following: "A normal body has the capacity to keep all cells functioning properly. It prevents any abnormal transformation and growth. Therefore, the natural task of this cancer therapy is to bring the body back to that normal physiology, or as near to it as is possible."[1]

Dr. Gerson's "secret" nutritional method steadily changes, by degrees. It brings an exceedingly sick and malfunctioning body to a state of subclinical illness, then advances that body to low-level wellness, followed by attaining homeostasis, next becoming a body exhibiting high-level wellness, and finally to being able to feel the joy of achieving the highest peak of physiological performance. Abstracted from two sources, the *Gerson Healing Newsletter* and Dr. Max Gerson's original book, *A Cancer Therapy: Results of Fifty Cases*, the following sections offer you a brief and simplified description of the Gerson diet from top to bottom. Later chapters will cover the methods of detoxification, which begin with juicing in chapter 9 and go on to coffee enemas in chapters 12 and 13. All of these procedures are equally vital for a sick person's recovery.

AN ABSTRACT OF THE GERSON THERAPY

From information we've already furnished, you know that in the years just prior to and following World War II, German-American physician Max Gerson, M.D., newly immigrated to the United States, proposed an empirically developed set of general dietary and medical measures. He used measures for the successful management of patients suffering from body system deterioration of all types, most especially tuberculosis, kidney diseases, diabetes, liver diseases, rheumatoid arthritis, stroke, gallbladder disease, nearly every addiction, and almost all of the over one hundred kinds of malignancies.

Dr. Gerson's therapeutic techniques involved having each patient use an integrated set of particular health care methods and managements, including focusing on the following (see Table 4-1):[2]

A. salt and water intake management through sodium (Na^+) mineral restriction and potassium (K^+) mineral supplementation,

B. superabundant intakes (hyperalimentation) of both macronutrients and micronutrients through the regular hourly preparation and drinking of raw, organically grown fruit and vegetable juices,

   C.   extreme limitation of fats consumed in foods,

   D.   temporary protein restriction through a basically vegetarian diet,

   E.   natural, supplemental thyroid administration,

   F.   production of bile by the liver (choleresis) by means of frequent self-administered coffee enemas.

THE CORE OF THE GERSON THERAPY

Dr. Gerson's dietary program, once established, was approved and employed by large numbers of medical authors who duplicated his results to cure migraine headaches and cutaneous tuberculosis (lupus vulgaris). It was also described in clinical journals published worldwide as a therapy for the various forms of pulmonary, gastrointestinal, and bone tuberculoses; cardiorenal insufficiency; skin conditions of many types including eczema, lichen planus, systemic lupus erythematosus (SLE), psoriasis, and pruritus; bronchitis and bronchiectasis; and nearly every liver and gallbladder condition.

By modifying the program, Dr. Gerson applied his therapeutic nutritional regimen to cancer, rheumatoid and osteoarthritis, cardiovascular diseases, multiple sclerosis, tuberculosis, migraine headaches, and much more, publishing results in American and German peer-reviewed journals. Table 4-1 reveals the core of Max Gerson's precise approach to changing an ill individual's physiology to a healthy one. By following the Gerson Therapy faithfully, a sick person can markedly improve his or her chances for illness reversal, resumption of good health, and assurance of continuing wellness.

Harold D. Foster, B.Sc., Ph.D., professor of geography at the University of Victoria in Victoria, British Columbia, Canada explained, "Gerson's Therapy drastically alters the mineral balance of the patient's body. Anyone undertaking this treatment rapidly loses sodium, while at the same time potassium and iodine body levels rise. Milk, cheese, and butter are forbidden, especially during the first months. Calcium is available through the carrot and green juices to the extent that osteoporosis can be reversed with the Gerson Therapy. The emphasis on fresh fruits and vegetables also means that the patient received high levels of anti-oxidants, especially betacarotene and vitamin C."[3]

THE GERSON THERAPY—IN HIS OWN WORDS

Here, in Dr. Gerson's own words (see the original edition of *A Cancer Therapy*), is a summary of his theory.[4]

> As science is not yet developed to the point of knowing all the enzymes, vitamins and many biological functions of hormones and minerals, it is safer to use foods raised, if possible, by an organic gardening process, thus obeying the laws of nature. [Today, more than forty-one years after he wrote these words, Dr. Gerson's concept is proven even more appropriate.] This observation helped the human race for thousands of years before any science was developed. In this way we bring in all known vitamins and enzymes, both the discovered and the undiscovered ones, and especially the unknown—"life stimulating substances"—given best as fresh as possible and not damaged by refining or preserving processes, such as canned [smoked, frozen, freeze-dried, dehydrated, irradiated, and otherwise manhandled] food. These contain all of the necessary substances in their proper quantity, mixture and composition, and are regulated by instinct, hunger, taste, smell, sight and other factors.

TABLE 4-1

The Core of the Gerson Therapy

The Gerson Therapy is a series of harmonious and cohesive medical treatments which have been observed to cure many individual cases of advanced cancer and other major health problems in mankind.

- The treatments consist of salt and water management which holds down the intake of Na^+ and increases the intake of K^+.
- A sick person's metabolism and cell energy production are stimulated by supplementing with natural thyroid hormone.
- Maximum digestibility of nutrients is achieved by hourly drinking fresh, raw vegetable and fruit juices and eating a basically vegetarian diet.
- Fat is restricted in order, to lower intake of disease promoters of all kinds.
- The restriction of protein tends to uplift a patient's immune response.
- Coffee enemas stimulate the bowel and liver enzymes to eliminate toxins across the bowel wall. It is a kind of intestinal dialysis.

Three-quarters of the foods [for illness-prevention] which should be consumed include the following:

All kinds of fruits, mostly fresh and some prepared in different ways; freshly prepared fruit juices (orange, grapefruit, grape, etc.); fruit salads; cold fruit soups; mashed bananas, raw grated apples, applesauce, etc.

All vegetables freshly prepared, some stewed in their own juices and others either raw or finely grated, such as carrots, cauliflower or celery; vegetable salads, soups, etc.; some dried fruits and vegetables are permitted but no frozen ones.

Potatoes are best when baked; the contents may be mashed with nonfat yogurt or salt-free soup; they should never be fried and preferably boiled in their jackets.

Salads of green leaves or mixed with tomatoes, fruits, vegetables, etc.

Bread should contain whole rye or some (up to 20 percent) whole wheat flour, or these may be mixed; it should be refined as little as possible. Oatmeal should be used freely. Buckwheat cakes and potato pancakes are optional, as are brown sugar, honey, maple sugar and maple candy. (No baking powder or baking soda may be used, even in cooking.)

Milk and milk products, such as pot cheese and other kinds of cheese which are not salted or spiced, buttermilk, nonfat yoghurt and butter. Cream and ice cream should be reduced to a minimum or restricted to holidays (ice cream is "poison" for children).

The remaining one-fourth of the dietary regimen, which allows for personal choice, may consist of meat, fish, eggs, nuts, candies, cakes, or whatever one likes best. Nicotine should be avoided; liquors, wine and beer should be reduced to a minimum in favor of fresh fruit juices; coffee and tea should be cut to a minimum with the exception of the following herb teas: peppermint, camomile, linden flower, orange flower, and a few others.

Salt, bicarbonate of soda, smoked fish and sausage should be avoided as much as possible, as should sharp condiments such as pepper and ginger, but fresh garden herbs should be used—onions, parsley leaves, chives, celery and even some horseradish.

As for vegetables and fruits, they should, I repeat, be stewed in their own juices to avoid the loss of minerals easily dissolved in water during cooking. It seems that these valuable minerals are not so well absorbed when they are out of their colloidal state.

All vegetables (except mushrooms and cucumbers) may be used. Especially recommended for their mineral content are carrots, peas, tomatoes, Swiss chard, spinach, string beans, Brussels sprouts, artichokes, beets cooked with apples, cauliflower with tomatoes, red cabbage with apples, raisins, etc.

The best way to prepare vegetables is to cook them slowly for one and one-half to two hours, without water. To prevent burning, place a heat distributing metal plate (asbestos mats have been replaced) under the saucepan. You may also use some stock of [special Hippocrates] soup or else onions or sliced tomatoes may be added to the vegetables. This also will improve the taste. Spinach water is too bitter for use; it generally is not liked and should be drained off. Onions, leeks and tomatoes have enough liquid of their own to keep them moist while cooking. (Beets should be cooked like potatoes, in their jackets and with water.) Wash and scrub vegetables thoroughly, but do not peel or scrape them. Saucepans must be tightly covered to prevent steam from escaping. Covers must be heavy or close fitting. (Use no pressure cookers.) Cooked vegetables may be kept in the refrigerator overnight. To warm them, heat slowly with a little soup or fresh tomato juice.

Dr. Gerson goes on to editorialize about his nutritional program's dietary summary. In conclusion, he additionally writes:[5]

The human body has a wonderful reserve power and many possibilities of adjustment, but the best defense apparatus is a 100 percent functioning metabolism and reabsorption in the intestinal tract in combination with a healthy liver. People may conclude, needlessly, that it is not important to place so much emphasis on nutrition. This may be so under normal conditions and if these persons are not damaged through heredity, civilization, sickness, trauma or other accumulations (nicotine and other poisons).

Civilization has partially taken away this natural bestowal. Experiments on test groups to produce different vitamin deficiencies by omitting food containing these vitamins showed that one third can be made deficient in about four months and two thirds in six months; only 5 to 6 percent resisted ten months of deficient feeding here in the United States. These nutritional experiments and others show that only a minority possesses a complete intact reabsorption apparatus and at the same time enough adjustment and reserve power for healthy and unhealthy periods in their lives.

It is not necessary for healthy persons to care so much about enough or too many carbohydrates and proteins, and their caloric value should be ignored. However, one cannot ignore the absolutely necessary minerals, vitamins and enzymes in their most natural composition and in sufficient amounts for a relatively long term and remain unpunished. The minerals have to be in the tissues where they belong, as they are the carriers of the electrical potentials in the cells; and there they enable the hormones, vitamins and enzymes to function properly. This gives the body the best working power and reserves for a sound metabolism and life.

REDISCOVERING THE WHEEL

A spate of popular consumer books—some hitting the best-seller lists—are now discussing Dr. Max Gerson's concept of diet and nutrition as the means of preventing and treating cancer. They are filling library and bookstore shelves today with what medical/nutrition specialists consider some kind of revolutionary concept. For them, it's new information. And none of the authors are giving our Dr. Gerson the credit due. Such books as Dr. Bob Arnot's *The Breast Cancer Prevention Diet* and *Eat to Beat Cancer* and *Dr. Gaynor's Cancer Prevention Program* make the case that anyone can eat to reduce the risk of degenerative diseases such as cancer. Such books lay out specific regimens to follow that are copycat versions of Dr. Gerson's original dietary approach to eliminating all types of illnesses, cancer in particular.

Moreover, some former professional/political persecutors of Dr. Gerson are rediscovering the wheel by talking about food as a means of therapy against cancer and other chronic illnesses. Grudgingly, pushed and pulled by the public's disillusionment with President Richard Nixon's lost "war against cancer," they are coming around to believing in the importance of diet and nutrition as cancer reducers.

When it comes to deciding whether we should improve our lifestyles by following the teachings of Dr. Max Gerson or sustain ourselves, if possible, on snack chips, Danish pastries, pizza, cheeseburgers, ice cream, and other junk foods, Gabriel Feldman, M.D., director of the prostate and colorectal cancer programs for the American Cancer Society, admits, "We don't need years of research. If people would implement what we know today, cancer rates would drop. It's that simple."

Dr. Max Gerson was correct in his medical/nutritional literary presentation of 1958 before the advent of fast food restaurants and supermarket convenience foods, and his intuitions are even more accurate today.

References for Chapter Four

1. Quoted in Walters, R. *Options: The Alternative Cancer Therapy Book* Garden City Park, N.Y.: Avery Publishing Group, 1992, pp. 189, 190.

2. Hildenbrand, G. "Bread, propaganda, and circuses." *Gerson Healing Newsletter*. 4(18/19):1, March/June 1987.

3. Foster, H.D. "Lifestyle changes and the 'spontaneous' regression of cancer: an initial computer analysis." *International Journal of Biosocial Research*. 10(1):17–33, 1988.

4. Gerson, M. A *Cancer Therapy: Results of Fifty Cases. Summarizing 30 Years of Clinical Practice and Experimentation. The Powerful Nutritional Therapy that Has Healed Thousands*. Bonita, Calif.: The Gerson Institute, 1958, pp. 22–24.

5. *Ibid.*, pp. 27–28.

Chapter Five

REMISSION—HOW IT HAPPENS

We should be paying more attention to the exceptional patients, those who get well unexpectedly, instead of staring bleakly at all those who die in the usual pattern. In the words of René Dubos, "Sometimes the more measurable drives out the most important."
Bernie B. Siegel, M.D., in *Love, Medicine and Miracles*

CURE OF LYMPHOMA BY USE OF THE GERSON THERAPY

Practicing as a chiropractor since 1955 in Amarillo, Texas, John Albracht, D.C., now age sixty-six, first underwent surgery for the removal of mixed-cell lymphoma in 1963. The laparotomy, performed then by surgeon Charles Y. Mayo Jr., M.D., son of the Mayo Clinic's famous founder, uncovered an irregular retroperitoneal tumor pushing up through the mesentery of the small bowel. Dr. Albracht's cancer was so large and extensive that it was considered inoperable, and Dr. Mayo Jr. merely closed up the incision. He sent his patient to receive twenty fractions of cobalt radiotherapy.

Following Dr. Albracht's radiation treatments, his residual mass shrank rapidly. At the time of his initial biopsy and laparotomy, Dr. Albracht was thirty years old.

He remained in remission for twenty-four years. On December 1, 1986, however, Dr. Albracht had a recurrence of multiple discomforting signs and symptoms of malignant disease. They consisted of severe gastrointestinal bleeding, excessive sweating (diaphoresis), muscle weakness, gastrointestinal gas, belching, indigestion, epigastric fullness, diarrhea, tachycardia, a low hemoglobin reading of 8 g/dL (normal is 14–18 g/dL), and a low packed red cell volume in blood (hematocrit) of 26 mL/dL (normal is 40–54 mL/dL). Four days later at the High Plains Baptist Hospital in Amarillo, gastrointestinal surgeon Gregorio Matos, M.D., performed a small-bowel resection with end-to-end anastomosis on the patient. The lymphoma involved one-third of the small bowel and extended to the mesothelium, including the whole jejunum down to the proximal ileum. Indeed, along with 7 feet of small bowel, the malignant tumor removed from Dr. Albracht's belly was the size of a cantaloupe.

Recommended followup by oncologist Karim Nawaz, M.D., was with massive amounts of five potent cytotoxic agents for a minimum of eight chemotherapies starting January 11, 1987. The patient tolerated two chemo treatments, but their adverse side effects were so awful—nausea and vomiting, diarrhea, abdominal cramping, severe abdominal pain, irritation, hoarseness, chest pains, shortness of breath, coughing, pain in the lower back, pain in the testicles, burning and swelling of both arms where the chemotherapy injections were placed, and a serious weight loss of 55 pounds in three weeks—that he voluntarily discontinued them.

"Dr. Matos used my case as a luncheon case study at the High Plains Baptist Hospital here. He told his study group that I had maybe three to six months to live," said Dr. Albracht.[1]

That's when this patient, still filled with abdominal disease, entered the Gerson Therapy hospital in Tijuana, Mexico, on Februrary 17, 1987. Dr. Matos and Dr. Nawaz continued to monitor his progress. They observed that his tumor mass, just to the right of the umbilicus, shrank steadily from 4 cm by 7 cm to nothing. By the close of 1987, with Dr. Albracht still following the Gerson dietary treatment for cancer, his mass was no longer detectable using any type of medical diagnostic method. The two conservative Amarillo cancer specialists, investigating the patient by use of lymphangiograms, bone marrow tests, laboratory tests, physical examinations, and more, considered him cured then and still do now.

Dr. Matos said to Dr. Albracht, "The way you were going downhill, your health was deteriorating. And I think you did the right things to bring your health back up, and your weight and strength, and to get some sunshine." Even now, Dr. John Albracht continues to maintain his Gerson Therapy eating and detoxification program. He still goes for regular five-month, follow-up checkups by Dr. Matos.[2]

Since his successful employment of the Gerson Therapy for reversing deadly malignant lymphoma, Dr. Albracht currently incorporates diet and nutrition into his practice of chiropractic. He admits to having used the Gerson dietary program as the sole means for saving and preserving his life. Yet some uninformed medical observers who are biased in favor of drug or radiation therapies may point to the patient's cured cancer and

comment with disdain, "Oh, that's just an example of a cancer's spontaneous regression." But Dr. John Albracht, whose life had been teetering in
the balance, knows the truth. There was no spontaneity to his cancer regression. He worked hard to achieve it in 1987 and now continues to do so
every day (see the photograph of Dr. Albracht with his wife).

THERE IS NO "SPONTANEOUS REMISSION" OF CANCER

In chapter 4, we briefly quoted from an article regarding cancer remission for patients resulting from lifestyle improvements. The information
came from a study conducted by Harold D. Foster, B.Sc., Ph.D., Professor
of Geography and a statistician with the University of Victoria in Victoria,
British Columbia, Canada. In 1988, Dr. Foster performed a thorough

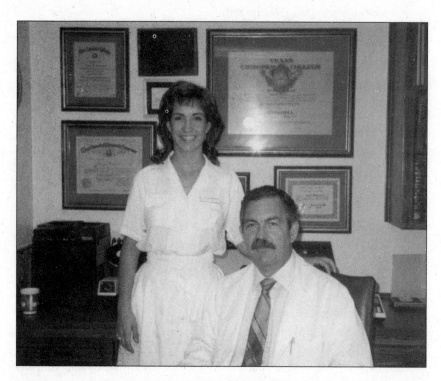

Dr. and Mrs. John Albracht

computer analysis of cancer patients who underwent so-called spontaneous regressions.

Spontaneous regression (or *spontaneous remission*) means that the cancer gets smaller or disappears completely (and with no new tumors developing) without any conventional treatment.[3]

The renowned pathologist William Boyd, M.D., collected a large series of such instances, all documented in great detail, in a book he published in 1961. Dr. Boyd estimated that approximately 1 in every 100,000 cases of cancer will show spontaneous regression. In his series, more than half of the proven cases of spontaneous regression came from four forms of tumor: (1) kidney (renal-cell) cancer, (2) melanoma (pigmented cancer of the skin), (3) neuroblastoma (a rare cancer of childhood), and (4) choriocarcinoma (a rare cancer of the placenta). As part of the other half of Dr. Boyd's cases, there were one or two examples of almost every other type of cancer.[4]

In his classic coauthored textbook *Spontaneous Regression of Cancer*, oncologist W. H. Cole, M.D., writes: "The term 'spontaneous' is an erroneous classification because there must be a cause of the regression."[5] Also, in his published writings and lectures, Max Gerson, M.D., has stated repeatedly that cancer regression does not happen spontaneously but that some specific improvement in the patient's physiology causes the cancer to react favorably.

"What is missing, therefore," says Harold D. Foster, Ph.D., "is an understanding on the part of those involved of why a major improvement in health is occurring." A wide variety of possible explanations have, of course, been put forward for spontaneous regression."[6]

Spontaneous Cancer Regression Analyzed by Dr. Harold Foster

Dr. Foster looked at the data on 200 recovered patients who had used various forms of alternative treatment, including the Gerson Therapy, Hoxsey's herbs, Kelley's dietary program, macrobiotics, the Moerman diet, and Jason Winters Herbal Tea. He discovered that more than half of these recovered chronic disease patients (with cancer striking most of them) had used some form of nutrition and lifestyle changes, including detoxification, such as coffee enemas, castor oil enemas, high colonic irrigation, dry heat saunas, or fasting. Eighty-eight percent of the patients had incorporated vegetarianism as their daily eating program, and 65 percent swallowed daily amounts of mineral supplements, with potassium and iodine being the most frequently taken. Additional nutrients ingested by them included niacin, digestive enzymes, bioflavonoids, red clover, and the vitamins A, B$_{12}$, and C.

Dr. Foster wrote that "spontaneous" cancer regressions "tended to occur most frequently in vegetarian nonsmokers, who did not use table salt, white flour, or sugar and who avoided canned, smoked, or frozen foods. Typically such individuals eschewed alcoholic beverages, tea, coffee, and cocoa, but instead drank freshly pressed fruit and/or vegetable juices. Many took vitamin and mineral supplements together with various herbs. The time interval spent by patients eating such special diets varied from one month to fifteen years, the median time period being forty-one months."[7]

Since there must always be a reason for cancer regression, confirmed Dr. Foster, he agreed with Dr. Max Gerson's original finding, saying, "There is really no such process as spontaneous regression." The data support his view that dramatic remissions occur "in association with major dietary changes, which must inevitably have resulted in alterations in the availability of bulk and trace elements to both the immune system and to tumors."

Dr. Foster affirmed that the Gerson therapy program was heavily represented among those cancer patients "who exceeded their anticipated lengths of survival by at least a factor of ten." In this group were persons who followed the Gerson protocol and recovered from brain tumors, lymphosarcoma, basal cell carcinoma, kidney sarcoma, spreading melanoma, breast cancer, spinal cord tumor, metastasized testicular cancer, and pituitary gland cancer. Recovered patients following the Gerson program were represented in nearly every category in Dr. Foster's study.[8]

The U.S. National Cancer Institute (NCI) and the Canadian Cancer Society (CCS) are promoting diets that they anticipate will reduce the incidence of cancer. Interestingly enough, many of the 200 patients who experienced cancer regression in Dr. Foster's study were following diets exactly like that advocated by Max Gerson, M.D. They were extreme forms of those now being championed by orthodox medicine, as represented by the NCI and the CCS.[9,10]

Creating "Spontaneous Regressions/Remissions"

Alternative methods of healing (considered unconventional by the standards of modern oncology) were applied by those investigated patients who experienced spontaneous regressions.

TABLE 5-1

Percentage Frequency with Which Particular Foods and Drinks Were Avoided by 200 Cancer Victims Who Underwent "Spontaneous Regressions"

Type of Food or Drink	*Percentage of Patient Sample*
All canned foods	80.0
All frozen foods	80.0
All smoked foods	80.0
White sugar	79.5
Meat	79.5
Pickles	75.5
Table salt (sodium chloride)	75.5
Alcoholic beverages	75.5
Spices	75.0
Eggs	70.0
Fish	67.0
Fats	65.5
White flour	65.5
Tea	65.5
Coffee	65.5
Chocolate	63.5
Oils	62.0
Milk	62.0
Nuts	59.5
Soybeans	49.0
Tomatoes	38.5
Shellfish	16.0

(Taken with permission from Foster, H.D. "Lifestyle changes and the 'spontaneous' regression of cancer: An initial computer analysis." *International Journal of Biosocial Research.* 10(1):17-33, 1988.

Of the recorded patients, 175 (87.5 percent) had made major improvements in their diets. Table 5-1 lists the foods which were typically avoided. As can be seen, these now healthy people closely followed the Gerson Therapy dietary recommendations (see chapters 7, 8, and 10). Eliminated from their meal planning were alcoholic, fatty, oily, dairy, canned, frozen, smoked, sweet, salted, spiced, and pickled foods. Eighty percent of the people who cured various cancers on their own discontinued eating these foods. In addition, tobacco, meat, and sugar were no longer ingested by 79.5 percent of the patients who later underwent

TABLE 5-2

Percentage Frequency with Which Particular Foods and Drinks Were Consumed by 200 Cancer Patients Experiencing "Spontaneous Regressions"

Type of Food or Drink	Percentage of Patient Sample
Broccoli	84.5
Leeks	84.5
Cauliflower	84.5
Onions	84.5
Legumes	84.5
Carrots	84.5
Brussels sprouts	84.5
Beet roots	82.5
Squash	82.5
Apples	81.5
Pears	81.5
Apricots	77.0
Whole grain cereals	75.0
Cantaloupe	73.5
Grapes	73.0
Tomatoes	72.5
Lentils	69.0
Grapefruit juice (freshly made)	58.0
Alfalfa and other sprouted seeds	57.5
Orange juice (freshly made)	57.0
Apple juice (freshly made)	57.0
Grape juice (freshly made)	55.0
Tomato juice (freshly made)	55.0
Carrot juice (freshly made)	53.5
Green leaf juice (freshly made)	51.5
Liver	46.5
Raisins	46.5
Almonds	32.0
Pineapples	26.0
Cottage cheese	24.5
Buttermilk (churned, *not* cultured)	24.5
Eggs	24.5
Wheatgrass	22.0
Yogurt	21.0
Olive oil	20.5
Sunflower seeds	19.5
Barley grass	18.5
Avocados	18.5
Kefir	16.5
Garlic	14.0

TABLE 5-2 (cont.)

Flax oil	7.5
Miso	4.5
Tamari	2.0

(Taken with permission from Foster, H.D. "Lifestyle changes and the 'spontaneous' regression of cancer: an initial computer analysis." *International Journal of Biosocial Research.* 10(1):17-33, 1988.)

"spontaneous" cancer regressions. As indicated below, spices, eggs, fish, oils and fats, tea, coffee, cocoa, chocolate, white flour, milk, and nuts were avoided as well by more than 50 percent of the patients.

In contrast, certain foods were consumed in large quantities by cancer patients seemingly undergoing "spontaneous regression." These are shown in Table 5-2. The most popular foods valued for their anticancer components proved to be fresh vegetables; namely carrots, beet roots, squash, broccoli, leeks, cauliflower, onions, legumes, and brussels sprouts. Such vegetables were the only foods specifically eaten by more than 80 percent of the spontaneously regressed patients. Also of note was that 57 percent of these fortunate (or informed) people followed the Gerson Therapy recommendation of freshly pressing and drinking apple, carrot, and orange juices. Freshly squeezed carrot juice, in fact, played a significant role in the diets of 53.5 percent of all patients in the sample. Grapefruit, grape, and tomato juices were also drunk by over half of those experiencing regressions. Other foods that were popular included whole grains, alfalfa sprouts, cantaloupes, tomatoes, lentils, grapes, and apricots.

SURVIVING AND THRIVING FORTY YEARS AFTER THE GERSON THERAPY

There is no shortage of confirmations that dietary improvements combined with detoxifying lifestyles help to eliminate cancer and other illnesses manifested by total cellular deterioration. Such confirmations include the statements of patients still living forty or more years after they had undergone the healing program advocated by Max Gerson, M.D. What follows is just such an example of surviving and thriving more than forty-two years after engaging in the Gerson Therapy to counteract bone cancer.

Carla Shuford (see photograph) is happy and healthy today, more than forty-two years after she was diagnosed with the metastatic cancer osteogenic sarcoma, at age fifteen.

Osteogenic sarcoma, a cancer of the bone tissue itself, is the second most common type of primary malignant bone tumor. Although most often seen in people aged ten to twenty years, an osteosarcoma of this type can occur at any age. About half of the tumors occur in or around the knee and within the femur, but they can originate in any bone. They tend to spread as secondary growths to the lungs. Usually, osteogenic sarcoma causes severe pain and swelling at the tumor sites.[11]

Carla Shuford was a victim of the disease but saved herself with the powerful nutritional and detoxification program advocated by Dr. Gerson. To help save the lives of other childhood cancer patients, she wrote her case history for publication in the bimonthly July/August 1998 issue of the *Gerson Healing Newsletter*.[12]

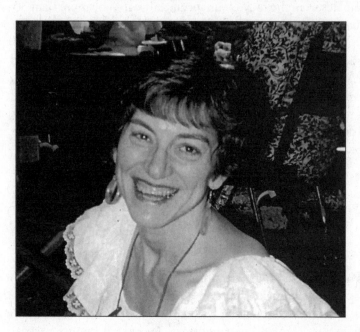

Carla Shuford

Here is Carla Shuford's story:

This year, on September 4, 1998, I will be celebrating my fortieth anniversary—an anniversary of life! I was diagnosed with cancer, and on that day forty years ago, my left leg was amputated at the hip. I had gone through seven months of pain before the tumor was discovered, so when the diagnosis of osteogenic sarcoma was confirmed in a biopsy report to John Preston, M.D. (the surgeon who had performed the biopsy), the prognosis was not good. The cancer had spread to my lymph system, and I was given six months to live.

At that time [early September 1958], radiation and surgery were the conventional methods of treatment. Radiation was not possible because of the tumor's location, and in desperation, the doctors decided to do radical surgery, offering a faint possibility that it could postpone my death by thirty to sixty days.

However, on the same day, and in fact, while the operation was being performed, something seemingly much less dramatic, but far more vital was taking place. My mother was talking [in person] to Dr. Max Gerson in his New York City office, making arrangements for me to begin his therapy immediately upon my hospital discharge.

The next five years were to be round-the-clock days of labor, as my parents devoted their lives to preserving mine, Gerson-style. We were poor dairy farmers from the mountains of western North Carolina, whose livelihood depended upon milking by hand our herd of thirty Jersey cows, and delivering the raw milk to our customers each morning.

Although it would have been preferable for me to be a resident of Dr. Gerson's New York clinic, circumstances made that impossible. Because of the extreme demands of time, energy, and the difficulty of acquiring toxin-free foods, along with the thoroughness and exactness that the program required, Dr. Gerson was reluctant for patients to handle the treatment at home, especially in the beginning stages. However, he was impressed with my mother's intelligence and untiring dedication to detail. In return for his trust, she made him the promise that she would follow his prescribed regimen to the letter.

So began five years of uncompromising observance to the Gerson Therapy by my mother, my father, and myself. In those days, the Gerson juicer was an enormously heavy machine (similar to a car jack), with a separate press and linen cloths to press the ground food in to prevent any chance of oxidation. We were all grateful that our arms had grown strong from years of milking cows, as it required equal strength to operate this equipment! As the juice had to be freshly ground and pressed with each feeding, my mother barely finished washing the machine and cloths, before it was time for the next round.

At that time too, the liver "juice" consisted of the liquid from grinding and pressing a calf's liver that had never been frozen. Our nearest source for the liver was in Asheville, forty miles away. My father's job was to meet the bus at 3:00 P.M. at the local station with our order of fresh liver.

While my father had converted to organic gardening in the early 1950s, none of the other local farmers had any interest in this pursuit. However, since the quantities of lettuce and carrots required for daily juicing, as well as the various roots and vegetables for the prescribed soup, were enormous [for me], my father needed the assistance of our neighbors. Different farmers agreed to allocate portions of their gardens to be pesticide-free. In those areas, they grew "Carla's carrots" and "Carla's lettuce" and "Carla's whatever."

The rest is history. Dr. Gerson died in the spring of 1959, less than six months after my mother had visited him. The doctors finally grew tired of requiring monthly chest X-rays that were consistently clear. Sloan-Kettering [Cancer Clinic] sent out a yearly survey to ask if I was still alive, and each year, to their amazement, it was returned. In 1988, I realized I had outlived their thirty-year study!

My father died in 1965. My mother died on January 18 of this year (1998), just three days before her ninetieth birthday. I am now an official senior, having turned fifty-five in April.

I eat only organic, unprocessed foods, with an emphasis on fruits, vegetables, and whole grains. I swim a mile each morning, and enjoy good health—other than the wear-and-tear that is attendant to a forty-year life on crutches.

I keep an updated "Gerson Folder" in my bureau drawer, so I will know what to do, should I ever need Doctor Max's help again. And perhaps most importantly, I look forward to celebrating my fortieth anniversary on September 4, 1998, as I once again give thanks to my mother, to my father, and to Dr. Max Gerson for MY LIFE!

Carla Shuford

References for Chapter Five

1. Hildenbrand, G. "Cure of a recurrent, inoperable, chemoresistant mixed cell lymphoma (retroperitoneal lymphocytic/histiocytic nodular diffused) through the Gerson cancer therapy." *Healing Newsletter.* 7(1-2):1–10, Jan./Feb. & Mar./Apr. 1992.

2. *Ibid.*, p. 10.

3. Bashford, E.F. cited by Rae, M.V. "Spontaneous regression of a hyper-nephroma." *American Journal of Cancer.* 24:839, 1935.

4. Buckman, R. *What You Really Need to Know about Cancer: A Comprehensive Guide for Patients and their Families.* Baltimore: The Johns Hopkins Univesity Press, 1997, pp. 242, 243.

5. Cole, W.H. "Opening address: Spontaneous regression of cancer and the importance of finding its cause." In *Conference on Spontaneous Regression of Cancer,* ed. by T.C. Everson, and W. H. Cole. Philadelphia: W.B. Saunders & Co., 1966, pp. 5–9.

6. Foster, H.D. "Lifestyle changes and the 'spontaneous' regression of cancer: an initial computer analysis." *International Journal of Biosocial Research.* 10(1):17–33, 1988.

7. *Ibid.*

8. *Ibid.*

9. Ross, Wk.S. "At last, an anticancer diet." *Reader's Digest.* 1222(733): 49–53, 1983.

10. Canadian Cancer Society. "Facts on cancer and diet: Your food choices may help you reduce your cancer risk." 1985.

11. *The Merck Manual of Medical Information: Home Edition.* Whitehouse Station, N.J.: Merck Research Laboratories, 1997, p. 223

12. Shuford, C. "Carla's story." *Gerson Healing Newsletter.* 13(4):5–6, July/ Aug. 1998.

Part Two

THE GERSON THERAPY IN ACTION

Chapter Six

HEALING MELANOMA WITH THE GERSON THERAPY

When a death-dealing skin cancer, melanoma, reaches the state of having spread, or metastasized, throughout the body, it is classified as a stage IV cancer. Such a circumstance is serious, unquestionably life-threatening, and carries no optimistic prognosis among conventionally practicing oncologists.

A *melanoma* (literally "black tumor") is a malignant mole, the most dangerous of all skin cancers and among the most malignant of all cancers. It can spread to nearly every organ and tissue and lead to death within a year after it recurs in distant sites (metastasizes). Although it is rare for a pregnant woman's tumor to spread to her fetus (see the case of Lana Matuseck near the conclusion of this chapter), melanomas lead the list among those tumors that do spread in this way.

Melanoma is most common in people in their forties to sixties. While not yet among the most common cancers, its incidence is rising faster worldwide than any other. In the United States alone, more than 40,300 cases occurred in 1997, and an even higher number are being counted for 1998.

Only one type of cell composing all melanomas exists—the malevolent pigment-producing cell called a *melanocyte*—but there are a few variants distinguished by their shapes, such as cuboidal or spindle-shaped. The behavior of each is generally similar in skin melanomas, although in eye melanomas their shape determines the behavior to a significant degree.[1]

MRS. DAEL MINTZ ARRIVES WITH STAGE IV MELANOMA

Arriving at a natural remedy hospital using the Gerson Therapy in Tijuana, Mexico, in June 1993, Dael Mintz, aged fifty-five, of Calabasas, California, had her life endangered by stage IV melanoma. Mrs. Mintz defied all the conventional medical odds. "Frankly, at the outset, we here at the Gerson Therapy treatment center in Tijuana thought that her prognosis was rather poor," admits Alicia Melendez, M.D., the Gerson Therapy–educated physician who specializes in treating cancers holistically.

"She had a severe case of metastasized melanoma, with tumor masses in her lungs and liver and lesions engulfing and compressing her mid-back and neck vertebrae. Dael's largest tumor measured 11.5 centimeters [cm] across; there was a mass of lumps just under the skin on her chest, and she had a tumor on her nose as well," relates Dr. Melendez. "Surgery followed by a skin graft had been unable to eliminate the nose tumor, and soon it grew to the size of a grape. A total of twenty tumors were found throughout her body (including her hip, spine, liver, bones, and kidneys) and her clavicle was visibly distended with clear signs of the cancer."

Conventionally practicing oncologists in California had given up on Mrs. Mintz. In fact, they predicted that she had less than six months to live. When melanoma is that far advanced, there is almost nothing regular drug-oriented (allopathic) medicine can do. Stage IV melanoma is resistant to radiation treatment, immunotherapy, and chemotherapy. None of these established procedures has been shown to bring about any good long-term results. All oncologists will tell you that stage IV skin cancer is among the most difficult malignancies to overcome. But it turns out that this was not the situation for Dael Mintz.

Over the next three weeks at the Gerson Therapy facility and then for eighteen months on her own, Mrs. Mintz followed the standard Gerson program of eating a specialized diet, consuming fresh vegetable juices, taking nutritional supplements, receiving remedial injections, going through detoxification, and giving herself coffee enemas. In addition, she received ozone topically for her nose lesions and took it rectally twice daily for general body detoxification. At the end of this three-week period, the patient still showed some lesions in and on her body, but she felt a great deal more energy. Overall, the Gerson Therapy doctors and staff evaluated her as being well on the road to recovery. She then returned home to treat herself.[2]

Stage IV Melanoma Remission, Regression, and Elimination

Dr. Melendez acknowledges that the severity of her patient's case was of great concern at first. "Her health at the time she had been admitted to our clinic was like a train plummeting down a mountain with an engineer who has had a heart attack. The melanoma was that far out of control. We needed to stop the train and push it back up the mountain," states the Gerson Therapy cancer specialist.

Within the next six months of her remaining on the Gerson program, Mrs. Mintz's clavicle returned to a normal appearance. After another six months, computerized axial tomography (CAT) scans she went through as a diagnostic procedure indicated that there was a substantial size reduction in her liver tumors; the scans also showed that most other organ metastases had disappeared. The woman's next CAT scan, six months later still (a year and a half from the start of her Gerson self-treatment), depicted a continued reduction in the liver tumor and only two (out of an initial five) lung tumors remained.

One year later, in June 1996, there were only two calcified nodules on her left lung and a single, 1-millimeter calcification on the right lobe of her liver remained. She was in remission, near to total regression, and approaching the end stage of complete elimination of her stage IV melanoma. This not uncommon occurrence for Gerson Therapy patients was confirmed repeatedly in two ways: by Dael Mintz consulting with her local oncologist and by return visits to the Gerson treatment center in Tijuana.

"Between June 1993 and June 1996, the tumor on her nose flattened out, developed a concave area in its center, and lightened in color," reported the patient's Mexican physician during the season that followed. "Dael feels very healthy, despite the lingering lesion on her nose. This last lesion, too, is drastically reduced from its original size and she believes it is gradually healing."

After the patient was on the Gerson program for two years, Dr. Alicia Melendez was able to pronounce her "almost completely clear of any cancer." Bearing in mind that the average life expectancy for someone with stage IV melanoma is under one year in almost all cases, for the patient still to still be alive to this point for seven years is highly impressive (see the photograph showing Mrs. Dael Mintz today).

At home in Calabasas, when Mrs. Mintz reported her recovery to her allopathic oncologist, he was "thunderstruck and amazed," she says. "He

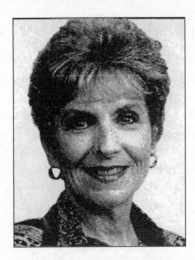

Mrs. Dael Mintz

was completely unable to understand what produced this turnaround in my presumably fatal melanoma. Fortunately, my oncologist had enough sense to encourage me to remain on the Gerson Therapy." She consults him periodically to confirm that melanoma is staying away.

We have described this deadly stage IV melanoma case history because Dael Mintz's skin cancer with its multiple metastases is even worse than most of the other melanomas studied as part of a broad-based retrospective investigation. We discuss the research below. A retrospective investigation or review is one that surveys past performance of some therapy. This examination reviewed how many melanoma patients lived at least five years (considered a "cure" by the American Cancer Society's oncological scientists).

The retrospective study reported here compared melanoma patients who first began the Gerson Therapy under medical supervision and then, like Mrs. Mintz, went on to self-administer the treatment at home. Our described melanoma patient and 152 other study participants who followed the Gerson Therapy with enthusiasm (153 in all) did exceedingly well regarding their five-year survival rates. Among them, 69 percent of the Gerson Therapy patients lived beyond five years. They were compared with those other melanoma patients taken from the medical literature (16,229 in all) who had undergone different courses of treatment. It's readily seen that the non–Gerson Therapy patients were less fortunate and died in greater numbers before the five-year mark (usually within a year).

THE MELANOMA RETROSPECTIVE REVIEW OF FIVE-YEAR SURVIVAL

The melanoma study was conducted by members of the Gerson Institute and the Cancer Prevention and Control Program at the University of California, both located in San Diego. This retrospective review described all patients, including nonresponders to therapy, and encompassed their melanomas in stages I and II (localized), stages IIIA and IIIB (regionally metastasized), stage IVA (distant lymph, skin, and subcutaneous tissue metastases), and stage IVB (visceral metastases). A peer-reviewed clinical journal article, "Five-Year Survival Rates of Melanoma Patients Treated by Diet Therapy after the Manner of Gerson: A Retrospective Review," was published in September 1995.[3]

The article's authors, G. L. Hildenbrand, L. Christeene Hildenbrand, Karen Bradford, and Shirley W. Cavin, summarized the clinical outcomes of melanoma patients treated with the nutrition-based cancer therapy in contrast with outcome rates reported in the medical literature. Over a fifteen-year period—from 1975 through July 1990—153 adult, white melanoma patients treated with the nutrition-based cancer therapy developed by Max Gerson, M.D. (who originally conducted his research at the University of Munich in the 1930s), were evaluated retrospectively. Although he published the results of his dietary program in Europe, Dr. Gerson publicized his findings even more extensively after 1936 when he immigrated to the United States.[4]

The Gerson Therapy melanoma patients studied ranged from twenty-five to seventy-two years of age. The Gerson program participants were treated with a lacto-vegetarian, low-sodium, low-fat, and low-protein diet. They received elevated amounts of potassium, fluid, and nutrients in the form of hourly administered eight-ounce glasses of raw vegetable juices and/or fruit juices. Their metabolism was increased by thyroid. The calorie supply was limited to from 2,600 to 3,200 calories per day. Coffee enemas as needed for dexotification, pain relief, and improvement of appetite were taken.

A few of the melanoma patients had been treated by private practice physicians, but almost all had been hospitalized at some facility providing the Gerson Therapy in the Tijuana area of Mexico. (Patient records were examined from four different Tijuana hospitals.)

This retrospective review revealed that 100 percent of the 14 Gerson Therapy Patients (GTP) with melanoma stages I and II survived for five years, compared with only 79 percent living that long of 15,798 stages I and II melanoma patients reported by oncologist C. M. Balch, M.D.[5]

Of 17 GTP with stage IIIA (regionally metastasized) melanoma, 82 percent were alive at five years, in contrast to just 39 percent of 103 stage IIIA melanoma patients taking therapy dispensed by the German health facility Fachklinik Hornheide.[6]

Of 33 GTP with stages IIIA plus IIIB melanoma, 71 percent lived five years, compared with 41 percent of 134 stages IIIA plus IIIB melanoma patients from the Fachklinik Hornheide.[7]

Of 18 GTP with stage IVA melanoma, 39 percent were alive at five years, compared with a mere 6 percent of 194 stage IVA melanoma patients from the Eastern Cooperative Oncology Group.[8]

Of 71 GTP not recorded statistically, after exclusions, the 153 total number of five-year survivors turned out to be clearly stage-related. Some patients were lost to follow-up because they died from causes other than melanoma or moved out of contact with the researchers and could not be reached.

The American Cancer Society has reported a 39 percent five-year survival rate for stage III melanoma.[9] Yet the assessable survival rate in stage III melanoma patients treated with Dr. Max Gerson's diet therapy is 71 percent.

Male and female survival rates were identical for stages I, II, IIIA, and IIIB melanoma, but stage IVA melanoma women (such as Dael Mintz) had a strong survival advantage over men. Survival impact was not assessed for stage IVB melanoma.

Various aspects of the Gerson Therapy program have been designated as the theoretical reasons for patient success against disease, yet no clearly defined mechanism has been identified. As will be understood from the chapters to follow, components of the Gerson Therapy program are dedicated to an improved oxidation process of the sick patient's cellular structures. Under this procedure, to more properly treat cancer and other degenerative diseases, the oxidation function must be increased markedly.[10]

It generally goes unrecognized by medical consumers that chronic illnesses replaced infectious diseases as the dominant public health issue in the 1920s, long before antibiotics appeared on the scene. There is a global pattern of chronic ill health related in particular to wrongly applied nutritional factors. The Gerson Therapy effectively corrects those human internal environmental factors which have gone awry.[11]

The first National Health Survey conducted in 1935 reported that 22 percent of Americans lived with a chronic condition of illness.[12] In 1987, nearly 30 percent of the population (upwards of 90 million Americans) suffered from one or more chronic conditions.[13] Based on trends during the preceding and succeeding decades, some 50 percent of the American population (perhaps 150 million people) are expected to be counted among the chronically ill before the year 2000 ends. These considerations are pertinent to Gerson Therapy. It is a main method for the permanent elimination of chronic degenerative diseases of all types but especially for the one hundred or more types of cancer.

Please note that the Medicare system's state of finances desperately needs the Gerson Therapy since in the Medicare program, more than 10 percent of beneficiaries consume about 72 percent of medical resources. That high percentage of chronically ill took up massive amounts of tax-payer money in 1998 and the situation is anticipated to worsen in each successive year.[14]

JULIE HEPNER HAS HER MELANOMA ELIMINATED BY THE GERSON THERAPY

Julie Hepner's good health ended in 1988 when she was only twenty-two years old. A mole was removed from her right shoulder by a dermatologist, and the biopsy he conducted determined that she had a melanoma. In the next four years Julie underwent seven surgical operations to remove a lump from her neck, a tumor from her brain, a cyst from her ovary, flesh from her tonsil, and 1 1/2 feet of colon. On each occasion, biopsies found melanoma.

After undergoing the colon surgery, Julie began the Gerson Therapy with assistance from her mother and regular consultations with metabolic physicians practicing medicine near her location who employ the Gerson Therapy. Despite a minor setback in 1993 when she moved into a newly painted and carpeted home and experienced environmental allergies, Julie has felt "great." This former melanoma patient has encountered no further recurrences of melanoma and to this day remains on a less intensive Gerson Therapy program. (See the photo on the next page, which pictures Julie Hepner as she looks today, eleven years after she was diagnosed with melanoma.)

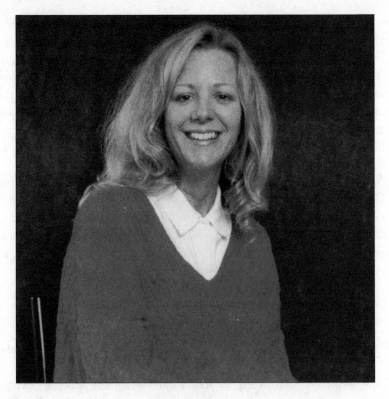

Julie Hepner

CAROL ASKHEW HEALS MELANOMA, ARTHRITIS, AND CHRONIC HEPATITIS C

Carol Askhew turned to the Gerson Therapy to deal with three different illnesses, beginning with arthritis, which had left both her father and her sister with multiple hip replacements. Although arthritis did affect her and was cured by application of the Gerson Therapy, melanoma was this woman's more serious health problem. Melanoma was what brought Carol to adopting the Gerson diet and detoxification metabolic program.

Her cancer happened after her father was diagnosed with melanoma. Carol became frightened for herself and had a biopsy performed on a lesion that had been frozen off several times before. When the results indicated melanoma, Carol Askhew entered a hospital administering the Gerson Therapy where she stayed for two weeks. She thrived on the pro-

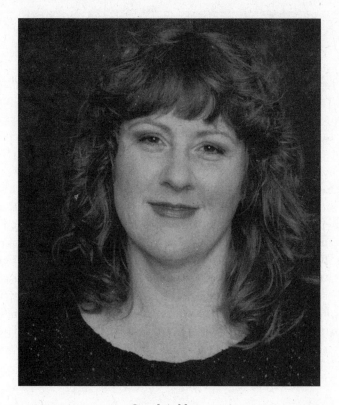

Carol Askhew

gram for as long as she followed it at home. Her arthritis and melanoma disappeared and have stayed away.

Then, in December 1995, a liver biopsy she required for the infection then invading her body indicated that this patient had stage III hepatitis C. Once again Carol Askhew returned to self-application of the Gerson Therapy and performed in accordance with its requirements. Her liver enzymes subsequently came back to normal levels where they remain today. Her health continues to improve. (See the above photograph, which shows how Carol Askhew looks today.)

Carol Askhew makes the following series of health-enhancing statements:

"There's nothing like losing your health to inspire you to do something to preserve it."

"Cancer is a symptom. Treat the cause."

"The Gerson Therapy saved my life."

"On the Gerson Therapy, I feel like I just get better and better."

KATHLEEN MONAGHAN ELIMINATES THE DEADLIEST FORM OF MELANOMA

After a mole and some lymph nodes were removed from her right arm, Mrs. Kathleen Monaghan was diagnosed with malignant melanoma, level IVB, the deadliest known form of skin cancer. Within a year, the melanoma had metastasized to her liver and adrenal glands where an additional tumor had developed. The patient's physicians then told the Monaghan family that she had only thirty days to remain alive.

The four authors of the above-described five-year retrospective survival survey made no attempt to assess the survival impact of the Gerson Therapy in stage IVB, because they were unable to find a single comparable treatment group worldwide moving through any treatment-reporting system. In other words, they did have stage IVB melanoma patients, all with gravely advanced disease, but there was no group of such patients who lived long enough anywhere else with which to make comparisons.

Despite family protests, Kathleen Monaghan entered a Gerson Therapy facility located in Tijuana, Mexico, in October 1993. There she embarked on the dietary/detoxification program with vigor and immediately felt rejuvenated.

MELANOMA OF THE EYE CURED BY USE OF THE GERSON THERAPY

Recently Charlotte Gerson received a telephone call from a woman who explained that she and her daughter had attended a Mexican cancer clinic that employs the Gerson Therapy in 1982. The mother went as a support person for her daughter, Lana Matuseck, aged twenty-six at the time. The daughter's body had paid the price for prolonged malnutrition during the time of her pregnancy, a year before. At the time of their 1982 visit across the Mexican/American border, they had brought along her one-year-old baby boy. During her period of pregnancy and beyond, Lana had been diagnosed with ocular melanoma of the left eye at the prestigious Health Sciences Center of Portland, Oregon.

Lana was lucky that, because of her pregnancy, she had not been treated with chemotherapy; however, by the time her baby was a year old, the woman had undergone seven surgical operations, each time to remove a quantity of the spreading melanoma around her left eyeball. Even so, additional melanoma tissue would appear in her eye socket, and each surgery sought to remove some more of the malignant tissue. Success was limited and the cancer kept returning.

At the Gerson Institute, it is especially painful for staff members to hear from young women such as Lana who are pregnant or with small children and are suffering from some type of cancer. Unfortunately, this is not a rare occurrence. In these situations, the same underlying physiological problems connected with all malignancies exist: body deficiency and toxicity.

In contrast, it's not possible for a healthy body to produce cancer. When all defenses, especially the immune syustem, are in place, the healthy body will naturally kill and eliminate cancer cells whenever or wherever they develop. Before a cancer establishes itself and becomes evident, therefore, a person's major immunological defenses weaken or disapper. Then one's immune system fails to work, the enzyme system becomes damaged, the pancreatic enzymes stop destroying foreign proteins (tumor tissue), the hormone system gets depleted, and minerals are . lacking.

Lana and many other young women today have bodies that are just barely maintaining balance and health under average conditions. However, when they become pregnant, their bodies are called upon to produce an entirely new person with its own organ system. This requirement puts a drain on a marginal body, just barely functioning. Both the mother-to-be and her fetus then must pay the elevated price of her chronic poor nourishment.

When the food intake contains the necessary ingredients (fresh, raw vitamins, minerals, and enzymes in assimilable form rather than in pharmaceutical preparations), the pregnant body receives the additional materials to accomplish this job as it has for thousands of years. Still, we often see that our modern typical American diet is seriously deficient in these live nutrients. Instead, it puts additional strain on a pregnant woman's body in the form of excess fats, proteins, and salt, along with food chemicals such as preservatives, dyes, emulsifiers, and worse.

Now comes the conundrum: nature always provides for the fetus, the new life, and will build a perfectly good body for the baby-to-be from available vitamins, minerals, and nutrients. If these are not being supplied to a woman in the form of appropriate nutrition, nature will take these required materials for the fetus out of the woman's already marginal body systems. Now the minerals, enzymes and nutrients for the pregnant woman's body become seriously depleted. With immune system defenses virtually gone, she manifests illness in the weakest part of her physiology. If the depletion and toxicity are serious enough, the result is likely to be a malignancy. Or, in other circumstances, illness might "only" result in tox-emia of pregnancy, kidney trouble, genitourinary disorder, or some other internal difficulty.

Originally all three of Lana's medical doctors—an internist, an oph-thalmologist, and an oncologist—concurred in a statement to her parents and husband that she would not live five months. But Lana, against odds, had exceeded that dire prediction. Nevertheless, the trio of doctors main-tained to the patient's mother that her daughter's situation was "hopeless and that there was nothing they could do to help stop the melanoma from killing her." Also they added that the type of treatment advocated on the Gerson program was "a waste of time, money, and hardship on the fam-ily."

By phone, Lana's mother further told Charlotte Gerson that when she was first seen by the Gerson Therapy physicians at the Mexican cancer clinic, the patient's affected eye was totally blind. She looked at the world only out of her right eye. But then, Lana Matuseck's parent reported, her daughter followed the Gerson Therapy faithfully. It was her only hope of recovery. Today, June 1, 1999, more than a decade and a half later, she is completely well and has been that way for over a dozen years. Mrs. Lana Matuseck has since delivered three more strong and healthy children, an-other boy and two girls. The whole Matuseck family lives a lifestyle ac-cording to the principles of Dr. Max Gerson.

At forty-one years of age, the ex-melanoma patient needs no corrective lenses and has full use of her vision in both eyes. Her formerly affected left eye has come back to 20/20 vision simply because she refused to ac-cept her three conventionally practicing, allopathic physicians' discourag-ing prognosis and instead has been following the Gerson Therapy these past sixteen years.

References for Chapter Six

1. Mitchell, M.S. "Melanoma." In *Everyone's Guide to Cancer Therapy.*, rev. 3rd ed., by M. Dollinger; E.H. Rosenbaum; and G. Cable, Kansas City, Mis-souri: Andrews McMeel Publishing, 1997, pp. 568, 569.

2. Gerson, C. "Successfully reversing stage IV melanoma: the story of Dael Mintz." *Healing Stories of the Gerson Therapy* from the *Alternative Medicine Digest.* Issue no. 18, May/June 1997.

3. Hildenbrand, G.L.; Hildenbrand, L.C.; Bradford, K.; Cavin, S.W. "Five-year survival rates of melanoma patients treated by diet therapy after the manner of Gerson: A retrospective review." *Alternative Therapies.* 1(4):29–37, September 1995.

4. Gerson, M. "Dietary considerations in malignant neoplastic disease; preliminary report." *Rev. Gastroenterol.* 12:419–425, 1945.

5. Balch, C.M. "Cutaneous melanoma: prognosis and treatment results worldwide." *Semin. Surg. Oncol.* 8:400–414, 1992.

6. Drepper, H.; Beiss, B.; Hofherr, B.; et al. "The prognosis of patients with stage III melanoma: prospective long-term study of 286 patients of the Fachklinik Hornheide." *Cancer.* 71:1239–1246, 1993.

7. *Ibid.*

8. Ryan, L.; Kramar, A.; Borden, E. "Prognostic factors in metastatic melanoma." *Cancer.* 71:2995–3005, 1993.

9. *Op. cit.,* Balch, C.M.

10. Ericson, R. *Cancer Treatment: Why So Many Failures?* Park Ridge, Ill.: GE-PS Cancer Memorial, 1979, p. 100.

11. Sydenstricker, E. "The vitality of the American people. In *Recent Trends in the United States.* New York: McGraw-Hill Co., 1993, chap. 2.

12. Philband, C.T. *National Health Survey: Preliminary Results.* Washington, D.C.: National Institutes of Health and the U.S. Public Health Service, 1937.

13. Hoffman, C.; Rice, D.; Sung, H.Y. "Persons with chronic conditions. Their prevalence and costs." *Journal of the American Medical Association.* 276:1473–1479, 1996.

14. Health Care Financing Administration. "Medicare: a profile." Washington, D.C.: Health Care Financing Administration, February 1995, chart PS-11.

Chapter Seven

SUCCESS WITH OTHER DISEASES

In this chapter, we will explore Dr. Max Gerson's nutritional eating program by relating some healing experiences of noncancerous Gerson Therapy patients.

EPILEPSY CURED BY SELF-APPLICATION OF THE GERSON THERAPY

By putting herself on the Gerson Therapy dietary program at home five years ago, Dallas, Texas, schoolgirl Jessica Kahn, then sixteen years old, was eventually able to permanently get rid of grand mal seizures. Epilepsy has finally stopped ruining her life, and now she has blossomed into a beautiful young woman who is active, vivacious, and completely recovered.

Epilepsy (falling sickness) is a chronic disorder characterized by paroxysmal brain dysfunction due to excessive neuronal discharge and is usually associated with some alteration of consciousness. The clinical manifestations of the mind/brain attack may vary from complex abnormalities of behavior including generalized or focal convulsions to momentary spells of impaired consciousness. These clinical states have been subjected by health professionals to a variety of classifications, none universally accepted to date among psychiatrists, neurologists, and other physicians who deal with mental and neurological processes of the disease.

Grand mal seizures cause the patient to fall to the ground unconscious with his or her muscles in a state of spasm. The lack of any respiratory activity or movement results in a bluish discoloration of the skin and lips (cyanosis). This "tonic" phase is replaced by convulsive movements when an involved patient may bite the tongue and urinary incontinence may occur (the "clonic" phase). Spasmodic movements die away and the patient may rouse in a state of confusion, complaining of headache, or he or she may fall asleep.

We asked Jessica Kahn to describe her health history. Here is what Ms. Kahn wrote:

When I was sixteen years old, I began to have grand mal seizures. At first they occurred once every three to four months, but my condition soon deteriorated. Eventually I was experiencing two or three seizures at a time, practically every week. Of course, they had me feeling depressed and devastated.

My father has had a mild seizure disorder for the past twenty years, and so I believed that my seizures were inherited and here to stay. I did consult neurology specialists and took EEGs [electroencephalograms] looking for my condition's cause and cure, but none of the doctors could figure out what was wrong. They didn't offer me anything more than anticonvulsive drugs. Not wanting to go down the orthodox medicine road and use toxic treatment, my family and I searched and experimented with several alternative therapies. All of them having failed, we decided to try the Gerson program because we had seen it work miracles with friends of ours who had once been affected by cancer.

I went completely on the program for eleven months; I was able to adjust my school day and my lifestyle, and I did manage to accomplish all of the juicing and purging required. Although my mother spoke to Charlotte Gerson on the telephone a couple of times, we did the Gerson Therapy "by the book." That old book written by Dr. Max Gerson so long ago became my bible—I memorized its pages word for word. During my eleven months on the Gerson program, I experienced only three seizures. They coincided with my anticipated healing crises, such as the one I went through after six weeks at the start of the Gerson Therapy.

It has now been over four years since I stopped the treatment and over five years since I experienced any kind of seizure! I am ever so grateful to the Gerson program and also to my family for being so persistent in searching out an epilepsy cure for me.

Jessica Kahn is graduating from college this spring and will be pursuing a career in the health care sciences. The general nutrition information this young woman acted upon as her road map to eliminating epilepsy and restoring neurological health is readily usable by all persons for overcoming any illness or for purposes of medical prevention.

PERMANENT RECOVERY FROM ADDICTIONS TO STREET DRUGS AND ALCOHOL

As they grew up, fourteen-year-old Rob (pseudonym) and his siblings engaged in a variety of antisocial activities. As a result, all three children became either alcohol-addicted or street-drug-addicted and led relatively unproductive lives. For example, Rob dropped out of high school early in his junior year due to his frequent double abuses of alcoholic beverages and marijuana. His mother, whose defeat of breast cancer you will learn about in chapter 14, says that her son never really was a "healthy" child.

To illustrate his physical weaknesses, Rob's mother describes his situation at the age of five when he was suffering from a rare bone disorder called Legg-Calve-Perthes disease. The illness manifests itself as a kind of perforation of the rounded head of the femur, or thigh bone, which rotates against the hip. When the woman first took her son for consultation with a physician, the M.D. dismissed the child's symptoms as "worries of an overly concerned mother." But she insisted on an X-ray examination of the boy's legs and hips, which confirmed the disease.

Embarrassed that he had missed the diagnosis, this physician advised her to take Rob for experimental treatment then ongoing at the University of California. But the mother refused to allow her child to be used as a human guinea pig. Rob did, however, need to wear a full leg cast from below the knee to his groin for months. During the course of such treatment, his mother describes how she learned about nutritional therapy, massage therapy, and reflexology "accidentally." She read about them while shopping in a health foods store. These and other holistic-type alternative methods of healing were subsequently utilized to treat Rob's Legg-Calve-Perthes disease. Medical care alternatives including dietary modifications, and not usual "orthodox" medicine, enabled the small boy to discard his long leg cast and recover naturally and permanently.

So, remembering their effectiveness for his leg and hip, Rob elected to use the diet and detoxification techniques of medical alternatives to clean up his body when he and his new wife considered having a baby. As it happens, he had married a girl who also used street drugs and alcohol to excess. The couple had watched while Rob's mother went through the Gerson Therapy program for curing her breast cancer, and the son was much admiring of his mother's personal healing efforts. He, but not his wife, therefore became an enrollee in the Tijuana, Mexico, hospital facility which then employed the Gerson Therapy.

In a matter of just a few weeks, Rob was completely free of his dependency on both alcohol and marijuana, with no withdrawal problems of any kind. He returned home "cleaned up" and told his wife that he was now ready to become a father. His wife, however, was not ready. While he now ate a strictly vegetarian diet and followed a highly regulated lifestyle, she did not. She seemed intolerant of a daily routine that allowed for no recreational drugs, no drinking, and no "fun." Therefore, one memorable weekend, she left him during his absence, taking every household effect with her—all of their jointly held assets.

Unable to cope with this psychological and financial trauma, Rob fell back into his old ways. During the summer of 1995, Rob went through a dramatic weight loss dropping 45 pounds, from 185 to 140. He literally lay on the floor of his now empty apartment, unable to move because of his total weakness.

In a moment of lucidity, this thirty-two-year-old addict realized that he was dying from self-inflicted wretchedness. His signs and symptoms of disease were variable and bizarre too. Rob had been suffering from what was later diagnosed as acute and chronic mercurialism (mercury poisoning), for his fingers swelled at night to twice their normal size and turned blue; he vomited repeatedly, and simultaneously, he had severe abdominal pains. Added to these discomforts were bloody diarrhea, inability to produce urine, mouth ulcerations, loose teeth, loss of appetite, and ringing in his ears. It turns out that the addict's mercurialism came from the dental amalgam fillings (comprising 50 percent mercury) that occupied cavities in twelve of his teeth. The amalgams' mercury content was leaching into his body and brain.

It was then that Rob finally gathered himself together and managed to muster enough energy to make his way to his mother's home in the San Diego area. That's when she recognized that her son was on the verge of death, confirmed by a physician at the University of California. And she put him on the Gerson Therapy at once. In just six weeks, Rob regained 20 pounds of muscle without exercising, freed himself of cravings, went through no agonizing symptoms of drug and alcohol withdrawal, and developed excellent muscle tone by strictly resuming his vegetarian diet. The young man's signs and symptoms of mercury poisoning disappeared along with his obvious addictions.

Of course, added to his Gerson Therapy, Rob sought out the services of a dentist who practices mercury-free, holistically, and biologically. The dentist removed Rob's amalgams, substituting dental composite filling materials. Rob is now functioning normally and has become a keen exponent of the Gerson Therapy. At 6 feet, 2 inches, he is back to his normal weight of 185 pounds and at the last report on March 30, 1999, is active and successful in his profession.

RECOVERY AFTER STROKE AND HEART ATTACK

At age eighty-seven, in December 1993, Rob's grandfather (on his mother's side) suffered a heart attack (myocardial infarction) at home. His grandfather's wife quicky called for an ambulance, but while he was waiting to be treated in the hospital emergency room he had a stroke that paralyzed him along the entire right side of his body. He could not move and lost the power to speak (aphasia) or to chew.

Myocardial infarction (MI) is death of a segment of heart muscle, which follows interruption of its blood supply and is usually confined to the heart's left ventricle. The patient experiences a "heart attack," sudden severe chest pain, which may spread to the arms and throat. The main danger is that of ventricular fibrillation (overly fast beating of the heart), which accounts for most of the MI fatalities. Associated complications are heart failure, heart rupture, pulmonary embolism, phlebothrombosis, pericarditis, shock, mitral incompetence, and perforation of the septum between the ventricles.

Stroke, formerly known as apoplexy, is a sudden attack of weakness affecting one side of the body, the consequence of an interruption of the flow of blood to the brain. The primary disease is in the heart or blood vessels; the effect on the brain is secondary. The stroke varies in severity from a passing weakness or tingling in a limb to a profound paralysis, coma, and death.

Rob's grandfather was hospitalized for the treatment of myocardial infarction and stroke near his Sacramento, California, home. During his confinement in intensive care for three weeks, he was administered lots of drugs. He was helpless to do anything for himself and, upon his discharge from the hospital, his wife was advised by the cardiovascular experts to put the sick old man into a nursing home. But Rob's mother wouldn't let that happen to her father whom she loved so much.

Although she was shocked by her dad's appearance as he slumped in his wheelchair, paralyzed, incontinent, speechless, head drooping to one side, and drooling, Rob's mother worked with him day and night. After learning of the Gerson Therapy, she put her father on the program, feeding him fresh vegetables and only a few juices at first, while he still took the prescribed drugs. Slowly but steadily she increased the intensity of her father's dietary treatment. With love, she prepared his vegetables, fresh raw organic juices, and Hippocrates soup and served them according to Dr. Gerson's recommendations. Slowly she decreased the many drugs he was taking.

In less than three weeks, her father was up and out of the wheelchair and walking around the yard. In three months, he was walking in a park across the street from his home. In August 1994, at age eighty-eight (eight months after the heart attack and its associated stroke), he walked into the Woodland office of the California Department of Motor Vehicles and applied for (and received) a driver's license. He lived to age ninety-three, when the complications of an accidental fall sent him to a hospital, where he died.

General Information about the Gerson Dietary Program

Dr. Gerson was a great admirer of the teachings of the Swiss physician and chemist Paracelsus (1493–1541), and he quoted the Paracelsus Arcanum, which emphasized: *Diet must be the basis of all medical therapy, yet diet should not be a treatment in itself.* Consequently, although the Gerson dietary program is the foundation for a total healing effect, other adjuvant aspects of treatment are incorporated too, such as coffee enemas, castor oil packs, ozone therapy, clay poultices, hydrotherapy, hyperthermia tub baths, live cell therapy, rectal ozone insufflation, dietary supplementation with specific nutrients, and other items.

In providing his nutritional eating program, Dr. Gerson was rather considerate of modern social mores, taste temptations, family feasts, holidays, personal living habits, cultural requirements, and the economic pressures that a sick or even a well person would have to face. Consequently, he divided the Gerson *preventive* dietary program into two portions: one-quarter of all the food to be eaten could be to one's choice; the three-quarters remaining must be taken for the purpose of protecting the functions of the highly essential organs—the liver, the kidneys, the brain, the heart, and so on.

Dr. Gerson did suggest that, in order to prevent disease, one should eat a good diet three-quarters of which is vegetarian, nutritious, and cell-building foods, while the other quarter could be "at choice." The authors believe that Dr. Gerson's liberalism with food percentages should be tempered at present. More than forty years later, because of modern usage of overly processed foods, doctor-prescribed and over-the-counter pharmaceutical products, toxic pesticides, herbicides, fungicides, and food-processing chemicals, plus additions of much greater amounts of carcinogenic, atherogenic, allergenic, mitogenic, and other synthetics, it is our opinion that Dr. Gerson's original food suggestions are too liberal.

Because he never anticipated how much industry and commerce would come to poison the people and reduce the food value of what's eaten, Dr. Gerson's humanitarian food proportions are no longer valid. We urge instead that a person newly recovered from illness, as well as any normal and healthy individual who wishes to remain that way, would be wiser to use 90 percent "defensive," highly nutritious foods, and possibly allow a mere 10 percent of their meals "at choice."

The fundamentals of Dr. Gerson's general dietary outline offered to patients, he said, were "written to prevent sickness, not to cure it." To achieve a complete cure, he added, a great deal more effort was required. As we've stated, Dr. Gerson included such procedures as medicinelike nutritional supplementation and liver detoxification, two mandatory programs that we will discuss at length in later chapters. His claim was, "It's safer to use foods in the most natural form, combined and mixed by nature and raised, if possible, by an organic gardening process, thus obeying the laws of nature."[1]

This chapter offers Dr. Gerson's philosophy of eating correctly. It lays down the general guideposts for spotting what's good and bad about the foods to be selected. However, the actual foods to be eaten at each meal on the Gerson menu plan don't make their appearance until the next chapter.

THE SCIENCE BEHIND DR. GERSON'S ANTI-DEGENERATIVE-DISEASE DIET

The anti-degenerative-disease diet developed during the 1930s by Max Gerson, M.D., was first officially recorded as a proven treatment program at the University of Munich. It was afforded extraordinary laboratory support through funding from both the Bavarian and the Prussian federal government.[2]

Dr. Gerson focused then on the experimental use of foods of dietary purity (unprocessed and totally natural). He added the adjunctive use of medications to remove tissue edema occurring in a variety of pathologies such as tuberculosis, arthritis, cardiovascular disease, and cancer. Edema is characterized by salt and water alterations in the tissues that were eventually defined and named in 1977 as *tissue damage syndrome*[3]—decreased cell potassium (K^+), increased cell sodium (Na^+), and increased cell water (cellular swelling).[4]

Nutritional treatment to provide cells with a high K^+, low Na^+ environment improves edema and leads to enhanced tissue resistance and immunities, which together bring about better healing outcomes for sick people such as tubercular patients.[5] This rationale of tissue damaged syndrome may be traced through all of Dr. Gerson's subsequent efforts in the management of degenerative diseases, particularly for those patients beset by cancer.[6]

Dr. Gerson's anti-degenerative-disease dietary program is individualized to meet the needs of every patient, but it does have uniform components. As we mentioned in chapters 1, 2, and 6, for most patients it is restricted in salt, fat, and protein. It furnishes large quantities of multiple nutrients, enzymes, phytochemicals, and other nourishing ingredients which act like nutraceuticals. At the same time, each day's thirteen hourly feedings of 8 ounces of raw vegetable and fruit juices offer the diet's participant an ultimate boosting of his or her immune system. Nothing else known to the mind of man could be healthier or more stimulating of medical preventive homeostasis than the Gerson Therapy.

Before the disruption of supplies that began in late 1985, raw veal liver was additionally offered as part of the Gerson dietary program. That practice of juicing and feeding calf's liver had to be discontinued in 1987 because of repeated instances of bacterial contamination by the pathological organism *Campylobacter fetus s. fetus*. Comparisons of patients from different time frames show that those sick people receiving uncontaminated calf's liver juice had experienced better survival outcomes overall.[7]

Served in three generous daily meals, Dr. Gerson's diet includes food consumption from 2,600 calories up to 3,200 calories per day. This is no small amount of food; it requires the ingestion of approximately 17 to 20 pounds of vegetables and fruits per day. The plant food comes from all of the required raw, organic material needed for the thirteen 8-ounce glasses of juices besides the solid foods of the three meals. Still, although massive in amount, there is some caloric restriction because of the naturalness and purity of quality of the foods.

The Gerson menu plan is patterned after the antitumor effect of calorie restriction first demonstrated in Germany in 1909[8] and again in the United States in 1914.[9] Although this natural way of eating—which we reemphasize as being mostly vegetables and fruits—was tailored mainly to correct the pathology of malignancies, it's a form of orthomolecular medicine that works toward improving the physical, mental, and emotional health states of any person undergoing a worsening of well-being. It also restores body weight to normal, causing weight loss in the obese as well as weight gain in underweight patients.

Orthomolecular medicine, as defined by the now deceased two-time Nobel laureate Linus Pauling, Ph.D., in his foreword for the book *Putting It All Together: The New Orthomolecular Nutrition,* coauthored by Abram Hoffer, M.D., Ph.D., and Morton Walker, D.P.M., is a relatively new term in medicine. It means that a therapeutic approach is designed to provide an optimum molecular environment for body functions. The orthomolecular method offers particular reference to the best concentrations of substances normally present in the human physiology, whether formed within the body (endogenously) or ingested from outside the body (exogenously).

Orthomolecular medicine is the use of completely natural remedies (vitamins, minerals, herbs, enzymes, nutraceuticals, etc.) without any application of synthetic or other pharmaceutical agents. Orthomolecular medicine, in fact, is the healthiest way to achieve a therapeutic effect for healing diseases of all types. It is totally different from the toximolecular medicine of currently popular allopathic drug treatment taught in most medical schools.[10]

WHAT'S DIFFERENT ABOUT THE GERSON DIET

Sometimes people wonder whether the Gerson diet is different from or similar to other nutritional treatment approaches. In some regards, it may be similar, but the Gerson diet is not the same as any other treatment. The macrobiotic approach, for example, recommends cooked foods almost exclusively and is high in sodium—just the opposite to Dr. Gerson's therapeutic basis of diet. Another dietary approach recommends large quantities of nuts and seeds. Still another stresses the importance of pH balance in foods. The Ann Wigmore diet prefers raw foods to the exclusion of any other edible form and recommends eating many nuts and sprouts.

These many diets have their supporters, and all have successfully treated some patients. There are numerous schools of thought about how diet affects health and the several different paths to wholeness. We acknowledge that *the approach you take to your own healing must be your own decision,* but we encourage you to choose one approach and stick with it, adding aspects from other techniques of treatment only when they are known to be compatible. The Gerson Therapy usually is not effective if its dietary guidelines are mixed with those from other treatments. While the Gerson diet is similar to, and has served as the foundation for many other nutritional healing programs, its guidelines activate specific biochemical processes that promote healing in a unique way.

The foods and juices consumed on the Gerson diet constitute its primary prescription for healing, comparable to a drug in allopathic treatment. Significant deviation from the diet can be as serious for a Gerson patient as missing an insulin shot can be for a diabetic, or as missing a chemotherapy or radiation appointment can be for a cancer patient undergoing an allopathic treatment.

All you need to know for optimum results from the Gerson Therapy is in this book. We have observed that the best results are achieved by following these guidelines to the letter. Of course, we recognize that sometimes it will be impossible to meet all of the guidelines, whether for logistical, financial, or other reasons, and many of those who must "cut corners" will still achieve fair to good healing with the Gerson method. Rare, mild deviation from the therapy does not seem to affect outcomes significantly.

You will not fail to heal simply because you miss one glass of juice a couple of times a month. You will not fail if you must make use of commercial produce occasionally instead of organic. If organic produce is unavailable, commercial vegetables may be juiced after you have washed them thoroughly to remove the coatings of pesticides, herbicides, and other standard poisons used by agribusiness. Nevertheless, commercial produce is still deficient in nutrients. You will reduce your chances of success if you cut too many corners. How many? There is no good answer to that question, because every patient, every diagnosis, responds differently to the Gerson Therapy.

On the other hand, many patients have followed the guidelines in Dr. Max Gerson's original book *A Cancer Therapy: Results of Fifty Cases* without medical assistance and have healed themselves. Still, the Gerson Therapy must not be considered a "paint by numbers" approach to healing. Some ingenuity on the part of the person endeavoring to heal is sometimes required.

ADJUNCTS TO THE DIETARY PROGRAM DEVELOPED IN MUNICH

The patient's metabolism is accelerated by the addition of iodine to his intake.[11] Dr. Gerson discovered that natural thyroid hormone derived from animal sources plus the use of Lugol's iodine solution along with mild exercise, all used together, improved the healing person's metabolism markedly.[12] Niacin, potassium salts (acetate, gluconate, and monophosphate), and crude liver extract with injectable vitamin B_{12} were given to support accelerated cellular energy production. These vitamin and mineral nutrients are still being utilized as supplements to the Gerson dietary program even today.

In his University of Munich experiments of the 1930s, Dr. Gerson found that temporary protein restriction aided edema absorption and favored improvement in his patients' overall health.[13] In his anti-degenerative-disease diet, especially as it involved cancer, a desirable protein repletion with nonfat, enzyme-predigested dairy products often occurs after at least six weeks. Therefore, enzyme-modified defatted milk such as yogurt or unsalted nonfat cottage cheese is allowed as part of the dietary therapy. Shorter periods of protein restriction are recommended for children and elderly patients.

The Munich investigations turned up the therapeutic usefulness of a variety of additional procedures which are currently employed for Gerson Therapy participants. For instance, here are some adjuncts to the Gerson degenerative disease diet which will be discussed at length in later chapters:

- Castor oil, a cathartic with no known adverse clinical side effects, should be administered to someone sick with acute or chronic damage, especially cancer patients, every other day for many weeks (see chapter 11).
- Enemas of boiled coffee are taken by the patient as needed, as frequently as every four hours throughout the day, for their ability to alleviate pain, detoxify, and improve nutritional condition (see chapter 12). Occasional nighttime enemas are suggested in special cases.

Coffee enemas work exceedingly well to overcome the inflammatory aches and pains of arthritis, cancer, and other painful body degenerations. In 1994, Dr. Peter Lechner observed statistically significant cancer pain relief from coffee enemas in a prospective matched control trial that he conducted at the Municipal Hospital of Graz, Austria.[14] Pain relief for all types of malignancies is theorized to occur from a dialysis across the gut wall through coffee enemas, for tumor tissue breakdown products such as the polyamines, toxic bound nitrogen, and ammonia.[15]

Also observed is that those cancer patients taking coffee enemas, large amounts of Vitamin C and other aspects of the Gerson Therapy are able to better tolerate aggressive treatments with cytotoxic agents currently recommended by many conventionally practicing and unenlightened oncologists.[16]

References for Chapter Seven

1. Gerson, M. A *Cancer Therapy: Results of Fifty Cases and The Cure of Advanced Cancer by Diet Therapy*, 6th edition. Bonita, Calif.: The Gerson Institute, 1999, 22.

2. Ward, P.S. *History of the Gerson Therapy.* Washington, D.C.: Office of Technology Assessment, 1988.

3. Cope, F.W. "Pathology of structured water and associated cations in cells (the tissue damage syndrome) and its medical treatment." *Physiological Chemistry and Physics.* 9(6):547–553, 1977.

4. Evans, W.E.D. *The Chemistry of Death.* Springfield, Ill.: Charles C. Thomas, 1963, pp. 23–25.

5. Gerson, M. *Diet Therapy for Lung Tuberculosis*. Leipzig, Germany: Franz Deuticke, 1934.

6. *Op. cit.*, Gerson, M., pp. 164, 166, 184, 197.

7. *Op. cit.*, Evans, W.E.D., p. 31.

8. Moreschi, C. "The connection between nutrition and tumor promotion." *Z. Immunitätsforsch.* 2:651, 1909.

9. Rous, P. "The influence of diet on transplanted and spontaneous mouse tumors." *Journal of Experimental Medicine*. 20:433, 1914.

10. Hoffer, A.; Walker, M. *Putting It All Together: The New Orthomolecular Nutrition*. New Canaan, Conn.: Keats Publishing, 1978 and 1997, pp. Iv, v.

11. Silverstone, H.; Tannenbaum, A. "Influence of thyroid hormone on the formation of induced skin tumors in mice." *Cancer Research*. 9:684–688, 1949.

12. Wesch, M.A.; Conen, L.A.; Wesch, C.W. "Inhibition of growth of human breast carcinoma xenografts by energy expenditure via voluntary exercise in athymic mice fed a high-fat diet." *Nutrition in Cancer*. 23:309–317, 1995.

13. Gerson, M. "Fluid rich potassium diet as treatment for cardiorenal insufficiency." *Munich med. Wochenschr.* 82:571–574, 1935.

14. Lechner, P.; Hildenbrand, G. "A reply to Saul Green's critique of the rationale for cancer treatment with coffee enemas and diet: cafestol derived from beverage coffee increases bile production in rats; and coffee enemas and diet ameliorate human cancer pain in stages I and II." *Townsend Letter for Doctors and Patients*. 130:526–529, 1994.

15. Gerson, M. "The cure of advanced cancer by diet therapy: a summary of 30 years of clinical experimentation" (posthumous publication). *Physiology of Chemistry and Physics*. 10(4):449–464, 1978.

16. Lechner, P.; Kronberger, I. "Erfahrungen mit dem Einsatz der Diät-Therapie in der Chirurgischen Onkologie." *Aktuel Ernährungsmedizin*. 2(15):72–78, 1990.

Chapter Eight

FOODS ON
THE GERSON DIET PLAN

After co-founding the Gerson Institute of Bonita, California, Charlotte Gerson has carried forward the specifics of what to eat and not to eat as part of the illness-fighting menu plan. Her father set down over half a century ago how to permanently overcome chronic degenerative diseases by use of dietary procedures. According to those original instructions, described in 1958 by Dr. Gerson in his book A *Cancer Therapy*, a sick person using the Gerson Therapy should include those eating guidelines now presented below.

FOODS THAT MAY BE CONSUMED
IN QUANTITY

- All kinds of fruits are acceptable, mostly fresh and some prepared in different ways; freshly prepared vegetable juices; fruit salads; cold fruit soups; mashed bananas, raw grated apples, applesauce, and some other fruits.
- The recommended fruits are apples, grapes, cherries, mangoes, peaches, oranges, apricots, grapefruit, bananas, tangerines, pears, plums, melons, papayas, persimmons, and so on, none of which should come from cans or frozen packages. Pears and plums are

more easily digestible when stewed. All fruit may also be stewed. Dried fruit may be eaten if unsulfured, such as apricots, peaches, raisins, prunes, or mixed fruit, all of which should be washed, soaked, and stewed. All berries, nuts, pineapple, avocados, and cucumbers are forbidden.

- All vegetables freshly prepared, some stewed in their own juices and others either raw or finely grated, such as organically grown carrots, cauliflower or celery; vegetable salads, soups, and so on. No frozen vegetables are allowed.
- Potatoes are best when baked; the contents may be mashed with yogurt or soup; they should never be fried but may be boiled in their jackets.
- Salads of green leaves may be mixed with tomatoes, fruits, vegetables, and other organically grown plant edibles.
- Unsalted bread may contain whole rye but only a small percentage of whole wheat flour. The grain should be organically grown.
- Buckwheat cakes and potato pancakes are optional, as are brown sugar (organic dried cane juice, i.e., Sucanat), honey, maple sugar, and 100 percent pure maple syrup. (Use *no* fats or baking soda when baking.)
- Oatmeal should be used freely.
- Milk products such as churned buttermilk, nonfat unflavored yogurt, and nonfat unsalted pot (cottage) cheese are allowed. After two years on a strict Gerson Therapy program, cream and ice cream can be used sparingly or restricted to holidays. (Dr. Gerson flat-out states: "Ice cream is 'poison' for children.")
- After the ill individual has recovered, allowing two years or more in some cases, the remaining 10 percent of the dietary regime (remembering from chapter 7 that Dr. Gerson's original food proportions have been modified to conform to the more unnatural methods used in growing and processing foods during modern times), which allows for personal choice, may consist of meat, fish, eggs, nuts, candies, cakes, or whatever one likes best.
- Nicotine should be avoided under any circumstances.
- Liquors, wine, and beer should be reduced to a minimum in favor of fresh fruit juices.
- Coffee and tea should be cut to a minimum with the exception of the following teas: peppermint, chamomile, linden flower, orange flower, and a few others.
- Salt, bicarbonate of soda, smoked fish, and sausage must be avoided

completely (see chapter 10 for a more complete explanation about salt).

- Sharp condiments such as pepper and ginger must be eliminated. But fresh garden herbs are recommended for regular consumption, including onions, garlic, parsley leaves, chives, horseradish, and celery.
- All vegetables may be consumed, stewed in their own juices to avoid the loss of minerals easily dissolved in water during cooking. Especially recommended for their mineral content are carrots, peas, tomatoes, broccoli, Swiss chard, spinach, string beans, brussels sprouts, artichokes, beets cooked with apples, cauliflower with tomatoes, red cabbage with apples, and raisins. Everything must be prepared without salt.
- Any cooking equipment made of aluminum is absolutely forbidden, as are microwave ovens, pressure cookers, and steam cookers.
- While following the Gerson eating plan for the first year and a half, don't eat any eggs, fish, meat, butter, cheese, and milk.

Altogether, because of the extensive juicing of vegetables, a follower of the Gerson eating plan takes in between 17 and 20 pounds of plant foods each day. You'll understand how and why this is done after reading our explanation of the juicing concept in chapter 9.

FOODS PROHIBITED ON
THE GERSON MENU PLAN

All foods eaten as part of the Gerson diet must be prepared *without* the use of the following categories of prohibited foods:[1]

Salt and Sodium

Salt and sodium in all forms, including table salt, sea salt, celery salt, vegetable salt, Bragg Liquid Aminos™, tamari, soy sauce, "lite salt," baking soda, sodium-based baking powders, and *anything* with "sodium" in its name, as well as salt substitutes, are forbidden. Skin contact with Epsom salts should be avoided. Combinations of herbs, often sold under names such as "instead of salt" or "salt-free seasoning," may be used in small quantities, if they contain permitted herbs without added salt or salt substitutes.

Oils and Fats

Oils and fats, plus any foods that contain them, are prohibited. This prohibition includes corn oils, olive oils, canola oils, and all other vegetable oils except flaxseed oil as specifically prescribed; also forbidden are butter, cheese, cream, and other dairy fats; all animal fats; all margarines or oil-based spreads; coconuts and avocados; all hydrogenated or partially hydrogenated oils; Olean, Olestra, and other "fat substitutes"; nut butters; and any other source of dietary fats, except as naturally occurring in allowed foods.

Proteins and High-Protein Foods

Proteins and high-protein foods are not allowed. These disallowed foods include all meats, seafoods, and other animal proteins; nuts and seeds; soy or other legume-based food products; all protein powders or supplements, including barley- or algae-based powders, unless specifically used when prescribed for protein supplementation.

In addition to the above three categories, there are certain other foods that must be "off-limits" until the ill individual is completely healed, and in some cases, even after full recovery. The "off-limits" foods include almost all packaged, prepared ("convenience") foods such as those frozen, canned, bottled, or boxed. They must be forsaken for health reasons. Restaurant food will almost always be *un*acceptable, because it is rarely organic and almost always is cooked with added salt, fats, or other additives inappropriate to the Gerson eating plan.

Because the Gerson approach to healing looks at everything that goes into, or on, the body as factors in the therapeutic process, the Gerson Therapy may appear more restrictive than other "natural" or "holistic" approaches. *By means of such attention to detail, the Gerson Therapy accomplishes healing even in some extremely advanced cases of pathology, or in diseases that otherwise are considered incurable.*

Sometimes it's tempting to deny the seriousness of one's own condition. A few sick people go through a thinking process that says, "Well, my malignancy isn't very advanced; it's only stage II cancer and not the worst kind, so I don't need to follow the diet as closely as someone near death." We believe this is a foolish form of thinking. Similarly, some Gerson Therapy patients are the recipients of well-meaning but uninformed advice from friends, relatives, and even medical practitioners who know little about the complex biochemical interactions occurring in a body combining the Gerson diet, medications, and detoxification. We advise that it's unwise to arbitrarily modify the true Gerson dietary therapy for the sake of personal convenience or to please somebody else's ego. Ask any person wanting to give you advice: "How many cancer patients have you healed with this advice?"

We strongly recommend that you refrain from adding to or changing the proven dietary guidelines without the advice of a certified Gerson Therapy practitioner. (Contact the Gerson Institute to be directed to a certified Gerson Therapy practitioner near your location.) Making even minor modifications of the Gerson Therapy protocol is poor practice. Why? Because the treatment procedure has shown itself repeatedly to success-fully achieve remission or cure of cancer and nearly every other chronic degenerative disease. Quite simply, used exactly as presented, the Gerson dietary program has shown itself to work!

THREE FOOD CATEGORIES: DESIRABLE, OCCASIONALLY ALLOWED, AND PROHIBITED

Desirable Organically Grown Foods

Sick or well, as a means of reversing pathology or to prevent its occur-ring, the food categories listed below are excellent sources of nourishment and may be consumed without limitations. The truly *desirable* foods are:

- All fruits and vegetables plus potatoes, except as listed under pro-hibited foods
- Fresh fruit and vegetable juices, as shown in chapter 9
- Raw fruit and vegetable salads (see below in this chapter)
- Special Hippocrates soup (see below for its preparation)
- Oatmeal

The desirable foods mentioned actually are necessary for their thera-peutic effects. They are easily and quickly digested. Eating large and fre-quent portions of them is encouraged on the Gerson diet. One may even eat them during the night when awaking hungry, to provide critical nutri-tion for rebuilding damaged tissues and maintaining necessary nourish-ment. As the body restores itself, many people become ravenous with hunger. There is virtually no limit to the quantity of these good foods that can be consumed, provided that it is high-quality, organically grown if possible, and fresh from the "desirable" list. We recommend keeping food available at the bedside for nighttime snacking (such as fruit, fruit salad, or applesauce).

Occasionally Allowed Organically Grown Foods

Unless otherwise prescribed by your Gerson-trained health professional, the following groups of foods, free of salt, salt derivatives, and oils and fats, may be eaten once per week:

- Breads made from whole rye, oat, or rice flour
- Organic popcorn (dry-popped, unsalted, and without fat)
- Brown or wild rice
- Yams and sweet potatoes
- Maple syrup, honey, raw brown sugar, and unsulfured blackstrap molasses up to a daily combined maximum of all sweeteners of 2 teaspoonfuls.

Very Occasionally Allowed Foods

Ingested not more than once or twice per month, the following food groups are permitted occasionally:

- Organically grown, frozen vegetables (if prepared without added salt, fat, or other prohibited ingredients)
- Sprouted beans or seeds (e.g., lentils, beans) other than alfalfa sprouts, which are forbidden.

Prohibited Foods

Whenever possible, we offer a brief explanation as to why the various foods cited under this prohibition category are not allowed on the Gerson dietary program.

- *All manufactured (processed) foods* such as those that are bottled, canned, frozen, preserved, refined, salted, smoked, or sulfured (except as specifically mentioned as being allowed) are forbidden.
- *Dairy products of all types* such as milk and milk products (including goat's milk) are forbidden. These prohibited items include cheese, cream, ice cream, ice milk, butter, and buttermilk, except as

specifically allowed under proteins. Dairy products are generally extremely high in fat. Cheeses may be 65 percent fat and high in sodium. The commercial buttermilks are "cultured" (produced from leftover milk, flavored, and thickened) and contain fat and sodium. When protein is prescribed, however, fresh, churned buttermilk without any additives may be taken after the sixth to twelfth week of healing. Unsalted, nonfat Quark is premitted when available.

- *Alcohol* should not be imbibed because it limits the blood's ability to carry oxygen and places strain on the liver to detoxify and remove it from the body. Alcohol is toxic.
- *Pineapples and berries* may cause an allergic reaction to the aromatic acids present.
- *Avocados* are too high in fats.
- *Cucumbers* in combination with the required juices to be taken daily are difficult to digest.
- *Spices* such as black pepper or paprika are irritants. Basil, oregano, and others are to be avoided because of their high aromatic acid content. Cayenne pepper, jalapenos, and so on are also irritants and can stop the healing.
- *Soybeans and soy products* including tofu, tempeh, miso, tamari, other soy sauces, Bragg's Liquid Aminos™, textured vegetable protein, soy milk, and all other soy-based products are disallowed. For a variety of different reasons including their high fat content, high sodium content, toxic inhibition to nutrient absorption, and/or elevated protein content, use of soy in all its forms must be avoided.
- *Dried beans and legumes* should not be used.
- *Sprouted Alfalfa and Other Bean or Seed Sprouts* are high in L-canavanine, an immature amino acid that is responsible for immune system suppression. Also, patients with no prior history of chronic joint pain have developed the sudden onset of arthritic symptoms upon ingesting alfalfa sprouts. Healthy monkeys have developed lupus erythematosus from alfalfa sprouts in their diet.
- *Oils and fats* of all kinds, with the exclusion of fresh, raw, organic flaxseed oil, are forbidden.
- *Refined white and brown sugars* are forbidden.
- *Wheat flour* (including whole wheat) is forbidden; also all types of pasta.
- *Beef, pork, poultry, eggs, fish, seafood, and all other meat or animal flesh products* are prohibited. These animal foods are high in pro-

tein, chemicals, perservatives, hormones, and salt and are difficult to digest, often have too much fat, and make additional work for the body's liver and excretory systems.

- *Black tea, green tea, and other nonherbal or caffeine-containing teas* are forbidden because of their undesirable aromatic acids and caffeine content. Dr. Gerson cited aromatics as interfering with healing by producing allergic reactions (see above as listed under *pineapples and berries*).

- *Candy, cakes, muffins, pastries, and other refined sweets* are prohibited because they contain health-threatening ingredients, such as fats, oils, refined sugars or flours, salt, soda, baking powder, or dairy products. Note, however, that some breads and pastries may be baked using permitted ingredients which will make the diet more interesting but must not be consumed on a regular basis.

- *The drinking of water* is not encouraged. Dr. Gerson believed that a Gerson Therapy patient should not drink water, because it dilutes the stomach acid and doesn't allow maximum gastrointestinal tract capacity for nutrition from fresh foods and juices. The juices provide adequate fluids.

- *Mushrooms* are not vegetables but fungi and contain complex proteins and are difficult to digest and offer little nutrition.

- *Coffee and coffee substitutes by mouth*, both with caffeine and decaffeinated, cause undesirable stimulation of the digestive system. Orally taken caffeine overly excites the central nervous system, while the essential oils disturb digestion. In contrast, when coffee is taken rectally, it offers an entirely advantageous effect on the liver where, aside from detoxification, it increases the production of glutathione S-transferase (a desirable enzyme).

- *Nuts and seeds*, including almonds, apricot kernels, sunflower seeds, flaxseeds, peanuts, cashews, and all other nuts and seeds, are prohibited because they are too high in protein and fat. In "roasting" salt is added, the fat is altered, and nuts and seeds become more harmful.

- *Hot peppers* (jalapenos, etc.) contain the same strong aromatics found in prohibited spices. Peppers tend to inhibit healing responses and should be avoided. Green, yellow, and sweet red peppers may be used without limitation.

- *Mustard and carrot greens.*

- *Baking powder and baking soda* contain sodium and alum (aluminum), which are highly toxic. Aluminum-free and sodium-free baking powders such as Featherweight™ (potassium-based powder) may be used occasionally.

- *Fluoride components* that are part of any item at all such as water, toothpaste, mouth gargle, hair dyes, beauty parlor permanents, cosmetics, underarm deodorants, lipstick, and lotions must be avoided under any conditions.

How to Prepare Foods on the Gerson Eating Program

Since foods of the Gerson eating program are easily digested, people following it generally require larger and more frequent servings. Eat as much of these foods as possible, even during the night if desired. The foods to be consumed include fresh and stewed fruit, juices of fresh fruits and vegetables, fresh raw and cooked vegetables and leaves, salads, special Hippocrates soup, potatoes, oatmeal, salt-free rye bread (limited to one or two slices a day), and herb tea.

Vegetable Preparation

We admit that by most standards of modern food preparation, Gerson Therapy meals are considered overcooked. Dr. Gerson believed that foods should be well done to make them tender, easy to chew, and digestible, which would help the weakened digestive system acquire the greatest amount of soft bulk plus nutrition in the most accessible form from the food consumed. The soft cooked victuals therefore provide a buffer for the considerable volume of juices and raw foods ingested. The modern "al dente" vegetable preparation is supposed to keep enzymes intact. That is not correct; all enzymes are dead at 140 degrees Fahrenheit. Very ample enzymes are provided on the Gerson Therapy through the raw juices, salads, and fruit.

All food must be prepared fresh; canned, bottled, boxed, or frozen foods always contain additives and inhibit restoration of the body. Absolutely no salt, soy sauces, or other sodium sources should be added to any consumed foods. All prepared foods containing salt, such as most breads, should be eliminated altogether.

It's not unnatural to tire of eating foods with the same soft consistency for every meal. In the early stages of treatment, people are encouraged to eat large quantities of foods and to cook them thoroughly. Raw fruit and salads with celery, green onions, and radishes provide crisp and chewy foods for variation from soft-cooked vegetables. Dr. Gerson did not want his patients to deviate from the cooking methods used, but as a patient progresses in health, it may be possible to include some foods cooked al dente for variation. Since exponents of the Gerson Therapy consider food to be medication, any changes in one's diet or cooking technique should be discussed with a trained Gerson Therapy health professional.

Cooked Foods

All vegetables, except those listed as prohibited, are recommended. Vegetables should be cooked with a minimum of water or soup stock (perhaps 2 or 3 tablespoonfuls) slowly on low heat, just at boiling, until well done. Usually such a procedure will take fifty to sixty minutes on the stovetop. To prevent burning, place a metal mat or ring between the burner and pot to help distribute the heat evenly. Vegetables can also be baked in covered glass dishes in an oven, where the heat is more even and burning is less likely. A tight-fitting lid should always be used to help retain moisture in foods, but no pressure cooking.

Onions, tomatoes, and squash contain a lot of water, generally don't need any added liquid for cooking, and can add flavor to the cooked foods. Celery is also good for flavoring.

Beets and potatoes can be boiled whole (without peeling) in water and peeled when done, or may be baked.

Potatoes can also be scalloped, mashed, made into potato salad, or prepared in a variety of other ways.

Spinach releases much water and oxalic acid in cooking. For this reason, the water left after cooking spinach is bitter and should be discarded.

Corn can be boiled in water or eaten raw.

Herbs and Spices

Inasmuch as the aromatics of herbs and spices, as with pineapples and berries, tend to interfere with the healing response, Dr. Gerson limited use of such aromatics to small quantities of the relatively mild ones such as allspice, anise, bay leaf, coriander, dill, fennel, mace, marjoram, rosemary, sage, saffron, tarragon, thyme, sorrel, and summer savory. Chives, onions, garlic, and parsley can be used in larger quantities.

Salads

It is essential that the patient eat as many salads of raw vegetables as possible. The following salad ingredients can be finely grated, chopped, or minced and mixed together or eaten separately:

- Apples
- Carrots
- Watercress
- Green onions
- Knob or branch celery
- Lettuce greens
- Cauliflower
- Endive
- Chives
- Chicory
- Radishes
- Green peppers
- Tomatoes

Salad Dressing

NEVER use bottled dressing. Dilute organic red wine or apple cider vinegar with water to taste for use as a salad dressing and add a little spray-dried organic cane juice (Sucanat), some herbs, onion, or garlic for taste variety. Lemon juice may be used in the place of vinegar. The prescribed flaxseed oil can be used as part of the salad dressing.

Hippocrates Special Soup

Created as a staple food item for nearly all of his degenerative disease patients, Dr. Gerson considered the Hippocrates special soup (invented by Hippocrates) extremely important to eat at both lunch and dinner. While much of the Gerson Therapy is directed toward cleansing the liver, the Hippocrates soup helps to cleanse the kidneys. Particularly after patients become used to eating without salt (usually within one to two weeks after starting the treatment), the special soup is a tasty start to every meal.

To make the Hippocrates special soup, the following vegetables should be thoroughly washed, not peeled, cut into cubes, covered with water, and cooked for two hours. Put everything through a food mill; allow only fibers and peels to remain. The result is a thick, creamy soup. Allow the soup to cool before storing in a refrigerator. Make only enough for about two days so that the excess, which loses its nutritional value after that time, will not be consumed. Here are the quantities of vegetables:

- 1 medium celery knob (root). If celery root is not in season, substitute 3 or 4 stalks of branch celery.
- A small amount of parsley
- 1 1/2 pounds of tomatoes (more if desired during the summer season)
- 2 medium onions
- 1 medium parsley root (rarely available; omit if not)
- 2 small leeks (if not available, substitute 2 additional medium onions)
- several cloves of garlic
- 1 pound of potatoes

Until the healing person is used to salt-free eating, raw pressed garlic may be added for giving a "kick" to this Hippocrates special soup and also to vegetables, salads, etc. Garlic is healthful and may be used any time in any amount.

Potatoes

High in plant proteins, potatoes are nutritional boons for any healing person. We recommend eating them for both lunch and dinner; replace them only rarely with organic brown or wild rice. Potatoes are of most nutritional value when baked. They can also be served boiled in their jackets, mashed with a little soup, peeled (after boiling), or cut up and mixed with salad dressing to make a potato salad. They can be baked in a casserole with onion, tomatoes, celery, and so on. If nonfat yogurt is prescribed after six to ten weeks on the Gerson diet, add onions, chives, or garlic to the yogurt for a tasty dressing for your baked potato, salad, or vegetable. Sweet potatoes may be served once a week.

Oatmeal

A large portion of oatmeal, cooked slowly from $\frac{1}{2}$ cup organic rolled oats and 1 (or a little more) cup of purified water, should be eaten every day for breakfast. Other cereals should not be used. Not only do oats supply good B complex vitamins as well as proteins; most importantly, they provide a soft cushion in the intestinal tract for the raw juices that follow. Harsh and grainy cereals cannot provide this. For variety, add raw grated apple, papaya, or other fruit; honey, 100 percent pure maple syrup, or unsulfured blackstrap molasses; raisins or other dried fruit, stewed prunes, or other stewed dried or fresh fruit.

Bread and Other Starches

You may use some salt-free and fat-free rye bread *only after consuming the full required meal*. Bread should not be the main part of any meal. When bread is dry, it can be grated and used in recipes requiring bread crumbs. Occasionally you may also use potato flour, tapioca, or cornstarch.

Sugars and Sweeteners

Use only organic brown sugar, maple syrup, organic light honey, or unsulfured molasses, and only up to 2 teaspoons a day of all combined sweeteners, and only when hypoglycemia and/or diabetes are not present.

Herbal Teas

Peppermint and some other herb teas are allowed and encouraged for various specific beneficial properties. Peppermint tea helps digestion; chamomile tea is soothing; valerian tea can help sleep. Tahebo, also known as pau d'arco, is a valuable anti-cancer tea and can be taken in any quantity at night.

Sample Menus

For *breakfast*, you should consume:

- 8 ounces of orange juice
- Large portion of oatmeal with choice of fruit sauce
- Organic 100 percent rye bread, unsalted and fat-free, toasted and spread with honey

Lunch should consist of:

- Salad of many mixed raw ingredients
- 8 ounces or more of warm Hippocrates special soup
- 8 ounces of apple-carrot juice in combination
- Baked potato (with yogurt dressing when permitted)

- Freshly cooked vegetables
- Raw or stewed fruit

For *dinner*, the menu is the same as for lunch.

We suggest that you vary meals by using different vegetables, a variety of methods of preparing potatoes, different kinds of salads, etc. Organic brown rice may be served once a week. Organic sweet potatoes may be served once a week.

See the Appendixes for the Patient Hourly Schedule.

Reference for Chapter Eight

1. *Gerson Therapy Practitioner's Training Seminar Workbook.* Bonita, Calif.: The Gerson Institute, 1996, pp. 120, 121.

Chapter Nine

THIRTEEN GLASSES

In 1981, when he was thirty-eight years old, acute infectious hepatitis struck Paul Schofield of Orlando, Florida. It took the form of fever, jaundice, and severe nausea. Mr. Schofield became so sick that he had to abandon his leatherworking craft and the rented shop where he sold saddles, belts, hats, and luggage of his own making. Day after day he felt weak to the point of collapse.

Hepatitis is an inflammation of the liver caused by viruses or bacteria and brought on by exposure to toxic substances, contaminated blood products, or immunological abnormalities. Acute infectious hepatitis may also be transmitted by food or drink contaminated by a carrier or patient, and it commonly occurs where sanitation is poor. After an incubation period ranging from two weeks to forty days, the patient develops abnormally elevated liver enzymes, fever, and sickness.

THE PATHOLOGY OF VIRAL HEPATITIS

A fairly common systemic disease, viral hepatitis is marked by liver (hepatic) cell destruction, necrosis, and autolysis, leading to anorexia, jaundice, and hepatomegaly (abnormal liver enlargement). More than 70,000 cases of the illness are reported annually in the United States. Today five specific types of viral hepatitis are recognized (but were unknown in 1981). The five forms of hepatitis are:

- *Type A* (infectious or short-incubation hepatitis). The incidence of hepatitis A is rising among homosexuals and for those persons with an immunosuppression related to an infection with the human immunodeficiency virus (HIV). The ingestion of seafood from polluted waters can cause it too.
- *Type B* (serum or long-incubation hepatitis). Also increasing among HIV-positive individuals, hepatitis B accounts for up to 10 percent of postransfusion viral hepatitis cases in the United States. It is also transmitted by human secretions and by feces, during intimate sexual contact, and from the transfer of viruses into food prepared by infected restaurant workers.
- *Type C* (undetermined as to specific organism type). This disease organism is mostly acquired by blood transfusion from asymptomatic donors. Of all the hepatitis viral diseases, type C hepatitis is on the fastest rise among modern-day Americans.
- *Type D* is found most frequently as a complication of acute or chronic hepatitis B, because this type D virus requires that sister organism's double-shelled surface antigen to replicate.
- *Type E* (formerly grouped with type C under the name *type non-A, non-B* hepatitis) primarily occurs among people recently returned from an endemic area such as India, Africa, Asia, or Central America.

Of the five viral hepatitis diseases, hepatitis B and hepatitis C are the most dangerous because they have a high risk of developing into liver cancer, and one of these types most likely had infected Mr. Schofield.

At the time of his infection, Mr. Schofield's skin showed a marked yellow discoloration, which persisted for three weeks; his medical doctor could offer no curative treatment because there was none known back then, in 1981, especially by those physicians who had exclusively practiced their particular allopathic-type (drug-dependent) medicine. There were no drugs to treat the condition. The only medical suggestion given to this patient was to rest a lot, take naps, and drink fluids like soda pop (which is toxic) or orange juice. Although he did this for no less than eight months, Mr. Schofield failed to improve in any way.

PAUL SCHOFIELD BEGINS JUICING ON THE GERSON THERAPY

A massage therapist from whom he received rubdowns recommended that the sick man read the book A *Cancer Therapy: Results of Fifty Cases*, which the patient did. The book's ideas seemed right and logical to him, so he set himself up with a Norwalk® Juicer, Dr. Norman Walker's famous hydraulic pressing device, and started the Gerson Therapy on his own. In proceeding with Dr. Gerson's instructions, Paul Schofield drank great quantities of juice, consisting of an 8-ounce glass of carrot and apple or green juice, every waking hour of his day—a minimum of thirteen glasses, and sometimes more.

"I immediately began to feel better. My liver enzyme test readings improved. They moved down from a pathological high of 2,400 to the normal range of 20. Within two months, when my physician reexamined me, his verdict was that I no longer remained infectious; my blood counts were normal," Paul Schofield said. "For several years, however, I occasionally suffered from flulike symptoms. At such times, I would immediately go back for a week to the full bevy of juicing required on the Gerson Therapy program.

"Sometimes drinking the juices for only a few days was sufficient for me to get rid of the hepatitis symptoms. Even after just one day of drinking thirteen glasses of juice my body, especially my liver, felt better. I learned that to eliminate any of the infecting viruses, Hepatitis A, B, C, D, and E, one must drink the fresh-made juices from organic vegetables and fruits," says this man who thrived on a self-help Gerson juicing and food menu plan.

Today, as indicated by his photograph, Paul Schofield is happy and thriving in good health. His hepatitis symptoms don't come on anymore; however, if they do, the man knows that he can banish them quickly by drinking fresh-made, organic vegetable and fruit juices.

SOME JUICING TIPS OFFERED PREVIOUSLY BY DR. GERSON

For the preparation of vegetable and fruit juices, Dr. Max Gerson recommended two machines: a separate triturator or grinder and a separate press. One of his juicing tips was that all parts of the juice machine that come into contact with ground foods should be made of stainless steel. Therapy exponents currently favor one machine in particular which uses these two processes.

As with Mr. Schofield, the juicing device most favored by Gerson Therapy patients is the Norwalk® Juicer. It was invented about 1936 by Norman W. Walker, D.Sc., and comes in two models, the 270-S Norwalk stainless finish and the 270 Norwalk woodgrain finish. (See the Appendix for a listing of names, locations, and other information advising as to where and how products and supplies recommended for use by Gerson Therapy followers may be found.)

Dr. Gerson required his recovering patients always to prepare fresh juices made from organic fruits and vegetables. He advised them never to attempt to prepare sufficient juice for the whole day in the morning. Also, as another tip discussed at length in his original text, Dr. Gerson advises not to drink water because the full capacity of one's stomach is needed for the juices and the Hippocrates special vegetable soup (see chapter 8). Components in the soup are readily absorbed through the gastrointestinal mucosa. Water filling up the stomach tends to dilute the action of that organ's gastric acids and digestive enzymes.

This chapter gives a complete description of the types of juicing machines along with the juicing process. As compared with Dr. Gerson's original text, here we provide much new information coming from those patients who have prepared their own juices at home and restored themselves to good health. A combination of the enzymatic effect of fresh, whole organic juices plus a therapeutic saltless diet (see chapter 10) with appropriate, limited, nutritional supplementation (see chapter 11) and the taking of coffee enemas (see chapters 12 and 13)—all assured means—results in renewed wellness that is long-lasting, natural, and safe. Juicing plant produce and swallowing the result is the most delicious way to good health.

RENEW WELLNESS BY DRINKING ORGANIC, FRESH-MADE JUICES

Juicing and imbibing such juice are integral aspects of the Gerson Therapy program. Unconditionally, the coauthors reaffirm: *For any ill individual as well as for someone in a state of good health, drinking fresh-made juices processed from organically grown fruits and vegetables frequently through each day is critical to renewing or maintaining wellness.*

An important note: While there are no federal standards for the commonly used combination term *organically grown*, it usually refers to produce planted and grown without chemical pesticides, herbicides, or synthetic fertilizers, on farm lands and in groves, orchards, or vineyards that have been free of such chemicals for from three to seven years.[1]

Along with providing sufficient fluid intake, fresh juices furnish nearly all of the nutrients—vitamins, minerals, enzymes, phytochemicals, herbals, and other vital food substances, including even proteins—required for your body to heal itself. Juice drinking is even more important for healing degenerative diseases than eating the same nutrients held in whole food. In fact, juices are food, of course, but in much more assimilable form for use by the gastrointestinal tract. Juice drinking allows for better digestion and greater absorption. By a person's conforming to the Gerson Therapy protocol and consuming thirteen 8-ounce glasses— about 104 ounces of juice daily—this vast amount of liquid plus three vegetarian meals offers the equivalent of between 17 and 20 pounds of food a day. Few people (possibly nobody) could consume that much solid edible material during usual waking hours. Drinking juices allows one to ingest massive amounts of nourishment in a short time.

Degenerative diseases often promote poor digestion for those persons victimized by them. Because of their intoxication from malfunctioning organs, the presence of decreased gastric acids, digestive dysfunction overall, and other such difficulties directly connective with the body's degenerations, such people are likely to suffer from the loss of appetite and an inability to eat at all or to hold and assimilate even small quantities of food. (Such a discomforting condition is known as *cachexia*.) Yet degenerative disease patients who suffer in this way often are able to keep themselves nourished rather well merely by drinking fresh made juices. The juiced nutrients are far more vital to one's body than the fiber contents of whole foods. Nevertheless, solid foods must be added to the patient's total intake.

JUICING HELPED DR. GERSON HEAL HIS PATIENTS

In order to bring about healing for his many tubercular, cardiovascular, cancerous, diabetic, arthritic, and other patients suffering from degenerative diseases, Max Gerson, M.D., sought out new methods for overcoming their subclinical malnutrition. Even obese persons can lack nutrients. For each ill individual, juicing at home is how Dr. Gerson met the challenge. And it was a technique which proved valuable. The juices made from raw foods and drunk by these very sick people provided the easiest and most effective means of giving them the highest-quality nutrition. This unique method of feeding that he developed during the approximately thirty-five year period from 1923 to 1958 produced the best clinical results ever witnessed in medical practice by that midpoint in the twentieth century.

Today, with the twenty-first century upon us, the coauthors are reluctant to make changes in a protocol that has been extremely effective for treating, reversing, or sending into near-permanent remission degenerative diseases of all types. These are the kinds of serious illnesses for which allopathic medicine has had very little to offer. Still, staff of the Gerson Institute are not close-minded. If some better method came along as a substitute for the high-dose nutrition made available by juicing or the other techniques perfected by Dr. Gerson, it would be adopted into the Gerson Therapy protocol.

During the course of his thirty years of active clinical practice, however, Dr. Gerson did change his protocol considerably. He repeatedly altered what the physician described as his "juice prescriptions" in response to his patients' blood test results, healing reaction responses, allergies, weight variations, and other metabolic conditions. The physiological responses of severely damaged or weakened individuals often required him to change the medications and juices on an almost daily basis, especially during their first weeks of following the Gerson Therapy. That is the situation for current patients as well.[2]

QUESTIONS AND ANSWERS ABOUT DRINKING JUICES

Drinking juices begets large numbers of questions for which there are few answers. For instance, we wonder at but cannot completely answer some of the following queries from those utilizing the Gerson Therapy:

When or how regularly should one drink the juices? Dr. Gerson advised that an ill individual should take 8 ounces at least once every hour, but it's not uncommon to find such a regimen difficult to accomplish.

What's to be done as a solution or compromise for being unable to follow the program exactly? Drink as much as you can, but keep trying to ingest more. In this situation for juicing and drinking, more is better.

How much juice should you drink? As mentioned, attempt to consume 104 ounces of fresh organic juice in twenty-four hours.

How soon after actually performing the juicing is the best time to drink down the juice? Unquestionably, the answer is "At once!"

Is it acceptable to store the juice for future drinking? The direct and uncompromising answer is "No!" But let's face it—if you work at a distance from home and can't lug around a 70-pound juicing machine, taking apple/carrot juices along with you in thermos-type storage containers (glass or stainless steel lined) or 8-ounce mason jars filled to the top is not all that bad. Do it if it's the only way you'll be getting your daily allotment of organic juices. Never keep or take along green juices (made from salad greens) for future ingestion because they oxidize quickly and lose their value.

Do we know what fruits and vegetables may best be combined or are incompatible? Our observation is that almost all of plant produce is compatible, although Dr. Gerson urged the use of specific combinations of carrot and apple, carrot only, and juice made from various greens. Avoid other juiced produce.

At which section of one's gastrointestinal tract is juice absorption best? The entire length of the intestinal tract (23 feet or 7 meters from the top opening of the stomach to the anus) goes to work on enzymes in juices and takes them into the bloodstream. But not too much nutrient absorption takes place in the stomach, large intestine, and rectum.

Is there a "vital force" taken into the body from juice drinking? It's strictly our opinion, but we say "Yes!" The live enzymes in vegetables and fruits may be absorbed into the physical, mental, and spiritual self and probably do invigorate one's soul. At least, we hope so.

Are the kidneys flushed more effectively if the recommended juices are consumed? Yes, physiological testing has shown that juice enzymes are cleansing agents—sometimes truly diuretic in nature. You can test this concept yourself by juicing large, white asparagus and drinking the product. Drinking celery juice is nearly as good a diuretic too. By drinking juices like these, you'll then urinate a lot, resulting in well-flushed kidneys and a swabbed-out urinary tract.

As stated, we do possess some opinions that come from our observations or good scientifically based answers for questions you may put forth, but not for all such questions.

Some Personal Rules about Juicing

Now we offer a bit of knowledge for you to assimilate. Since the therapeutic enzymes in freshly produced plant juices do oxidize out of existence and into free radical destruction by exposure to the oxygen in air for any prolonged period, we must offer two parts of one definite rule to follow. Although compromises may be inevitable, the ensuing two-part rule comes from representatives who offer telephone advice when you call for it at the Gerson Institute:

1. If at all possible, try to freshly prepare each of your 8-ounce glasses of juice and drink them down immediately. This is especially important for the very ill patient.
2. In the morning, do *not* prepare all juices for drinking during the day in order to store them for later use, because before the day's end you'll probably be swallowing deficient juice with many nutrients missing.

Types of Juicing Devices

Partly on an intuitive belief but mostly observing results in his patients, Dr. Gerson presumed that the method of juice extraction decidedly affected the concentration of nutrients his patients took into their bodies. Forty years after his death, we know from analyses of juices produced by each type of juicing device that some machines are better than others for the production of quality drinking liquids. Also, the clinical results experienced by patients using each type of juicer provide further support for Dr. Gerson's original presumptions.

Although there are six types of juicers manufactured, which we will describe briefly, our preference focuses on one particular product type. We will cite the lesser machines first and move on to the best kind to use for the Gerson Therapy program—discussed near the end of this section.

Below are descriptions of the forms of juicing mechanisms which do produce vegetable and fruit juices but, compared to the sixth one that we prefer, a few of them hardly provide anything really drinkable in acceptable qualities and quantities.

1. Masticating Juicers

Masticators, as the term describes, chew up the vegetables or fruits and extract their juices in one step. The juice quality is fairly good, but the amount of vegetable or fruit pulp remaining is excessive with some of the plant enzymes being left behind in so much pulp. While the juice produced by masticators is richer in nutrients than that from centrifugal juicers (see below), it is less nourishing than what's acquired from the type of triturator or grinder/press that we prefer (see the sixth device to be described). Also, a masticating juicer heats up inside its grinding chamber, which tends to damage the enzymatic quality of the resulting juice. Manufactured brands of masticating juicers include the Champion®, the Green Power®, and the Royal®. Their prices are moderate and range between U.S.$225 and U.S.$700.

2. Centrifugal Juicers

By far the most common and least expensive of the juice extractors, centrifugal juicers are also the least desirable for fulfilling requirements of a patient on the Gerson Therapy.

A centrifugal juicer works by pushing the vegetable or fruit part against a rotating disk whose teeth reduce it to pulp. Centrifugal force then throws the plant pulp against a basket screen through which the juice is strained, while the pulp remains behind. Such a mechanism sounds just right, but there are problems with the centrifugal procedure.

a.   The produce does not get ground finely enough, particularly in the green leafy sort of vegetable.

b.   The centrifugal force is less effective than the pressing action of other juicers in extracting juice. Such inadequate pressing causes minerals and phytochemicals in the pulp to remain in the pulp; thus, the juice that's rendered is lower in healing enzymes and other nutrients.

c. Dr. Gerson said about centrifugal juicers, "When the grinding wheel rotates against a resistance with insufficient access of air, positive electricity is produced and induces negative electricity on the surrounding wall. The exchange of positive and negative [ions] kills the oxidizing enzymes and renders the juice deficient." He went on to say that his patients who utilized centrifugal juicers did not experience healing successes with their self-administration of his therapy.[3]

Among the centrifugal juicers, those with a vertical-wall basket such as the original Acme Juicerator® (which may no longer be manufactured) presents an enzyme deficiency problem. In contrast, centrifugal juicers with angled-wall juicer baskets (currently popular because of vast amounts of promotion and advertising) such as those found in the Juiceman®, the Braun®, the Hamilton-Beach®, and others don't have such a serious problem. Even so, centrifugal juicers offer an overall lack of nutrients and a reduced quantity of juice when compared with other types. As with the masticator juice machines, the centrifugal types are moderately priced.

3. Wheatgrass Juicers

Being small and highly specialized devices, wheatgrass juicers are designed specifically to extract the chlorophyll-laden juice of wheatgrass. The Gerson Therapy does not use wheatgrass inasmuch as most patients find it to be extremely harsh for assimilation by the stomach. Besides, the desirable components in wheatgrass are already found in the Gerson green leaf juice, which is recommended for ingestion two to four times every day and is much easier on the digestive tract.

4. Citrus Juicers

Used for orange or grapefruit juicing exclusively, a citrus juice apparatus is a reamer-type device that cannot be used for any other type of fruit or vegetable. One should never use a citrus juicer that presses the skin. Dr. Gerson believed that citrus was the least important juice for achieving a therapeutic effect and added it primarily for the patient's convenience as a start to his or her day. Spurred by the media hype of the Florida and California orange juice industries (remember O. J. Simpson and the slogan his former fans called out to him: "Juice! Juice! Juice!"), many people drink orange juice as their first act in the morning.

Even so, orange juice has been described by nutritionists as bringing on too much mucus formation when large quantities are consumed. In our opinion, it may be better for you to replace grapefruit and orange juices with either apple juice or carrot juice. Citrus juices should not be used by patients suffering from collagen diseases such as rheumatoid arthritis or lupus erythematosus.

5. Blender/Liquefiers

Certain liquefying machines like the Vita-Mix® Total Nutrition Center are powerful blenders and not really juicers at all. They grind the produce into a fine pulp, but they don't extract its juice. Since there is no reduction of bulk with a blender/liquefier, to derive the nutrients equivalent to those in 104 ounces of freshly produced organic plant juice, a person would need to ingest an alarming quantity of produce. According to our calculations, it would amount to at least 6 pounds of carrots, 8 pounds of apples, and four heads of lettuce every day, in addition to eating three regular meals. That's much too much bulk food for anyone to take into one's digestive tract in a twenty-four-hour period, especially very ill people with little appetite and disturbed digestive systems.

Yet any juicer is better than no juicer at all. Even the less effective type of juice machine will furnish more nutrients than might be consumed in the equivalent quantity of produce.

But don't let price be the governing factor in choosing your juicing device. At the Gerson Institute, observations have repeatedly been made that some patients rigorously following the Gerson Therapy by use of a lower-cost centrifugal juicer have failed to experience either reductions in tumor masses or healing reactions even after many weeks on the program. However, when they switched to the grinder/press juicer we're about to describe, their healing reactions occurred rapidly, and many saw dramatic improvements in their conditions. Be advised, therefore, that the choice of an appropriate juicer may be a life-or-death matter.

Among the various kinds of juice machines marketed today, we prefer only a couple of brands coming from the one particular extractor type to which we have alluded. We'll now discuss this sixth kind of juicer.

6. The Triturator (Grinder)/Press Combination

Possessing a grinder or triturator for turning vegetables and fruits into a fine, juicy pulp and a hydraulic press for extracting the juice's enzymes from this pulp, the particular juicer—a triturator (grinder)/press combination machine—is the most acceptable choice for people suffering from serious degenerative diseases, especially for cancer patients. It is the juicer type of our preference. After grinding (the definition of "trituration"), juice is extracted from vegetable or fruit pulp by being squeezed under high pressure of as much as 2,000 pounds per square inch (PSI).

Dr. Gerson recommended this type of machine above all others and suggested to his patients that they mix the pulp of different vegetables or fruits together thoroughly before pressing to enhance the extraction of certain nutrients. Such a course of action is possible only with a juicer that separates the grinding and pressing functions. Research indicates that Dr. Gerson's selection of a grinder (triturator)/press type of machine produces as much as fifty times higher amounts of certain essential nutrients such as the lycopene in ripe tomatoes or the proanthocyanidin in the seed membranes of grapes, both of which have proven anticancer qualities.

Taken from a triturator/press type of device, the vegetable or fruit juice is much fuller-bodied than that produced by other kinds of juicers. Moreover, it is free of pulp and furnishes about a 35 percent greater quantity of juice from the same amount of raw produce that might have been put through other juicing machines. Green leafy vegetables offer up even more quantity when processed by a triturator (grinder)/press extractor. You can see that we favor such a juicing device over others, and, in fact, both authors own and use this type of machine many times daily.

But the triturator (grinder)/press extractor is expensive. And only two manufacturers produce it, the Norwalk® Juicer Sales and Service Company and the K & K Company. According to the model chosen, prices for the two kinds of triturator (grinder)/press extractor are the most expensive of all the juicers. They range in retail cost from U.S.$800 to U.S.$2,095. From a survey we conducted, no less than four out of every five Gerson Therapy patients have chosen to invest in a triturator (grinder)/press extractor for participating in their self-administration of personal treatments or for merely enjoying the deliciousness of freshly squeezed organic vegetable and fruit juices.

When considering your investment in a juicer, therefore, know that the higher-priced triturator (grinder)/press machine produces more juice from less produce than other types and most likely offers greater value in the long run. Given the quantity of produce used by an individual on the Gerson Therapy, the more expensive juicer will, in our judgment, probably pay for itself in less than a year.

How to Juice without Undergoing a Nervous Breakdown[4]

Whatever the juicing apparatus one uses, to produce various juices without undergoing a nervous breakdown, particularly during the beginning weeks of the Gerson Therapy program, we have some helpful hints to offer.

The patient or the patient's support person will be spending three to five hours of each waking day in front of the juicer producing the healing liquids that impart nourishment to body parts, tissues, and cells which have been lacking them. (That's one of the reasons the patient's immune system is performing in a lesser manner than it's supposed to.) So, here is our series of what we anticipate will be helpful suggestions:

- Place the machine in a location that's pleasant to view—in front of a picture window, next to the sound of music, close to favorite photographs, and so on.
- Since wash water for the juicer will be required regularly, have the machine's location be near the sink.
- Because the juice goes in undesirable directions on occasion, it's a good practice to place the device on a large cafeteria tray to save your countertop from excessive washing.
- It's not uncommon for vegetable pulp (especially carrots and green leafy items) to end up on the ceiling—especially during the first weeks of the juicing regimen. But this occurrence may be minimized by holding the flat of your hand over the open-mouth tube into which the produce is fed. Without letting your fingers get ground with the vegetables, this action will stop produce splatters and feedback.
- Wear a large apron to protect your clothing from such splatters too.
- Figure in advance how many carrots, apples, greens, peppers, chard, red cabbage, and other produce will be required for each day's juicing. Then scrub and wash them in advance, cut them into smaller pieces, and bag them in sufficient quantity for each session of juicing.
- Consider making your clothes washer into a giant "salad spinner" by putting greens for the day into a mesh bag and running them through the "damp dry" cycle on the washer for twenty seconds to get rid of the excess water.

- Use small pillowcases wrapped inside a large garbage bag to hold all of the day's greens and keep them from getting limp before use.
- Purchase vegetables and fruits several times each week to ensure their freshness. Don't let them sit around for an entire week before they are turned into juice. This suggestion relates to green leafy items in particular. Still, you may need a second refrigerator.
- Of course, acquire only organically grown produce, and at all costs avoid plant life that's come in contact with chemicals such as pesticides and herbicides. Chemicals on fruits and vegetables are a major reason that degenerative diseases of all types cause disability and death. Degenerations are known to some members of every family in the form of pathological symptoms.
- Inasmuch as some organic produce becomes unavailable when it goes out of season (such as apples), it's advantageous to arrange in advance with your produce distributor for you or the support person to buy and pay for a couple of months' supply (but greens won't keep), to be held in the distributor's cooler until needed by the patient.
- If you can afford it, install your own walk-in cooler for the advance storage of out-of-season produce.
- After each juicing, try to disassemble the machine and wash its separate parts. It's tempting to do this after every third or fourth juicing, but be aware that bacteria or other unwelcome microorganisms may lodge on the food debris.
- Use of a sink disposal unit and a sink sprayer hose makes it easier to clean the juicing apparatus.
- For a press-type juicer such as the Norwalk®, rinse off pulp from the pressing cloths, wring them out, place in Ziploc® bags, and store them in the freezer. Such an action keeps them microorganism-free.
- Once a week, boil the pressing cloths in purified water.
- If, after some time, the juice taste is "off" or "pulp explosions" occur too frequently, the fault probably will lie with overused cloths. It's time to replace them because the cloths' pores become clogged with fibers from the pulped juice.
- If work or travel make it difficult to produce fresh juices during the day, here is the procedure to follow. Acquire a glass-lined or stainless steel vacuum bottle (Thermos®) and fill it with juice completely to avoid excess air exposure. Avoid storing green juices, but carrot/apple juice may be stored.

From our observations over a quarter of a century of advising on the Gerson Therapy, we've arrived at some insights. A main one is that degenerative disease patients who make and consume juices throughout the day have a higher rate of healing success than those people who regularly prepare juices several hours in advance of drinking them.

Numbers of recipes have been devised by exponents of the Gerson Therapy juicing program. Patients and other supporters of the Gerson Institute have created various formulations for juice combinations. For instance, there are recipes for carrot/apple juice, carrot juice by itself, citrus juice, green leaf juice, and many additional ones. Most of these recipes are presented in chapter 22. Our final suggestion is to check out this last chapter of our book and use its recipes to your advantage.

References for Chapter Nine

1. Winter, R. A *Consumer's Dictionary of Medicines: Prescription, Over-the-Counter, and Herbal, plus Medical Definitions*. New York: Crown Trade Paperbacks, 1993, p. 343.

2. The Gerson Institute. *Gerson Therapy Practitioner's Training Seminar Workbook*. Chula Vista, Calif.: The Gerson Institute, 1996, pp. 17, 18.

3. *Ibid.*, p. 19.

4. The Gerson Support Group. *The Little Juicing Book*. Chula Vista, Calif.: The Gerson Institute.

Chapter Ten

THE GERSON SALTLESS DIET

In April 1997, Celia Collins, aged fifty-eight, a professional puppeteer, arrived at the Gerson clinic in Sedona, Arizona (now closed), diagnosed with breast cancer. Her pathology was described in medical records she had brought with her as "an infiltrating ductal carcinoma (closed margins) of the right breast 1.5 centimeters in diameter and involving three lymph nodes." The tumor was classified by the woman's oncologist as stage II cancer at grade III (most aggressive) and non-estrogen-receptive. In April 1997, the computerized axial tomography (CAT) scan that Mrs. Collins had undergone also showed some areas that doctors declared they needed to "watch" on her liver and lung.

She chose to receive a lumpectomy breast procedure, after which the attending oncologist recommended that six months of chemotherapy be carried out. But her breast surgeon did not agree. He said that in his experience such a series of toxic chemical treatments had never prolonged anyone's life and he would not suggest that she accept chemotherapy. The oncologist also wanted Mrs. Collins to take seven weeks of radiation therapy with some extra radiation "swats" for the closed margins. The breast surgeon did not express enthusiasm for radiotherapy either.

"I was staggered by being confronted with the oncologist's negative choices. They just did *not* add up and so I began to look for some options. I selected the Gerson Therapy rather than accept the chemo and radiation," Mrs. Collins stated for publication. (To see this former cancer patient, you may view her photograph on the facing page).

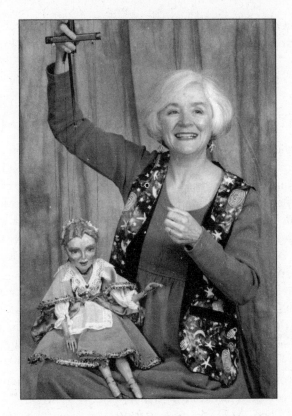

Celia Collins

She was intrigued with Dr. Gerson's saltless diet, for the woman had for years suspected that most of us take in too much salt by excessive seasoning. And she often experienced cellular edema (swelling) from the sodium chloride added to foods. So Mrs. Collins thought she would adapt well to the Gerson therapeutic saltless eating program. Thus, she immediately embarked on the full menu plan of the Gerson Therapy.

"The decision made, my daughter and I took off for the Gerson Healing Center in Sedona where we involved ourselves in the healing atmosphere. It was so refreshing and invigorating. Everyone was exceedingly positive, happy, and encouraging, even the cleaning lady. The care, the wonderful saltless food, the other patients and staff . . . were all special and good. As a result, my healing took place swiftly. I underwent another CAT scan in September 1997, after being on the Gerson Therapy for six months, and all of the scans were reported as clear of cancer—my lesions are gone. And it's official from my breast surgeon too, who additionally reported on my diagnostic tests. He said that I am free of cancer without having taken any chemotherapy or radiation," said Celia Collins. "I'm so happy!"

WHY THERE IS NEED OF A SALTLESS DIET

A main therapeutic concept put forth by Dr. Max Gerson is that elevating the cancer patient's potassium level while restricting sodium in the diet acts against tumor formation.[1] Dr. Gerson was a strong exponent of eating a saltless diet to eliminate the retained sodium (chemical symbol Na), chloride (indicated as Cl), and water (H_2O), together with toxins and poisons from the tissues all over the body. Dr. Gerson wrote that NaCl (salt) excretion increases in tuberculosis, cancer, and other chronic diseases after two to three days on a saltless diet.

This increased salt excretion stays at the higher level for up to two weeks, when it drops to normal on the saltless diet. Sometimes purgative flare-ups in the form of nausea, diarrhea, and nervous disturbances occur. They have been identified as "healing reactions" by the Gerson Institute. Such reactions come from greater bile secretion and stimulation of the visceral nervous system. After each flare-up, the reacting patients feel easier and improve both physically and mentally.[2]

Freeman Cope, M.D., writing in the peer-reviewed journal *Physiological Chemistry and Physics*, said: "The high potassium, low sodium diet of the Gerson Therapy has been observed experimentally to cure many cases of advanced cancer in man, but the reason was not clear. Recent studies [this was in 1978] from the laboratory of Dr. F. G. Ling and associates indicate that high potassium, low sodium environments can partially return damaged cell proteins to their normal undamaged configuration. Therefore, the damage in other tissues, indicated by toxins and breakdown products from the cancer, is probably partly repaired by the Gerson Therapy through this mechanism."[3]

Much more needs to be explained about ingesting no salt and adding potassium, sodium's mineral antagonist. We discuss potassium below. Not only does elevated blood pressure improve from high potassium usage and reduced sodium intake, but the saltless diet is responsible for reversing both acute and chronic illnesses of all types such as arthritis, diabetes, multiple sclerosis, cardiovascular disease, autoimmune diseases, chronic fatigue syndrome, and many others. In fact, each of the fifty-two disorders listed in this book which react positively to Dr. Gerson's dietary program, exemplified by patient case histories, respond exceedingly well to avoiding the ingestion of salt. Too much sodium consumption can be a killer!

ALBERT SCHWEITER SAYS THE WHITE MAN'S SALTED DIET HARMS BLACK AFRICANS

In 1954, the much heralded humanitarian, concert organist, medical missionary and Nobel laureate Professor Dr. Albert Schweitzer, M.D., wrote that the black Africans residing all around the area of his Lambaréné hospital in Gabon, French Equatorial Africa, had been altering their dietary practices and adapting to the salted diet of white people. Dr. Schweitzer's medical efforts on their behalf were being made more difficult because of the people's elevated salt intake.

"Many natives, especially those who are living in larger communities, do not now live the same way as formerly—they lived almost exclusively on fruits and vegetables, bananas, cassava, ignam, taro, sweet potatoes and other fruits. They now have begun to live on condensed milk, canned butter, meat-and-fish [salted] preserves and bread," Dr. Schweitzer wrote. He traced the appearance of cancer, appendicitis, and other degenerative diseases among black Africans to this dietary change.[4]

"Based upon my own experience, going back to 1913, I can say, if cancer occurred at all [then], it was very rare but that it has become more frequent since. . . . It is obvious to connect the fact of increase of cancer with the increased use of salt by the natives," the Nobel laureate continued. "For the past forty years, practical experience was gathered about the effects of salt limitation upon diseases of the kidneys. It was shown just here that radical limitation of salt intake, which corresponds to the usual saltless nutrition, decreases the burden on the [black Africans'] diseased kidneys. As soon as the diseased kidneys are not over-irritated and over-burdened by the excessive intake of chlorides in nutrition, they recover in an amazingly short time and . . . eliminate more NaCl on a saltless diet than on the salt-rich diet!"

When salt is removed, however, need something else be substituted? Some nutritional supplements, especially potassium, are in order. While the composition of all nutritional supplements used as part of the Gerson Therapy is the subject of our chapter 11, potassium's efficacy is discussed immediately below.

THE USEFULNESS OF POTASSIUM FOR HUMAN METABOLISM

Potassium (chemical symbol K) is a mineral element needed by all plants and animals to live and thrive. It is the essential mineral required within all tissues and cells in the body for normal smooth function and for all their activities. Since it is required in the cells, not in the fluids, it is referred to as the "intercellular" mineral. Potassium is contained in all foods, particularly in fruits, vegetables, and whole grains. Animal sources, such as fish and meat, also contain potassium, but the plant-based material is easier to absorb.

Potassium is absorbed from foods through the intestinal tract; any excess is released in the urine. The kidneys play an important role in determining how much potassium is released or absorbed into the system. If the kidneys are irritated by chemicals, drugs or other problems, they may release too much potassium, contributing to a deficiency. Potassium can also be lost through vomiting, diarrhea and surgical drainage, as well as laxatives and diuretics (agents that increase the flow of urine). Loss through the skin is rare but it can result from sweating during too much exercise or when overheated.[5]

Part of the Gerson Therapy involves consuming a diet not only loaded with high-potassium foods but also supplemented with elevated doses of the mineral itself. In fact, from the Faculty of Life Sciences at Bar-Ilan University in Ramat-Gan, Israel, Professor Jacob Shoham, M.D., Ph.D., commented about potassium quantities in his friendly and informed September 28, 1998, letter of inquiry to Charlotte Gerson. Dr. Shoham wrote, "Potassium obviously is a central pillar in the whole structure of Dr. Gerson's therapy. We are dealing here with enormous amounts of K— about 20 grams in the [supplemental] potassium solution during the first four weeks, reduced to half thereafter, about nine to ten grams in the juices, and probably two to three grams in the food, all together about thirty grams per day during the first weeks and then twenty grams per day subsequently."

Dr. Jacob Shoham was concerned about the possibility of hyper-kalemia, an overabundance of potassium in a person's metabolism, which could possibly occur from a patient's conforming to the Gerson Therapy recommendation of K supplemention. Yet adverse signs or symptoms of hyperkalemia are not an effect from the high dose of potassium supple-mentation. Several Gerson Therapy patients have accidentally, through misinterpretation of labeling, self-medicated with potassium at levels ap-proximately thirty-two times the recommended dosage of K for periods of up to three weeks. They did this without undergoing any significant ad-verse effects. Over time, from experience of users, elevating K intake to neutralize too much sodium (Na) in the tissues appears to be safe and ef-fective. Excess K is easily excreted by normal kidneys.

Also, more than forty years ago, Dr. Gerson answered the hyperkalemia question in his celebrated book. He declares: "The content of potassium in the serum is, in many cases, misleading." Then he goes on to say, "It [potassium in serum] does not give any definite indication of an increas-ing or decreasing amount of K present in the *tissues* of essential organs.... More coincident examinations of K made at the same time in serum and tissues and in different stages of the [cancerous] disease, are necessary for such decisions."[6]

Dr. Gerson advises that hyperkalemia occurs from seven specific sources: (1) "loss of fluids—blood, in majority of cases dehydration"; (2) "Epilepsy—most cases"; (3) "Cancer patients more often in the period before they go over to the terminal stage (on the way to elimination)"; (4) "Never in cancer patients during restoration time"; (5) "Addison's dis-ease"; (6) "Anuria—uremia (inability of liver and kidneys to excrete excess potassium in solution—lost from essential organs)"; (7) "Acute and chronic asthma, and other degenerative allergies."[7]

Potassium belongs to a chemical group that is associated with both phosphoric acids and carbohydrates, and the three substances readily combine with colloids; therefore, Dr. Gerson suggests that we may speak of these four grouped ingredients of the metabolism as the *potassium group*. Na is part of its own chemical group, the *sodium group*.

We take in an enormous amount of sodium, not necessarily with the foods we prepare ourselves but with those we purchase already packaged, es-pecially those mixed ingredients that people eat in restaurants. Dining out-side the home is an unhealthy way to eat and live. It's an underlying source of degenerating illnesses such as high blood pressure, stroke, and cancer.

In his monthly newsletter *Health & Healing*®, Julian Whitaker, M.D., writes, "The way to bring your sodium-potassium ratio back into balance is to eat lots of vegetables, legumes, whole grains, and fruit. These wholesome foods naturally have an excellent sodium-to-potassium ratio of at least 1:50." Dr. Whitaker adds that some fruits, such as oranges, offer a good mineral proportion of 1 part sodium to 260 parts potassium. Bananas have an even more ideal sodium-to-potassium content of 1:440."[8] However, bananas are too high in sugars, especially for cancer patients. They may be eaten only in moderation.

POTASSIUM SUPPLEMENTATION ON THE GERSON THERAPY

At the Gerson Therapy hospitals, when patients are beginning their therapeutic programs, blood tests and urinalyses are performed once a week. This would be the case when someone is under the care of a Gerson certified practitioner as well. Monitoring of blood and urine values of patients on a continuous basis is of great importance.

Monitoring laboratory tests should be repeated about every six weeks, depending upon the severity of an individual's disease process. In the early stages with the debilitated patient, every four weeks would be recommended. These laboratory studies must accompany numerous clinical examinations. One of the most important laboratory tests involves the determination of the blood serum's potassium levels. K levels for sick Gerson patients will often fall between 5.9 and 6 milliequivalents per liter (mEq/L). Normal ranges for non-Gerson patients generally record at 3.4 to 5.1 mEq/L.[9]

Particularly in the initial stages of treatment, Gerson patients ingest significant potassium supplementation of up to 150 mEq/day. Even in the presence of elevated potassium serum levels, it's necessary to continue K supplementation. Dr. Gerson tells us that K ions are indispensable in certain enzymatic reactions and K plays a role in tissue protein synthesis. Normally, muscles, brain, and liver possess much higher K content than Na content. As long as K remains normal, Na is diminished, and that's maintaining a healthy state.

At the Gerson Therapy hospitals, after blood testing upon the patient's hospital admission, 10 percent potassium solution is administered immediately. The K administration takes the form of 4 teaspoonfuls ten times daily added to all juices, and this dose usually continues for three to four weeks. Then the amount of K is reduced to half. Presenting a warning, Dr. Gerson says, "The combination of the blood level with the clinical observations teaches us that the restoration of the potassium content in the organs is a difficult and long-drawn-out process."[10]

A compound solution of potassium salts is made from 33 grams (g) each of potassium acetate, monophosphate, and gluconate, diluted in 32 ounces of distilled water. As stated, dosages vary from 1 to 4 teaspoonfuls (tsp), representing from 3.5 to 14 grams of K per day. This medication is added in equal amounts to each of the carrot/apple, greens, and orange juices (but not to the pure carrot juices) daily, about 1 to 4 tsp per juice drink.

Further information about nutritional supplementation with potassium compound salts is provided in chapter 11. We place emphasis on medicating with potassium because it forms a keystone for achieving healing benefits from use of the Gerson Therapy. This K medication is primary to the treatment of tissue damage syndrome (the penetration of Na into tissues), found in all cancers and in most other degenerative diseases. It combines with the other medications and dietary regimen to increase cellular K levels, reduce intercellular edema, and restore normal cell function.

As we alluded before, patients have experienced some misunderstandings using this high-dose K medication, even though instructions are provided on the container. You must dilute the contents of the container holding the concentrated K powder into 32 ounces of water. Spoon the diluted liquid you have created into the juices. Do not spoon the powder itself into the juices or you will be mixing in an overabundant dose. No adverse side effects occur at this usual dosage, except perhaps for an irritation in the throat due to the strong potassium salts. Eating oatmeal gruel heals the potential throat irritation.

Store the potassium solution in a glass container rather than in plastic or metal. It needs no refrigeration but should be held in a dark closet (pantry) or stored in a brown- or amber-colored bottle or jar. One quart of potassium solution will last from one to three weeks, depending on the prescribed dosage. Discard any of the remaining potassium solution and replace it if, after some time has elapsed, it becomes cloudy.

POTASSIUM COMPOUND FOR ONE'S ENEMA SOLUTION

The same potassium solution that is added to juices for drinking may be applied directly to enemas for the relief of abdominal spasms that occur from colon contractions. The dosage of this potassium compound consists of 2 to 3 tsp of K solution placed into each enema. At times, lesser amounts of water combined with the potassium compound for enemas may be required simply because the abdominal spasms may be too great to accept any increased liquid pressure into one's colon. Discontinue adding potassium compound to the coffee enema after six to eight days or it will cause irritation of the colon.

TISSUE DAMAGE SYNDROME FROM CELLULAR POISONING

According to a 1977 published report by Freeman Cope, M.D., a pioneering physician and research physicist, medical science has learned that cellular structures become poisoned by exposure to carcinogens, atherogens, antigens, allergens, and other offending pollutants in our surroundings. The cellular pollutants may cause oxygen starvation, trauma, generalized insult, or other tissue damage of the cells that takes the form of a syndrome, a series of symptoms and signs that manifest themselves in a repeated pattern. Any part of the body can undergo *tissue damage syndrome*, a cycle of cellular destruction, which Dr. Cope defines as "the damaged configurational state in which the cell proteins lose their preference for association with $K+$ rather than $Na+$, and the water content of the cell increases (the cell swells)."[11]

As described by Dr. Cope, the tissue damage syndrome presents an ill patient's dysfunctional cells with this series of pathological symptoms:

1. The damaged cells lose potassium.
2. The involved cells readily accept sodium.
3. The cells swell with too much water.

The symptom that may be recognized most readily by the attending health professional is then labeled *cellular edema*. Cellular edema does not allow for the manufacture of energy in the form of adenosine triphosphate (ATP). ATP is the energy storage compound of the body; it's the energy currency that results from burning sugar through oxidation. ATP gets manufactured, then it's used up, is manufactured again, and becomes used once more on a continuous basis. During the course of this metabolic process, ATP liberates bursts of energy for cellular use. ATP is an adenosine molecule possessing three strong phosphate bonds that contain the required energy. The cell must have ATP or it dies. If enough cells die, tissue dies. If too many tissues die, an organ or body part dies. If too many organs die, the person dies.

When an excessive amount of water is present in the cell, the production of ATP is inhibited or stops altogether. At the same time, protein synthesis and lipid (fat) metabolism stops. On the Gerson Therapy, the damaged cell is confronted with less sodium, is allowed to bind with potassium, is delivered of its excess water content, and is improved in its mitochondrial function. Certain organelles, those tiny chemical factories inside of each cell called *mitochondria*, perform the energy functions of burning sugar with oxygen, synthesizing protein, and metabolizing fats.

To eliminate the excess cellular water which shows up as edema, before Dr. Freeman Cope described and named tissue damage syndrome, Max Gerson was treating the condition as far back as the 1920s. Dr. Gerson eliminated sodium from the diet, fashioned an eating program that was high in potassium, supplemented the diet with additional potassium, and developed the means to remove from the bloodstream toxins that inhibit normal cellular enzyme functions, metabolism, and respiration.

To paint a defining picture of just what tissue damage syndrome is, think of Dr. Cope's discovery in this way. See the cell as an industrialized nation with its mitochondria as the nation's industrial cities. They are the cities of industry. When a cell (as the nation) has lost potassium, gained sodium, and swollen with water, it's equivalent to all of its cities' sewers backing up. Then the industrial cities are shut down in their function. Energy cannot be made by the cities of industry to clean out the sewers. The entire industrialized nation (that damaged cell) becomes over-polluted, becomes severely dysfunctional in every facet of its existence, and dies. Tissue damage syndrome has been the responsible agent for cellular death.

By eating the saltless diet and supplementing with elevated doses of potassium, clinically undiscernible but laboratory-measurable tissue damage syndrome can be avoided. During the time that Dr. Max Gerson was writing his life-saving book, A *Cancer Therapy: Results of Fifty Cases and*

The Cure of Advanced Cancer by Diet Therapy: A Summary of 30 Years of Clinical Experimentation, this information was published in the American Cancer Society's health professionals' journal *Cancer*.[12] There is no better means of removing the puffy malfunctioning sphere of partial metabolites and cellular edema from diseased tissue materials than application of the Gerson Therapy's saltless and high-potassium diet.

References for Chapter Ten

1. Regelson, W. "The 'grand conspiracy' against the cancer cure." Commentary, *Journal of the American Medical Association*. 243:337–339, Jan. 25, 1980.

2. Gerson, M. A *Cancer Therapy: Results of Fifty Cases and The Cure of Advanced Cancer by Diet Therapy: A Summary of 30 Years of Clinical Experimentation*, 6th edition. Bonita, Calif.: The Gerson Institute, 1999, pp. 164–166.

3. Cope, F.W. "A medical application of the Ling association-induction hypothesis: the high potassium, low sodium diet of the Gerson cancer therapy." *Physiological Chemistry and Physics*, NMR. 10:465–468, 1978.

4. Schweitzer, A. *Briefe aus dem Lambarenespital (Letters from the Lambaréné Hospital)*. Africa, 1954.

5. *The Mosby Medical Encyclopedia*. New York: New American Library, 1985, p. 589.

6. *Op. cit.*, Gerson, M., 1990, p. 93.

7. *Ibid.*

8. Whitaker, J. "Minerals, Part 3: Lower your blood pressure with the 'K factor'. *Health & Healing®* 9:1–3, June 1999.

9. The Gerson Institute. *Gerson™ Therapy Practitioner's Training Seminar Workbook*. Bonita, Calif.: The Gerson Institute, 1996, p. 31.

10. *Op. cit.*, Gerson, M., 1990, pp. 208, 209.

11. *Op. cit.*, Cope, F.W., 1978.

12. Waterhouse, C.; Craig, A. "Body-composition and changes in patients with advanced cancer." *Cancer*. 11(6), November/December, 1957.

Chapter Eleven

NUTRITIONAL SUPPLEMENTS ON THE DIET

L iving in upstate New York, forty-two-year-old Tom Powers Jr. saw a mole on his right temple as he stood at the mirror shaving. As a result of Mr. Powers' telephone description, his family doctor asked him to have it biopsied right away and made the appointment with a pathology laboratory. By means of a special instrument that pierces directly through the skin, a small cylindrical specimen was removed by punch biopsy. Immediately thereafter, Tom Powers learned that he had been struck by malignant melanoma.

As described in Chapter 6, *malignant melanoma* is a highly dangerous tumor consisting of melanocytes, the melanin-forming cells. It usually occurs in the skin, eye, and mucous membranes, often developing from excessive exposure to sunlight. Spread of this skin cancer to other parts of the body, especially to the lymph nodes and liver, is common. Melanin or its precursors (melanogens) are excreted in the urine, and the skin may be deeply pigmented.

While Tom Powers waited, deciding what to do, metastatic melanoma growths recurred, this time in three places: first on the biopsied operation site, then on his chest, and finally on the left arm. These cancer resurgencies popped out just eight days after the biopsy had been performed. It was apparent that the patient's circumstances were life-threatening.

"I consulted four different medical doctors, who agreed that neither surgery, radiation, nor any known form of chemotherapy, alone or in combination, offered hope for a cure of this type of cancer at this stage in its development. In unvarnished terms, my situation was viewed as terminal," Tom Powers Jr. wrote. (Mr. Powers' photograph may be viewed below.)

The patient and his family learned from friends and a Gerson program participant that the Gerson Therapy is highly successful as a treatment for malignant melanoma. (We suggest, again, that you refer to chapter 6 for the percentages of Gerson treatment success according to the melanoma tumor's staging.)

"The fact that my cancer had metastasized did not rule out the chances of complete remission for me. I had avoided radiation therapy or chemotherapy and this was in my favor; it meant that my immune system had not been artificially suppressed and would respond better to this metabolic treatment plan with its highly specialized nutritional supplements," advised Mr. Powers. "The supplements consist of potassium salts, thyroid, Lugol's iodine solution, pancreatic enzymes, and niacin, plus medicinal injections with vitamin B_{12} and liver. Castor oil taken orally and by enema is used as a liver organ detoxifier rather than as a nutritional supplement.

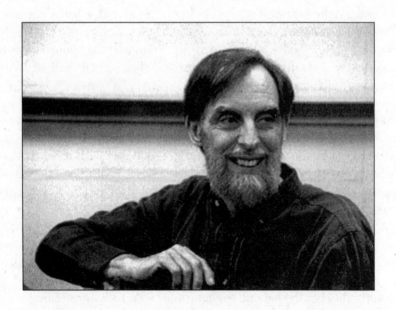

Tom Powers Jr.

"On May 14, 1982, I began the Gerson Therapy and became expert at treating myself at home. Dr. Gerson's genius, to my eternal gratitude, had his nutritional supplementation working beautifully. Remission occurred. By July 1, 1982, all visible tumors were gone. They just faded away and the skin appeared normal once again. I had no further surgery. I had no chemotherapy or radiation therapy. When my family physician saw me next in September 1982, he was deeply impressed to find the disease in permanent remission. I remained on the Gerson Therapy for twenty months. I have had no recurrence of the cancer in the fourteen years since," concluded Tom Powers Jr.

According to guidelines presented by the American Cancer Society, this patient has experienced a "cure." From Tom Powers Jr., the last report that he furnished about his prolonged remission or cure of malignant melanoma arrived at the Gerson Institute during December 2000. To date, he has flourished in excellent health for eighteen years.

NUTRITIONAL SUPPLEMENTS ADVOCATED BY DR. GERSON

As mentioned by Tom Powers, there are just a few nutritional supplements used in the Gerson Therapy. Iodine supplements in the form of Lugol's solution are utilized, for example. Lugol's solution (as described in the U.S. Pharmacopeia), often incorporated into medicines, consists of 5 grams of iodine and 10 grams of potassium iodide per 100 milliliters (mL) of purified water.

Raw liver juice had been an integral part of the Gerson vegetable-and-fruit-juice-drinking procedure until 1989. Then, because of bacterial and parasitic contamination of most commercially available domestic animal livers from calves, the practice of drinking raw liver juice had to be discontinued. Liver injections can be continued by the patient instead. Also, supplementing with coenzyme Q_{10} helps to replace some of the raw liver substances. (Chapter 12 discusses about the importance of detoxifying or cleansing the liver.)

In addition to liver detoxification, pancreatic enzyme tablets are always prescribed along with potassium compound, potassium iodide, thyroid extract, niacin, and hydrochloric acid as well as pepsin, a digestive enzyme. Niacin forms part of the coenzyme NADH, which detoxifies the body of cancer-causing pollutants.

That's all! In general, no other nutritional supplementation is required because the organically grown vegetarian eating plan is massively packed with natural nutrients. A degenerative disease patient participating in the Gerson program becomes well once again and remains that way merely from eating what nature offers as our bounty. We will explain everything there is to know about the Gerson Therapy's form of nutrition, supplementation, and detoxification starting immediately after this next section.

THE GERSON HIPPOCRATES SOUP

One of the main recommendations in Dr. Gerson's nutritional program to counter all types of acute and chronic diseases is that a person should eat a daily quantity of vegetable soup—not Heinz's™ or Campbell's™ (both loaded with salt), but soup that you make from scratch. (We furnish the recipe for preparing Dr. Gerson's special Hippocrates soup near the end of chapter 8 as a discussion of the eating plan.) As we've stated, the Gerson special Hippocrates soup is a staple for all patients for both lunch and dinner because it aids the kidneys to accomplish their job of detoxification.

In addition to the Hippocrates soup itself, fresh vegetables are mandatory, stewed in their own juices. The soup stock becomes loaded with nutrients. (In Dr. Gerson's time, neither he nor any member of the nutritional science community had as yet identified the phytochemicals present in certain vegetables.) Such phytochemicals ingested in this manner are easily absorbed and assimilated. As you've been advised, informed nutritionists usually refer to phytochemicals of this type as *nutraceuticals*, because they produce a pharmaceutical-like effect in the body, almost like the individualized components of nutritional supplements, but more easily assimilated.

Such good eating along with detoxification, as by giving oneself enemas made from organic coffee, keeps the gut free of disease-producing waste products, the liver clean, and the whole body system vigorous. What could be better for managing your day? As you'll learn by reading chapter 12, the only really healthy way to ingest coffee is by use of an enema bottle applied for its assigned purpose.

ADJUNCTIVE SUPPLEMENTATION WITH THYROID MEDICATION

In the next section you will learn that iodine is a trace element required in the manufacture of thyroid hormone, and this is important because iodine deficiency is a source of thyroid gland pathology. When such pathology occurs, symptoms of long-term health difficulties appear (including a disturbed immune system), and thyroid medication may be required. Thyroid medication, in fact, is an integral part of the adjunctive nutrient supplementation in the Gerson Therapy.

The thyroid gland adds iodine to the amino acid tyrosine to create the several thyroid hormones. Because they regulate metabolism in each body cell, a deficiency of thyroid gland hormones can affect virtually all body functions. The severity of symptoms in adults ranges from extremely mild deficiency states as in *subclinical hypothyroidism* to severe deficiency which sometimes may become life-threatening as in *myxedema*.[1,2]

Deficiency of thyroid hormone may come from defective hormone synthesis or lack of stimulation by the pituitary gland, which secretes the thyroid-stimulating hormone (TSH). When thyroid hormone levels in the blood are low, the pituitary secretes TSH. If thyroid hormone levels are decreased and TSH levels are elevated in the blood, this usually indicates defective thyroid hormone synthesis, known as *primary hypothyroidism*. If TSH levels are low and thyroid hormone levels are also low, an endocrinologist will likely recognize that the patient's pituitary gland is responsible for the low thyroid function. Such a situation is referred to as *secondary hypothyroidism*.[3,4]

Because thyroid hormone enhances production of mitochondria, the tiny chemical factories or organelles in each cell which produce cellular power (ATP), Dr. Gerson made use of pure, desiccated thyroid gland as an adjunctive supplemental medication for underactivity of the thyroid gland. The Gerson Institute continues to recommend such a thyroid product, consisting of desiccated pork thyroid gland, supplied in a dose of $1/2$- or 1-grain tablets made by the West Pharmaceuticals/Jones Medical Laboratories. The normal initial treatment dosage for a cancer patient is 1.5 to 5 grains per day, tapering down to 1 to 3 grains daily after three to ten weeks. The use of synthetic thyroid is not recommended, because only the natural material relieves symptoms of hypothyroidism on a permanent basis.

If thyroid causes the patient's heart to race up to 120 beats per minute (tachycardia), overdosage with thyroid may be suspected, and this medication should be discontinued, at least temporarily, and subsequently reduced. Also, no thyroid medication is given during menstruation.

Adjunctive to supplementation with desiccated porcine (pig) thyroid is the mineral iodine, which is a main chemical component of human thyroid hormone. In the Gerson program, iodine is nutritionally supplemented in the form of a solution (Lugol's) which has standard usage in orthodox medicine.

Nutritional Supplementation with Lugol's Solution

Named after its inventor, the French physician Jean Guillaume Auguste Lugol, who lived from 1786 to 1851, Lugol's solution is a deep brown liquid, with the odor of iodine. It consists of the mineral iodine (chemical symbol I) and potassium iodide (KI) dissolved in purified water. Each 100 mL of Lugol's solution contains 4.5 to 5.5 grams of iodine and 9.5 to 10.5 grams of potassium iodide. Orthodox medicine, following *United States Pharmacopeia* guidelines, uses this concentration, administered orally, as a souce of the iodine mineral in preparation for a patient undergoing thyroid surgery. It is also referred to as *compound iodine solution.*[5]

Lugol's solution works with potassium, the main base ion of intracellular fluid. Acting together, Lugol's solution and potassium are biochemically synergistic medications that increase cellular energy of normal cells, reduce intercellular edema, restore normal cellular functions, and elevate cellular potassium levels. Being synergistic, they interact to produce increased activity that is greater than the sum of the effects of the two substances given separately to patients.

Max Gerson, M.D., applied a half-strength Lugol's solution consisting of 5 grams of potassium iodide plus 10 grams of iodine with water added to make 200 mL. The typical dosage for cancer patients not pretreated with chemotherapy is three drops, six times per day. This is reduced after two or three weeks to one drop six times a day. Patients treated with chemotherapy as well as those with other degenerative diseases start with one drop six times per day. After five to six weeks, this dosage is adjusted to three or four drops per day.[6]

Lugol's solution becomes a critical factor in the control of the oxidation rates of cells when it is administered correctly by adding it, with potassium (see the section immediately below), to the orange and carrot/apple juices. It shouldn't be added to the green juice or pure carrot juice. Accuracy and appropriate dosages of Lugol's solution are essential for the success of the Gerson Therapy.

The half-strength dosage is taken only during the first three to four weeks of treatment in the following manner: put three drops in each of six orange and carrot/apple juices so that one is consuming eighteen drops or six times three drops of Lugol's solution daily. As mentioned, *do not* put Lugol's solution in any of the green juices.

After the startup period, reduce the Lugol's solution dosage to only one drop in each of six juices daily for eight weeks. Then lower the dose to only one drop in each of three juices per day for the duration of treatment.

When a patient is being treated at a Gerson Therapy hospital or by a certified Gerson-trained physician in private practice, the Lugol's solution is premixed at half strength to a 5 percent dilution. The product must be used as supplied and not diluted further.[7]

The Lugol's solution works by causing iodine to invade cancer tumors when inflamed. This situation may be especially significant for inflammatory skin cancer such as inflammatory breast disease (carcinoma) and melanosarcoma before healing sets in and again later in inflammatory flare-ups. The solution's iodine is necessary in the control of normal cell differentiation. The larger dose such as is used in the beginning weeks of the Gerson Therapy is favorable for inhibiting excessive growth of tumor tissue.[8]

A similar physiological response to Lugol's solution occurs from the oral ingestion of potassium compound salts, which cancel out the toxic products of sodium compound salts. Potassium ions are the neutralizing factors for sodium ions and actually react like antidotes to them.

POTASSIUM COMPOUND SALTS

Dr. Gerson discovered that patients with chronic degenerative illnesses exhibit a marked decrease of potassium (K), one of the elemental substances important in enzyme production as well as muscle contraction and strength. According to his research, the beginning of all chronic disease is the loss of K^+ ions from the cells and invasion of sodium (Na^+) ions into the cells—and with it water. Such a situation (as we learned in chapter 10) brings on edema and the resulting cellular/physiological malfunctions that go with it—loss of electrical potentials in the cells, improper enzyme formation, reduced cell oxidation, other symptoms of tissue damage syndrome (TDS), and worse. The building of almost all the body's enzymes by the cells requires K as a catalyst (activating agent). In contrast, Na permeating the tissues inhibits (slows or stops) enzyme production. To stimulate enzymatic action, therefore, it's mandatory to eliminate excess Na and substitute K for the cells' use. At the same time, detoxification procedures will remove accumulated intermediary substances and other interfering poisons.[9]

Besides detoxifying with coffee enemas (see the next chapter), the best way to simultaneously pull sodium from the tissues and infuse them with potassium is by drinking voluminous amounts of fresh fruit and vegetable juices. The juices contain large quantities of K and cell-cleansing enzymes. More than the juices alone, however, a solution of potassium compound salts added to these juices ensures that K in quantity is ingested and assimilated.

As discussed in chapter 10, a solution of potassium compound salts is made from 33 grams each of potassium acetate, potassium monophosphate, and potassium gluconate, diluted in 32 ounces of distilled water. Typical potassium dosages vary from 1 to 4 teaspoonfuls ten times per day of the prepared solution, representing 3.5 to 14 grams of potassium daily. Such a quantity of medication is added every day in equal amounts to each of the juices, including carrot/apple, orange, and the greens but not the pure carrot juice.[10]

The primary benefit these potassium compound salts offer is for their treatment of TDS, found in all cancers, and in most other degenerative diseases. The K compound combines with the other medications and dietary regimen to accomplish similar effects to that of iodine. Potassium compound salts solution, which needs no refrigeration, should be stored in a dark glass bottle, not plastic or metal. Discard it if it becomes cloudy with age.[11]

As stated, K is synergistic with I, and together they reduce swelling in the tissues, in part by pushing out Na.

ACIDOL PEPSIN

A general name for several enzymes of the gastric juice created in the stomach, *pepsin* catalyzes the hydrolysis of proteins to form polypeptides. The stomach's parietal (wall) cells secrete enough hydrochloric acid

(HCl) from the blood to acidify the food predigested by saliva to a low pH of from 3.0 to 1.5. This acidic pH temporarily deactivates the plant enzymes, and the predigested food passes to the lower or pyloric portion of the stomach (the pylorus), from which the stomach lining's chief cells also secrete pepsin. In the pylorus, pepsin continues the digestion of protein. Adequate HCl is required to activate pepsin from its inactive enzyme form pepsinogen inside the chief cells, and to maintain the stomach pH below 3.0, the optimum pH at which pepsin does its work.[12]

Acidol pepsin is the most important of the three gastric enzymes by its speeding along the hydrolysis of proteins with preferential cleavage at the amino acid residues of phenylalanine, tryptophan, tyrosine, and leucine. Acidol pepsin is secreted by the gastric mucosa in the form of pepsinogen and has an optimum pH of 1.5 to 2.0.[13]

Acidol pepsin capsules (betaine HCl and pepsin) are part of the Gerson Therapy medications for purposes of aiding digestion of foods and juices. They are the source of the supplemental hydrochloric acid that was administered by Dr. Gerson and remain actively used today. Take them before each meal in a dosage of two capsules three times a day, as a source of HCl.

Niacin (Vitamin B₃) Supplementation

Acting as a coenzyme in several important biochemical functions, *niacin* or *vitamin B₃* is involved in the metabolism of lipids (fats), gastrointestinal tract functions, workings of the nervous system, and promotion of healthy skin growth. An overwhelming number of scientific studies show that niacin is effective in reducing both cholesterol and triglyceride levels in the blood; moreover, vasodilation (opening of the blood vessels promoting increased circulation) is another cardiovascular benefit derived from niacin usage. It also significantly increases high-density lipoproteins (HDL). Niacin reduces the incidence of gastrointestinal cancer and the risk of gallbladder disease.[14]

The Optimum Daily Intake (ODI) for vitamin B₃ nutritional maintenance supplementation varies from 25 mg to 300 mg daily; for therapeutic purposes, however, Dr. Gerson had his patients take six 50-mg tablets of niacin daily for six months. In advanced cases of cancer or other degenerative diseases he used 50 mg of niacin every hour around the clock (1,200 mg of niacin). By today's standards in accordance with the practice of orthomolecular medicine as first recommended by a candidate for the

Nobel Prize in Medicine for 2001, Canadian orthomolecular psychiatrist Abram Hoffer, M.D., Ph.D., 1,200 mg of niacin is a usual dose.[15,16]

Ingesting such an elevated dosage of niacin can create a skin-flushing effect with temporary and harmless redness, heat, and itching. Dosing with niacin should be discontinued during menstruation or any type of bleeding.

Note: The nicotinic form of niacin is being recommended here as a medication for the Gerson Therapy and not the niacinamide ("no-flush") form, which shows almost no beneficial effect for most degenerative diseases except the arthritides such as osteoarthritis. If the niacin flush irritates the patient, take the tablet after meals or let it dissolve under the tongue. It should not be discontinued because it provides vasodilation which improves blood circulation, elevates skin temperature, increases oxygenation, promotes cellular nutrition, and produces an overall detoxification effect. This also is a factor in protein digestion.

PANCREATIN

An enzymatic secretion of the pancreas, the vital substance *pancreatin* contains three specific groups of enzymes for the digestion and absorption of food. They are *lipases* for absorption of fats and fat-soluble vitamins, *amylases* for the breakdown of starch molecules into smaller sugars, and *proteases* for the reconstruction of protein molecules into single amino acids. Each of these enzyme groups contains separate enzymes; for instance, the proteases offer up trypsin, chymotrypsin, and carboxypeptidase. The proteases also aid in the breakdown of tumor tissue, scar tissue, or other damaged areas.

Supplementation with some or all of these pancreatin-derived enzymes is employed in the treatment of impaired digestion, malabsorption, nutrient deficiencies, and abdominal discomfort. They are useful for overcoming the symptoms of digestive disturbances such as celiac disease; cystic fibrosis; food allergies; the yeast syndrome; autoimmune disorders like rheumatoid arthritis, lupus erythematosus, scleroderma, multiple sclerosis, and many types of cancer; sports injuries and trauma; and viral infections such as herpes zoster and AIDS.[17]

In lectures to medical consumers, Dr. Gerson explained, "Pancreatin [as an uncoated tablet] is given four times a day, three tablets each time. So they [the cancer patients] always have plenty of trypsin, pepsin, lipase, and diastase in their systems. The blood can carry this around and digest the tumor masses wherever they may be."[18]

In following the current Gerson Therapy protocol, the recommended dosage of pancreatin for debulking a malignant tumor usually is three 325-mg tablets four times a day. While a few people don't tolerate pancreatin well, most benefit, with less digestive trouble, gas spasms, and weakness. (It should not be given to sarcoma patients.) Encouraged for use is a pancreatin tablet made without cereal fillers that's manufactured by the Key Company of St. Louis, Missouri.

FLAXSEED OIL

With the Latin name *Linum usitatissimum*, the fresh *oil of flaxseeds* is the richest edible product known containing the important omega-3 fatty acid *alpha-linolenic acid* (a-LNA), which is mandatory for physical health. Flaxseed oil is a primary therapeutic agent for fatty degeneration in cardiovascular disease, cancer, diabetes, and other pathologies. Moreover, its LNA and other components regulate blood pressure, platelet, kidney, immune system, and arterial functions; reinforce the body's inflammatory response; and play roles in calcium and energy metabolism. Adjunctive conversion cofactors for turning LNA into series 3 prostaglandins requires that one's diet or nutritional supplementation should provide vitamins B_3, B_6, and C, plus the minerals magnesium and zinc.[19] (*Prostaglandins* are hormonelike fatty acids that act in tiny amounts on internal organs and the autonomic and central nervous systems.)

Dr. Gerson placed much value on the work of German lipid researcher Johanna Budwig, Ph.D. (still living in her early nineties), who recommends flax oil for enemas in colon cancer and bowel obstruction. Research in North America has finally discovered the value of flax oil's LNA in treating smaller tumors, metastases, inflammatory conditions, high triglycerides, cardiovascular conditions, diabetes, weight loss, and other degenerative illnesses.[20]

The Gerson Therapy requires a participant to use organic, cold-pressed flax oil, such as that manufactured by Omega, Arrowhead Mills, Barleans, or other branded names produced by the Organo process. But users should never heat the oil as in putting it on a steaming hot potato or other vegetable or cooking with it; heating alters the fatty acid chains in its chemical bonds and actually renders the flax oil harmful to the body. Also, don't consume whole flaxseeds because of other components in them that interfere with the healing process.

Flaxseed oil assists the body to utilize vitamin A. During the first month of following the Gerson Therapy, take 2 tablespoonfuls of flax oil per day. After the first month and during the balance of treatment, limit your use of flax oil to 1 tablespoonful daily. Flax oil is best taken at lunch or dinner as part of the salad dressing or on potatoes and vegetables.

BEE POLLEN AND ROYAL JELLY

There are two types of flower pollen: an exceedingly light kind sent haphazardly on the winds and another heavier form delivered mechanically by bees and other insects. *Bee pollen*, therefore, is the heavier, non-airborne substance derived from the male seed of flowers known as *entomophile pollens*, which hitch a ride on honeybees who forage among flower blossoms. Entomophile pollens depend solely on insect transport for spreading flowers' fertilization. Because they are not airborne, the entomophile pollens in bee pollen do not produce the widely disseminated pollen-induced allergies.

Bee pollen contains massive amounts of nutritional ingredients, including ten amino acids, ten minerals, fifteen vitamins, ten nutraceuticals, antibiotics potent against *E. coli* and proteus microbes, and human-growth-stimulating substances. All over our planet, scientists and medical researchers praise the nutritive properties of bee pollen.[21]

The Gerson Therapy incorporates bee pollen into its program, especially for those patients coping with cancer. Then, 2 to 4 teaspoonfuls per day of bee pollen are used at the point of treatment progress when proteins are reintroduced into the patient's diet, starting from approximately the tenth or twelfth week. Noncancer patients can begin taking bee pollen earlier, about the sixth week. Despite bee pollen's being a nonallergenic substance, some patients may exhibit allergies to it, so the initial dosage should probably be as little as ½ teaspoonful per day.

Royal jelly is the rich substance fed to the queen bee for the whole of her life and plays an essential role in the making of a queen. It is exceptionally rich in hormones, twenty amino acids, sugars, acetylcholine, DNA, RNA, fatty acids, gelatin, collagen, gamma globulin, antibiotics, and B vitamins, plus vitamins A, C, and E.[22]

As an optional nutritional supplement that may be added to the

Gerson Therapy if desired, the recommended dosage of royal jelly is 100 mg in capsules taken one hour before breakfast. Do not take royal jelly with hot food.

VITAMIN B₁₂ INJECTIONS AND CRUDE LIVER EXTRACT

Required for proper digestion, absorption of foods, the synthesis of protein, and the metabolism of carbohydrates and fats, *vitamin B₁₂* certainly is an appropriate nutritional supplement for inclusion in the Gerson Therapy. It is particularly effective for the treatment of anemia. Also, it aids in normal cell formation and cellular longevity, prevents nerve damage, maintains fertility, and promotes normal growth and development by maintaining the fatty sheaths that cover and protect nerve endings.[23]

Vitamin B₁₂ is administered by intramuscular injection into the gluteus medius muscle, 0.1 cc (100 mcg) once daily for four to six months or more. It is accompanied simultaneously (in the same injection syringe) by 3 cc of *crude liver extract*. Dr. Gerson found that such liver therapy brings about the restoration of new red blood corpuscles (reticulocytes) and helps the body make the correct use of amino acids. He found crude liver extact was indicated in intoxication during pregnancy; tuberculosis of the lungs and other organs; arthritis deformans in more advanced stages; mental diseases and bodily asthenias; spastic conditions, especially angina pectoris; and malignancies.

Dr. Gerson reports that "leukemias and myelomas need greater doses of liver juice [which is no longer available] and vitamin B₁₂. . . . In the case of all of these diseases, we have cause to assume the concomitant damage to the liver has occurred as a result of permanent intoxication or functional disorders of the neighboring organs."[24]

VITAMIN C

Inasmuch as the Gerson diet contains large amounts of natural vitamin C, a routine daily supplementation with this vitamin should not be necessary; however, *vitamin C* is the prime nutrient when it comes to overall support of the immune system. Vitamin C is used supplementally as a tool for fighting infection, and as part of a pain-relieving triad of natural and nontoxic medications. It also offsets free radical pathology created by the administration of chemotherapy or radiation therapy.

The Gerson Therapy's dose of vitamin C comes in orally administered crystalline (powdered) form such as Bronson's Vitamin C in an amount of 1 to 1.5 grams per day. *Never* use calcium or sodium ascorbate, since these two particular products will bring about serious detrimental effects. High doses of intravenous vitamin C are associated with long-term survival in patients with a variety of cancers, even after the tumors have metastasized.[25]

CHROMIUM PICOLINATE

This supplement has been found to be helfpul in overcoming age-onset and, to some extent, also Juvenile Diabetes. It is also given to such patients.

CHARCOAL TABLETS

Used as a controlling mechanism for diarrhea, gas absorption in the intestinal tract, and externally in clay poultices, *charcoal tablets* are made from 10 grains of highly reamed wood charcoal. The number of tablets taken (dosages) is variable depending on the extent of symptoms.

OX BILE POWDER AND CASTILE SOAP

For purposes of emulsification, *ox bile powder* and *castile soap* are products applied to mix one liquid into another, making a suspension of castor oil. Thus, as described in chapter 13, ox bile powder and castile soap tend to bring the castor oil enema into solution.

POLARIZING TREATMENT

Developed by the noted Mexico City cardiologist and researcher Demetrio Sodi-Pallares, M.D., an intravenous solution known as *GKI* is infused intravenously as an addition to the Gerson Therapy. GKI consists of 1 liter of 10 percent dextrose in water, 20 mEq of potassium chloride, and 15 units "lente" insulin. Up to a maximum of 3 liters of GKI are administered to the patient over twenty-four hours to bring about the reduction of intercellular edema, increase cellular uptake of postassium, stimulate anaerobic and aerobic glycolysis (particularly in the Krebs cycle and oxidative phosphorylation), lower intercellular acidosis, and promote protein synthesis. It is a nontoxic but potent analgesic. Polarizing treatment is a recent add-on to the Gerson Therapy protocol.

GKI, the basic polarizing solution, is described in *Merck's Manual of Standard Medical Procedures*, a standard medical text. Dr. Sodi-Pallares reports that in many patients who are deficient in potassium, it is necessary to provide GKI as a transport mechanism to help potassium travel through the cell membrane. He achieved this by using glucose (G), a potassium solution (K), and a small amount of insulin (I), which are injected together intravenously. Polarizing treatment promotes healing in the diseased heart and in tissues damaged by cancer and other degenerative illnesses. Patients with edema do experience an accelerated reabsorption and release of the tissue fluids that they have accumulated.[26] Since the Gerson Therapy provides ample potassium as well as glucose in juices, one can use just 3 units of lente insulin in some patients to produce the same result.

AMYGDALIN/LAETRILE

Laetrile, the purified form of *amygdalin,* which occurs naturally in apricot pits and many other foods, was thought to cure cancer, but over time we have learned that it does not do so by itself. Laetrile is a cyanogenic glycoside (meaning that it contains cyanide), but it is nontoxic. It has been used by some Gerson Therapy facilities as an analgesic for the relief of pain and for other anticancer properties. While it is not a standard part of the Gerson Therapy protocol, Gerson patients may request laetrile from their physician for use in their treatment. It has come into more common use and is more effective when applied with hyperthermia, hot tub baths, and hot fomentations.[27]

References for Chapter Eleven

1. Petersdorf, R., et al., eds. *Harrison's Principles of Internal Medicine.* New York: McGraw-Hill, 1983, pp. 614–623.

2. Mazzaferri, E.L. "Adult hypothyroidism." *Postgraduate Medicine.* 79:64–72, 1986.

3. Barnes, B.O.; Galton, L. *Hypothyroidism: The Unsuspected Illness.* New York: Thomas Crowell, 1976.

4. Langer, S.E.; Scheer, J.F. *Solved: The Riddle of Illness.* New Canaan, Conn.: Keats Publishing, 1984.

5. *Dorland's Illustrated Medical Dictionary,* 28th ed. Philadelphia: W.B. Saunders Company, 1994, p. 1543.

6. *Gerson Therapy Practitioner's Training Seminar Workbook.* Bonita, Calif.: The Gerson Institute, 1996, p. 49.

7. *The Gerson Handbook,* 4th ed. Bonita, Calif.: The Gerson Institute, 1996, p. 6.

8. Gerson, M. A *Cancer Therapy: Results of Fifty Cases and The Cure of Advanced Cancer by Diet Therapy.* Bonita, Calif.: The Gerson Institute, 1990, p. 205.

9. Gerson, C. "Restoring the healing mechanism in other chronic diseases." In Gerson, M., A *Cancer Therapy: Results of Fifty Cases and The Cure of Advanced Cancer by Diet Therapy.* Bonita, Calif.: The Gerson Institute, 1990, pp. 391–399.

10. *Op. cit., Gerson Therapy Practitioner's Training Seminar Workbook,* p. 47.

11. *Ibid.,* p. 48.

12. Lee, L.; Turner, L. *The Enzyme Cure: How Plant Enzymes Can Help You Relieve 36 Health Problems.* Tiburon, Calif.: Future Medicine Publishing, 1998, p. 20.

13. *Op. cit., Dorland's Illustrated Medical Dictionary,* p. 1254.

14. Lieberman, S.; Bruning, N. *The Real Vitamin and Mineral Book.* Garden City Park, N.Y.: Avery Publishing Group, 1997, pp. 97–99.

15. Hoffer, A.; Walker, M. *Putting It All Together: The New Orthomolecular Nutrition.* New Canaan, Conn.: Keats Publishing, 1996.

16. Hoffer, A.; Walker, M. *Smart Nutrients: A Guide to Nutrients That Can Prevent and Reverse Senility.* Garden City Park, N.Y.: Avery Publishing Group, 1994.

17. Murray, M.T. *Encyclopedia of Nutritional Supplements.* Rocklin, Calif.: Prima Publishing, 1996, pp. 394–399.

18. *Op. cit.,* Gerson, M., 1990, p. 411.

19. Erasmus, U. *Fats That Heal, Fats That Kill.* Burnaby, British Columbia, Canada: Alive Books, 1997, p. 282.

20. *Ibid.,* pp. 282, 283.

21. Brown, R. *The World's Only Perfect Food: The Bee Pollen Bible.* Prescott, Ariz.: Hohm Press, 1993, pp. 131–145.

22. *Ibid.,* pp. 211–218.

23. Balch, J.F.; and Balch, P.A. *Prescription for Nutritional Healing.* 2nd ed. Garden City Park, N.Y.: Avery Publishing Group, 1997, p. 16.

24. *Op. cit.,* Gerson, M., 1990, pp. 79–81.

25. Null, G. *The Complete Encyclopedia of Natural Healing.* New York: Kensington Books, 1998, p.102.

26. *The Gerson Handbook: An Adjunct of A Cancer Therapy—Results of Fifty Cases by Max Gerson, M.D. Practical Guidance, Resources, and Recipes for Gerson Therapy Patients,* 4th ed. Bonita, Calif.: Gerson Institute, 1996, p. 7.

27. *Ibid.,* p. 50.

Chapter Twelve

LIVER DETOXIFICATION WITH COFFEE ENEMAS

Kent Gardner, aged forty-six, a taxidermist living in Phoenix, Arizona, discovered that he had only an 8 percent chance of five-year survival because cancer of both the esophagus and larynx had struck him. Expanding in Mr. Gardner's throat was a golf-ball-sized malignant tumor that imminently endangered his life.

"I bought the Gerson Therapy book [A Cancer Therapy: Results of Fifty Cases], read it two times in less than twenty days, and decided, what do I have to lose? I knew I was dying. The coffee enemas were a mental hurdle I had to overcome, but once I experienced one of them, I could feel a difference in the boosting of my health and realized their importance," Kent Gardner wrote for the Gerson Healing Newsletter. (Mr. Gardner's photograph may be viewed on the facing page).

"After about one and a half months, the swelling was way down, and the tumor was dead," he continues. "Reducing in size weekly, it was rotting in my throat. Frankly, it felt like hell! This thing now rotting produced a constant, horrible smell unlike anything I had ever experienced—even after working for twenty-four years as a taxidermist!

"Still doing the Gerson Therapy faithfully, about two and a half months later, as I was locking my car to walk into a local hardware store, the dead tumor fluttered [vibrated] for about two seconds, then as I swallowed I felt it break free. I sort of staggered into the store, feeling panicked. I broke into profuse sweating and started losing consciousness. I fell

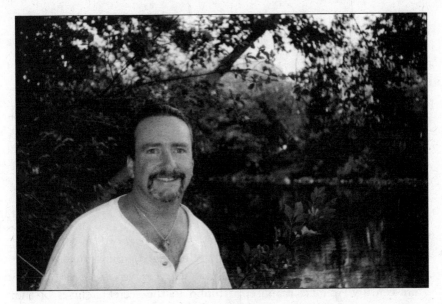

Kent Gardner

to my knees in a series of convulsions, and I knew I was in trouble," Mr. Gardner asserts.

"Thinking about this situation later, I realized the tumor had fallen into my stomach, where it mixed with digestive juices, producing ammonia poisons and gases. I should have tried to throw it up, but ego, and not being able to think clearly, didn't allow me to vomit publicly. To this day," admits Mr. Gardner, "I don't remember or know how I managed to make it back to my car and then drive home, which was a twenty-minute ride. For the next five days I was totally bedridden.

"I took three coffee enemas a day; my wife helped me, doing all that was necessary. The tumor's toxic effects were manifold—headaches, vomiting, bad abdominal cramps, flulike aches and pains of the joints and muscles, fever, sleeplessness, fast pulse, dry mouth, no appetite, constipation, and many other troubles," the taxidermist states. "I was in an awful state of absolute illness!

"But on the sixth day I felt better and was able to walk around. I have been walking on water ever since. Because of that experience, I have done my homework and am experientially educated far beyond my I.Q., concerning the human body and nutrition," Kent Gardner says. "All living cells and organisms on this planet need water, food, and air. It is the quality, not the quantity, that determines perfect health, or disease. You can't trash and pollute your body and expect to have perfect health. What all of us need are daily coffee enemas, something I do on a regular basis—cancer or not."

ORIGINS OF COFFEE ENEMAS AS GERSON THERAPY

The much disputed, ridiculed, and controversial coffee enemas have an unusual origin in becoming a primary component of the Gerson Therapy.

Certainly enemas are not new; they were transcribed as part of the *Manual of Discipline*, recorded two thousand years ago, comprising one of the books in the Dead Sea Scrolls. Also, *The Essene Gospel of Peace*, a third-century Aramaic manuscript found in the secret archives of the Vatican, strongly advises about the taking of enemas in the following manner:[1]

I tell you truly, the angel of water shall cast out of your body all uncleannesses which defiled it without and within. And all unclean and evil-smelling things shall flow out of you, even as the uncleannesses of garments washed in water flow away and are lost in the stream of the river. I tell you truly, holy is the angel of water who cleanses all that is unclean and makes all evil-smelling things of a sweet odor. . . .

Think not that it is sufficient that the angel of water embrace you outwards only. I tell you truly, the uncleanness within is greater by much than the uncleanness without. And he who cleanses himself without, but within remains unclean, is like to tombs that outwards are painted fair, but are within full of all manner of horrible uncleannesses and abominations. So I tell you truly, suffer the angel of water to baptize you also within, that you may become free from all your past sins, and that within likewise you may become as pure as the river's foam sporting in the sunlight. . . .

Seek, therefore, a large trailing gourd, having a stalk the length of a man; take out its inwards and fill it with water from the river which the sun has warmed. Hang it upon the branch of a tree, and kneel upon the ground before the angel of water, and suffer the end of the stalk of the trailing gourd to enter your hinder parts, that the water may flow through all your bowels. Afterwards rest kneeling on the ground before the angel of water and pray to the living God that he will forgive you all your past sins, and pray to the angel of water that he will free your body from every uncleanness and disease. Then let the water run out from your body, that it may carry away from within it all the unclean and evil-smelling things of Satan. And you shall see with your eyes and smell with your nose all the abominations and uncleannesses which defiled the temple of your body; even all the sins which abode in your body, tormenting you with all manner of pains. I tell you truly, baptism with water frees you from all of these. Renew your baptizing with water on every day of your fast, till the day when you see that the water which flows out of you is as pure as the river's foam. Then betake your body to the coursing river, and therein the arms of the angel of water render thanks to the living God that he has freed you from your sins. And this holy baptizing by the angel of water is the Rebirth unto the new life.

So enemas have been used for general purposes of detoxification since ancient times. However, the use of coffee to increase the effectiveness of treatment and to reduce pain probably dates back only to the time of the First World War. A Gerson Therapy exponent, Dr. Jerry Walters, tells the following story about the original administrations of enemas containing the coffee beverage:

During World War I, Germany was surrounded by the Allies' military forces, and many imported materials were short or missing for German citizens. Among other things, morphine was running very low in supply. Also there was hardly any coffee available to drink. Moreover, painkillers, anesthetics, and other drugs were lacking too. When soldiers were sent back from the front lines, severely wounded, and in need of surgery, there usually was just a bit of anesthesia available—perhaps only enough to get them through the surgical operation.

When the anesthesia wore off, obviously the pain set in for the wounded soldier. In many cases, after the doctors finished operating, they ordered plain water enemas for the patients. But the nurses were desperately looking for something more to help the soldiers deal with their pain.

It happened that there was always coffee brewing, available only for the surgeons to drink. They often had to work around the clock, and needed to be kept awake by caffeine in the beverage. Sometimes, a little of their black coffee was left over. Apparently, some nurse had the idea that, since the coffee was doing the surgeons good, perhaps it would also help the soldiers. So the nurses poured a quantity of the leftover coffee into the soldiers' enema buckets. The soldiers receiving coffee enemas reported that these were doing them some good, and that their pain was much relieved.

These reports coming out of the First World War aroused the interest of two researchers, Professor O. A. Meyer, M.D., and Professor Martin Heubner, M.D., at the German University of Goettingen's College of Medicine. (Please see Dr. Max Gerson's lecture describing this occurrence, reproduced in its entirety in Appendix II of *A Cancer Therapy: Results of Fifty Cases.*) During the 1920s, these two medical professors further examined the effect of caffeine when given rectally to rats. They observed that the caffeinated enemas stimulated the laboratory animals' bile ducts to open, and the professors then published their findings in the German medical literature.

For some time after learning of this research by Professors Meyer and Heubner, Dr. Max Gerson used a combination of the two drugs, caffeine and potassium citrate, in the form of drops that were added to the enema water. But he found later that a solution simply made by boiling coffee grounds was more effective and was much more easily available to everybody who wanted to take coffee enemas. Thus, Dr. Gerson incorporated a program of detoxification using coffee enemas into the Gerson Therapy, and the same procedure remains today.[2]

THE BENEFICIAL ACTION OF A COFFEE ENEMA

Enemas made from drip-grind boiled coffee have proven themselves an advantageous means of restoring the liver. The caffeine drug in coffee administered as an enema definitely detoxifies the liver and is a primary therapeutic approach of the Gerson Therapy. "This treatment should be followed strictly, both in the clinic and later at home, for at least two years. . . . The liver is the main organ for the regeneration of the body's metabolism for the transformation of food from intake to output," writes Dr. Gerson.[3]

During a 1985 conference on cancer treatment conducted by the late alternative treatment cancer specialist Harold Manner, Ph.D., held at King of Prussia, Pennsylvania, Dr. Manner discussed the internal workings of a coffee enema. He announced to the audience that he learned about these physiological actions from Dr. Max Gerson, who had expounded on the subject in the same way at least thirty years before. He gave Dr. Gerson full credit for developing this liver detoxification technique for the treatment of cancer. The next few paragraphs are paraphased from Dr.

Manner's description of the body's cleansing mechanism that occurs when the coffee enema is administered.

While the coffee enema is being retained in the gut (for an optimum period ranging from twelve to fifteen minutes), all of the body's blood passes through the liver every three minutes. The hemorrhoidal blood vessels dilate from exposure to the caffeine; in turn, the liver's portal veins dilate too. Simultaneously, the bile ducts expand with blood, the bile flow increases, and the smooth muscles of these internal organs relax. The blood serum and its many components are detoxified as this vital fluid passes through the individual's caffeinated liver. The quart of water being retained in the bowel stimulates the visceral nervous system, promoting peristalsis. The water delivered through the bowel dilutes the bile and causes an even greater increase in bile flow. There is a flushing of toxic bile which is further affected by the body's enzymatic catalyst known to physiologists as glutathione S-transferase (GST).

The GST is increased in quantity in the small bowel by 700 percent, which is an excellent physiological effect, because this enzyme quenches free radicals. These quenched radicals leave the liver and gallbladder as bile salts flowing through the duodenum. The bile salts are carried away by peristalsis in the gut, traveling from the small intestine, through the colon, and out the rectum.

In 1990, the Austrian surgeon Peter Lechner, M.D., and his colleagues, who had been investigating Dr. Gerson's cancer treatment, discussed the benefits of increasing quantities of GST in the gut. It was then that Dr. Lechner reported:[4]

- GST binds bilirubin and its glucuronides so that they can be eliminated from the hepatocytes (liver cells).
- GST blocks and detoxifies carcinogens, which require oxidation or reduction to be activated. Its catalytic function produces a protective effect against many chemical carcinogens.
- GST forms a covalent bond with nearly all highly electrophilic (free radical) substances, which is the precondition of their elimination from the body. The intermediate products of potential liver poisons (*hepatotoxic cytostatics*) also belong in this category of forming free radical pathology.

Before the above published finding, Dr. Lechner had decided in 1984 that the coffee enema had a very specific purpose: lowering serum toxins. His medical report states, "Coffee enemas have a definite effect on the colon which can be observed with an endoscope. Wattenberg and coworkers were able to prove in 1981 that the palmitic acid found in coffee promotes the activity of glutathione S-transferase and other ligands by manyfold times above the normal. It is this enzyme group which is responsible primarily for the conjugation of free electrophile radicals which the gall bladder will then release."[5]

Starting in the late 1970s, the laboratory owned and supervised by biochemist Lee W. Wattenberg, Ph.D., identified two salts of palmitic acid, cafestol palmitate and kahweol palmitate (both present in coffee), as the potent intensifiers of glutathione S-transferase. Such enhancement turns this enzyme into a major detoxification system that catalyzes the binding of a vast variety of electron acceptors (the electrophiles) from the bloodstream to the sulfhydryl group of glutathione. Because the reactive ultimate carcinogenic forms of chemicals are electrophiles, the glutathione S-transferase system becomes an important mechanism for cleaning away any existing cancer cells (carcinogenic detoxification).[6,7,8]

This detoxifying of cancer cells has been demonstrated innumerable times by experiments on laboratory mice wherein detoxification of the liver increases by 600 percent and the small bowel detoxifies by 700 percent when coffee beans are added to the animals' diet. Analogous results take place within humans who are giving themselves coffee enemas.[9,10,11]

COFFEE ENEMAS CAUSE EXCRETION OF CANCER BREAKDOWN PRODUCTS

The coffee enema has a very specific purpose in the treatment and reversal of degenerative diseases. As stated by Dr. Peter Lechner, it lowers the quantity of blood serum toxins, literally cleaning the poisons out of fluids nourishing normal cells. Invariably, some small quantities of poisons are contained therein. Each cell is challenged by toxins, oxygen starvation, malnutrition, or trauma which collectively alter the cell's molecular configuration and cause it to lose its preference for potassium. As explained in chapters 10 and 11, sodium competes with potassium for association sites in damaged cells.

Loss of cellular potassium and increase of cellular sodium results in decreased electron flow through the damaged cell, which some biochemists refer to as a *macromolecule*. This injured macromolecule becomes unattractive to paramagnetic ions and a subsequent disorganization of water molecules may take place. Because bulk-phase water, structured in a high-energy state, is the main mechanism controlling cellular water content and purity, any disturbance in water structuring will result in the cell's swelling with excess water and extracellular solutes. When the internal environment of the macromolecule becomes polluted with excess water and extracellular materials, mitochondrial production of ATP (adenosine triphosphate) is greatly impaired. The result is that macromolecules cannot produce sufficient energy to repair themselves unless the challenge is removed.

Endogenous serum toxins can be generated within macromolecules by bacteria and by malignant cells. It's been observed that surrounding almost any active malignancies are spheres of damaged normal tissue in which water structuring is impaired by the chronic insult of tumor toxins. Energy production and immunity are depressed in these macromolecules, which are swollen with excess salt and water. Such damaged tissue possesses a decreased blood circulation because oversized edematous cells crowd together inside the capillaries, arterioles, and lymph ducts.[12]

Teaching that improved blood circulation and tissue integrity would prevent the spread and cause the destruction of malignancies, Max Gerson, M.D., held it as axiomatic that no cancer could exist in the presence of normal metabolism. Dr. Gerson's favorite example of this fact was that the tissues of healthy laboratory animals receiving transplanted malignant tumors quickly kill these tumors by the process of inflammation which arises in the healthy animal hosts. They defend themselves against such foreign proteins. In order to cause transplanted malignant cells to "take" in the experimental animals, laboratory technicians must first damage the animals' thyroid and adrenal glands. Of course, Dr. Gerson's efforts were directed toward healing and normality. His desire was to create a near-normal metabolism in tissues surrounding his patients' existing malignant tumors.

Enzyme systems in the liver and small bowel are responsible for conversion and neutralization of the four most common tissue toxins, polyamines, ammonia, toxic-bound nitrogen, and electrophiles, all of which can cause cell and membrane damage. Such protective liver and gut enzyme systems are massively increased in their beneficial effects by coffee enemas. Twenty years after his death, editors at the highly scientific journal *Physiological Chemistry and Physics* complimented Dr. Gerson by reprinting one of his works. They affirmed, "Caffeine enemas cause dilation of bile ducts, which facilitates excretion of toxic cancer breakdown products by the liver and dialysis of toxic products from blood across the colonic wall."[13]

PAIN RELIEF RESULTS FROM TAKING COFFEE ENEMAS

Prior to the reported findings of both Dr. Lee W. Wattenberg and Dr. Peter Lechner, medical journalist Mark F. McCarty, in 1981, wrote in the journal *Medical Hypotheses*,[14] "At the Senate Select Subcommittee hearing on cancer research in 1946,[15] five independent medical doctors who had had personal experience with patients treated by Dr. Gerson, submitted letters indicating that they had been surprised and encouraged by the results they had seen, and urged a widespread trial of the method including taking coffee enemas. One of these doctors claimed that 'relief of severe pain was achieved in about 90 percent of cases'."

Observations so recorded back in 1946 were the truth then and remain correct today in the same way. While the use of coffee as an enema often evokes astonishment and mirth in persons who don't use enemas as well as in those who emphatically prefer to drink their coffee at the nearby Starbucks™ beverage shop, these same people would benefit immensely from receiving coffee through the rectum. They could get rid of their pain and other discomforts, whatever the source, by accepting the value of this detoxification method. From the patient's point of view, no matter which degenerative disease is causing symptoms, the coffee enema means relief from confusion, general nervous tension, depression, many allergy-related symptoms, and, most importantly, from severe pain.[16]

COFFEE ENEMAS STIMULATE BILE FLOW

The coffee enema is in a class by itself as a therapeutic agent. In no way does the oral administration of beverage coffee have the same effect as its rectal administration. On the contrary, drinking coffee virtually ensures reabsorption of toxic bile. While other agents classed as stimulators of bile flow (choleretics) do increase bile production from the liver, they hardly enhance any detoxifying by that organ's enzyme systems. Choleretics do nothing to ensure the passage of bile from the intestines out the rectum. It's a physiological fact that bile is normally reabsorbed up to ten times by the body before working its way out of the intestines in feces.

The enzyme-intensifying ability of the coffee enema is unique among choleretics. Because it does not allow reabsorption of toxic bile by the liver across the gut wall, it is an entirely effective means of detoxifying the bloodstream through existing enzyme systems in both the liver and the small intestine. Inasmuch as clinical practice has taught clinicians utilizing the Gerson Therapy that coffee enemas are well tolerated by patients when used as frequently as every four hours in a twenty-four-hour period, the coffee enema should be categorized in the medical literature as the only nonreabsorbed, effective, repeatable choleretic agent. Such a classification could go far to bring about the healing of pathologies that require quick absorption and no reuse of bile.

SUMMARIZING THE PHYSIOLOGICAL BENEFITS OF COFFEE ENEMAS

Dr. Gerson hypothesized on the physiological actions and effects of coffee enemas and observed their clinical benefits.

Introducing a quart of boiled coffee solution into the colon will accomplish the following physiological benefits:

- It dilutes portal blood and, subsequently, the bile.
- Theophylline and theobromine, major nutraceutical constituents of coffee, dilate blood vessels and counter inflammation of the gut.
- The palmitates of coffee enhance glutathione S-transferase, which is responsible for the removal of many toxic radicals from blood serum.
- The fluid of the enema itself stimulates the visceral nervous system, promoting peristalsis and the transit of diluted toxic bile from the duodenum out the rectum.
- Because the stimulating enema is retained for up to fifteen minutes, and because all the blood in the body passes through the liver nearly every three minutes, coffee enemas represent a form of dialysis of blood across the gut wall.

Coffee enemas are safe when used within the context of the combined regime of the Gerson Therapy. Dr. Gerson's stated intention in supplying a sodium-restricted, high-potassium, high-micronutrient diet of fruits, vegetables, and whole grains was to supply all nutrients, known and unknown, which are necessary for cell respiration and energy production. High-potassium, low-sodium environments tend to return cell macromolecules to normal configuration states and to improve water structuring and water content. The addition by Dr. Gerson of supplemental potassium salts as acetate, gluconate, and phosphate (monobasic) to the diet, in which malate is supplied by frequent use of apples, improves the efficiency of the tricarboxylic acid (Krebs) cycle in mitochondrial energy production. The Krebs cycle is a series of enzyme reactions in which the body uses carbohydrates, proteins, and fats to yield carbon dioxide, water, and energy for organ functions.

Animal protein restriction, employed by Dr. Gerson as a temporary aspect of treatment for his degenerative disease patients, was observed even in the late nineteenth century to aid in the reduction of cellular edema. Administration of high loading doses of thyroid hormone and Lugol's solution result in multiplication of mitochondria, which have their own DNA and RNA and replicate independently of the cell. Thyroid is known to improve cell oxidation of sugars and therefore ATP production so that cell energy is markedly increased.

These numerous treatment mechanisms, including coffee enemas, proposed by Dr. Max Gerson achieve the following. They:

- Reduce blood serum toxins to eliminate chronic challenge to damaged normal cells (macromolecules),
- Improve cell potassium ion content,
- Reduce cell sodium content,
- Reduce cell swelling through improved water structuring,
- Increase cell mitochondria count and activity, and
- Supply micronutrients necessary for cell energy production and repair.

For a person attempting to cope with any form of chronic or acute illness occurring from some degenerative process, the contribution of low blood serum toxin levels by the regular administration of coffee enemas is basic to achieving increased cell energy production, enhanced tissue integrity, improved blood circulation, boosted immunity, better tissue repair, and cellular regeneration. All of these beneficial physiological effects have been observed clinically to result from the administration of the combined regime of the Gerson healing program. Unquestionably, taking coffee enemas is among the most vital aspects of the Gerson Therapy.

References for Chapter Twelve

1. Szekely, E.B. *The Essene Gospel of Peace.* London: International Biogenic Society, 1981, pp. 15, 16.

2. Gerson, M. "The cure of advanced cancer by diet therapy: a summary of 30 years of clinical experimentation." Appendix II in A *Cancer Therapy: Results of Fifty Cases,* 6th ed. Bonita, Calif.: The Gerson Institute, 1999, pp. 407, 408.

3. *Ibid.,* p. 247.

4. Lechner, P.; Kronberger, I. "Erfahrungen mit dem Einsatz der Diät-Therapie in der chirurgischen Onkologie." *Aktuel Ernährungmedizin.* 2(15):72–78, 1990.

5. Lechner, P. "Dietary regime to be used in oncological postoperative care." *Proceedings of the Oesterreicher Gesellschaft für Chirurgie.* June 21–23, 1984.

6. Chasseaud, L.F. "The role of glutathione S-transferase in the metabolism of chemical carcinogens and other electrophilic agents." *Advanced Cancer Research.* 29:175–274, 1979.

7. Jakoby, W.B. "A group of multifunctional detoxification proteins." *Advanced Enzymology and Related Areas of Molecular Biology.* 46:383–414, 1978.

8. Sparnins, V.L.; Wattenberg, L.W. "Enhancement of glutathione S-transferase activity of the mouse forestomach by inhibitors of benzo[a]pyrene-induced neoplasia of forestomach." *Journal of the National Cancer Institute.* 66:769–771, 1981.

9. Sparnins, V.L. "Effects of dietary constituents on (G-S-T) glutathione S-transferase activity." *Proceedings of the American Association of Cancer Researchers and the American Society of Clinical Oncologists.* 21:80, Abstract 319, 1980.

10. Sparnins, V.L.; Lam, L.K.T.; Wattenberg, L.W. "Effects of coffee on glutathione S-transferase (G-S-T) activity and 7-12-dimethylbenz(a)anthracene (DMBA)-induced neoplasia." *Proceedings of the American Association of Cancer Researchers and the American Society of Clinical Oncologists.* 22:114, Abstract 453, 1981.

11. Lam, L.K.T.; Spanins, V.L.; Wattenberg, L.W. "Isolation and identification of kahweol palmitate and cafestol palmitate as active constituents of green coffee beans that enhance glutathione S-transferase activity in the mouse." *Cancer Research.* 42:1193–1198, 1982.

12. Cope, F.W. "Pathology of structured water and associated cations in cells (the tissue damage syndrome) and its medical treatment." *Physiological Chemistry and Physics.* 9(6):547–553, 1977.

13. Gerson, M. "The cure of advanced cancer by diet therapy: a summary

of 30 years of clinical experimentation." *Physiological Chemistry and Physics.* 10(5):449–464, 1978.

14. McCarty, M. "Aldosterone and the Gerson diet—a speculation." *Medical Hypotheses.* 7:591–597, 1981.

15. Subcommittee of the Committee on Foreign Relations of the United States Senate, 1946. Seventy-ninth Congress, Second Session, Hearings on Bill S. 1875, pp. 95–126. Washington, D.C.: United States Government Printing Office, July 1, 2, and 3, 1946.

16. Hildenbrand, G. "A coffee enema? Now I've heard everything." *Gerson Healing Newsletter.* no.13, May/June 1986, p. 99.

Chapter Thirteen

COFFEE ENEMAS AND HOW TO TAKE THEM

Broadly known almost as a hallmark of the Gerson Therapy, the technique of giving or receiving coffee enemas for program participants has reaped its share of denigration. Numbers of critics, general detractors, and outright slanderers have condemned the practice; yet rectal self-injection with a quart of liquid containing coffee beverage is therapeutic and healing.

Exemplifying disparagement of coffee enemas was the editor of the *Journal of the American Medical Association*, Morris Fishbein, M.D. Now deceased, Dr. Fishbein was an avowed enemy of Max Gerson, M.D. and anything to do with his treatment program. Publicly and privately, in speaking of alternative methods of healing, then known as "unconventional cancer therapies," Dr. Fishbein used to repeatedly offer the tired joke: "How do you want your coffee enema, with cream or sugar?"

ADDRESSING THE TOPIC OF COFFEE ENEMAS

But even with a supposed medical oddity relating to its coffee enemas, the Gerson Therapy has won worldwide respectability. For instance, in a letter dated March 8, 1999, the Earl Baldwin of Bewdley, a member of the House of Lords in England, invited Charlotte Gerson to address members of the English Parliament about the Gerson Therapy. Peers and MPs attended her presentation before the Parliamentary Group for Alternative and Complementary Medicine on May 19, 1999, and her lecture was a great success.

Furthermore, Dr. Gerson's daughter accepts invitations to address medical school classes as well, and there are many from which to choose. It is difficult to describe the incredulous facial expressions which ripple across the audience of medical students when the topic of coffee enemas is introduced. Embarrassed sniggering invariably may be heard from several seats in the lecture hall. And then a wise guy student will be heard to heckle aloud, "How do you take your coffee?" Snatching a page from Dr. Fishbein's book, Charlotte Gerson doesn't miss a beat when she swiftly answers: "Black—*without* cream and sugar." Laughter relaxes the entire classroom and Charlotte goes on to explain this detoxifying aspect of her famous father's treatment program.

Responses from the audience of budding doctors will typically be: "Boy, I'll bet you get a buzz out of that!" Or, "Couldn't you just drink three or four cups of coffee?" Or, "Why go to all that trouble just for a caffeine high?" And eventually, the most significant question gets asked from active student thinkers whose medical interests are piqued, "What does a coffee enema do?"

Since the full answer was given in our prior chapter, you know the correct response already. If not, please return to read chapter 12.

Dr. Gerson Summarizes the Coffee Enema Procedure

In a succinct manner, Dr. Max Gerson summarized the best procedure for self-administration of a coffee enema. He had written down the simple steps in abbreviated form for easy following. Those directions were recorded in his famous text for the medical consumer, and the Gerson Institute has carried forward with refinements to his method as described in its volume of educational literature.

Dr. Gerson suggests that the individual assume a specific body position when taking a coffee enema. He writes: "To make enemas most effective, the patient should lie on his right side, with both legs drawn close to the abdomen, and breathe deeply, in order to suck the greatest amount of fluid into all parts of the colon. The fluid should be retained ten to fifteen minutes."

As was described by now-deceased Harold Manner, Ph.D., in chapter 12, within twelve minutes nearly all the caffeine from the coffee is absorbed through the bowel wall and into the hemorrhoidal veins. From these blood vessels it flows directly into the portal veins and then into the liver. Dr. Gerson advises for cancer patients and other very sick people that during the first months of treatment, enemas may be taken as frequently as every four hours, day and night, for their optimal effect. Some terminal cancer patients save their lives and restore health by taking five coffee enemas each day for months at a time.[1]

In his writings, the formulation that the much-respected German-American physician had offered as the best coffee enema concentration is the following:

1. Drop 3 rounded tablespoonfuls of ground (drip) coffee (not instant) into one quart of water.
2. Let the solution boil three minutes and then simmer fifteen minutes more.
3. Strain the solution.
4. Fill a quart glass container with the liquid and let cool to body temperature.
5. Use this solution at body temperature for purposes of bowel infusion.

The daily amount of coffee liquid can be prepared at one time, or a more concentrated coffee solution may be made and then diluted down to the required strength for repeated separate enemas during consecutive applications.

COFFEE ENEMA IMPROVEMENTS OVER HALF A CENTURY

Detoxification of the body is one of the most important life-enhancement contributions of the Gerson Therapy. The coffee enema is the basic procedure employed; but since the colon is a highly absorptive organ, enemas can be applied for various reasons. As you learned in the

last chapter, enemas go back to the ancients, and are described in literature through the ages.

During the past half century or more since Dr. Gerson first instituted
coffee enemas as part of his treatment program, many improvements
have been added as refinements to the actual enema procedure. This section will describe some of those new methods that the Gerson Institute
has incorporated.

Self-administration of the regular coffee enema has been modified
slightly and is now made as follows:

1. Take three rounded tablespoonfuls of drip-grind coffee and add
    them to a quart of boiling water (use distilled water if your drink-
    ing water is furnished from a fluoridated water source; use filtered
    water if you reside in an average drinking water area).
2. Let the mixture boil for three minutes uncovered and allow it to
    simmer for another fifteen minutes more covered.
3. Strain the solution through a fine strainer to catch floating coffee
    grounds. Or employ a coarser strainer lined with a filter cloth, such
    as an old, used piece of white sheeting or a piece cut from a knit
    undershirt. Add enough hot water to refill a glass container up to
    the 1-quart level. (Some water will have been lost in boiling and
    straining.)
4. Prepare yourself to instill this coffee solution into the rectum
    when it cools to body temperature.

Procedure for Instilling
the Coffee Enema

The patient should lie either on the padded floor (use a cushioning
mat) or on a mattress protected with a plastic sheet, either setup covered
for comfort with a towel. Rather than the floor or a bed, some patients use
a camp bed or the famous enema bench. This enema bench is made up of
a table, about the size of a 4-foot-by-2-foot cocktail table, covered with a
3- to 4-inch-thick layer of foam rubber, which, in turn, is covered with
some Naugahyde or plastic for easy cleaning.

In fact, if you are able to get up and down easily, most often a clean
bathroom floor works best for giving yourself an enema. If that is the case,
you may prefer to put some soft padding on the bathroom floor, cover it

with plastic and a towel (a lawn chaise pad is excellent), plop down a pillow, and lie down on that padded floor. Be sure, in any case, that you or the patient you're assisting are comfortable and warm.

The patient should lie on his or her right side, with legs pulled up in a relaxed position. If, due to pain, the patient is unable to lie on the right side, it is acceptable to lie on one's back, also with legs pulled up. Lie on the left side only as a last resort because the coffee enema goes deeper into the bowel most effectively from the right side. Take your time letting gravity force the fluid into your rectum and bowel. Have the bottom of an enema bag or bucket elevated only about 18 inches above the tube's end that is penetrating one's anus.

The enema once fully infused into the colon should, ideally, be held for from twelve to fifteen minutes. By that time, almost all the available caffeine has been absorbed. It is not suggested to hold it longer than fifteen minutes, since the liquid will also be absorbed into the system. If a person cannot hold the enema for twelve minutes, he or she should do the best they can without trying desperately to retain the fluid, which could bring on abdominal cramping. If she or he can only manage say six to nine minutes, do release the liquid at that shorter interval. Eventually, holding the coffee enema inside the bowel for twelve minutes does become quite comfortable. It merely takes practice, and some people have taken three or four months before achieving the ideal time period.

A COFFEE ENEMA FOR THE BEDFAST PATIENT

Occasionally, a patient is bedfast and cannot get up for an enema or go to the bathroom. In that case, assistance from a support person is required. Then, proceed as we have described above:

1. Cover the mattress and bed clothing with plastic and a towel.
2. Have the patient take the enema while lying in bed.
3. Hold the quart of fluid if possible for from twelve to fifteen minutes, and provide the patient with a bedpan.
4. If incontinence is a complication, the enema has to be introduced while the patient is lying on the bedpan.

As we've mentioned—and it's an important point—the enema bucket or bag should not be more than 18 inches (50 cm) above the body so the coffee does not flow into the bowel under too much pressure. The reason for this becomes all too apparent rather quickly. An excessive height could cause excessive pressure and easily set up counterperistalsis with cramping.

If cramping occurs, stop the flow of liquid, either by pinching the tube closed or by lowering the bucket or bag to the level of the body for a little while. Then resume the enema's flow.

A number of patients, at the start of the treatment, have reported experiencing difficulty getting a full quart of liquid into the colon. If that becomes the situation for you or your loved one, start with whatever amount is most comfortably received. Let the patient take and hold that lesser amount; expel it, and then accept the rest of the enema.

Some people are able to take a full quart of coffee solution from the start, but at the time of going through their first healing reaction, they can't even take half that amount. This may come from toxic pressure produced by the liver. It requires the same sort of procedure as just described: take as much liquid as is comfortable to hold; expel it, and then take the rest.

VARIATIONS TO THE COFFEE ENEMA SOLUTION

There are many variations to the coffee enema. Some patients, if suffering from an irritated bowel, colitis, diarrhea, bleeding, or cramping, may find it more comfortable to use half a quart of the regular coffee and add half a quart of chamomile tea. This combination is soothing to the intestinal tract and usually helps to clear the above symptoms.

In case of serious diarrhea, it may be necessary to eliminate the coffee and use only chamomile tea. Usually, as symptoms clear away, some coffee concentrate can slowly be added to the herb tea, starting with 2 to 4 ounces, then 6 to 8 ounces (always maintaining the quart quantity as the ideal measurement), until the patient can again handle the full coffee enema.

Chamomile tea rather than coffee is also useful at the start of the Gerson Therapy. During that time, when patients are required to receive five coffee enemas a day, the last one at 10:00 P.M. may tend to keep them awake. In that case, we recommend that such individuals replace the last coffee enema with chamomile tea. Usually, in three to four days, the 10:00 P.M. coffee enema no longer causes loss of sleep.

In a few special cases (during severe reactions, in heavy tumor absorption, or in case of pain striking during the night), Dr. Gerson also suggested a nighttime enema. If the patient cannot sleep because of pain or discomfort, it's better for the patient to get up and out of bed at 2:00 or 3:00 A.M. to take a coffee enema rather than to toss and turn and not sleep anyway. Instillation of that coffee enema often allows the individual to go back to sleep. It may be surprising to some, but these middle-of-the-night enemas never seem to keep the patient awake.

Very-early-morning enemas are also extremely important for drug addicts who wake up with nightmares due to toxicity or from withdrawal symptoms. Here is a tip learned recently: before taking the nighttime or first morning enema, it is wise to eat a piece of fruit or have some applesauce or fruit salad (placed on the night table by the patient's bedside) to raise the blood sugar a little.

More Explicit Information on the Castor Oil Treatment

Besides self-administering the coffee enema, another important feature of detoxification is the castor oil procedure. To accomplish an exceedingly intensive cleansing technique, Dr. Gerson prescribed a castor oil treatment for the cancer patient to be conducted every other day. (This castor oil procedure does not apply to cancer patients who were previously treated with cytotoxic or other chemotherapy drugs. They should *not* take castor oil.)

Here is how a candidate should proceed with the castor oil treatment:

1. At about 5:00 A.M. drink 2 tbsp of castor oil, followed by a cup of black coffee with 1 tsp of organic brown sugar (Sucanat).
2. At 6:00 A.M. take the usual coffee enema.
3. At 10:00 A.M. replace the coffee enema with a castor oil enema.

Make the castor oil enema in the following manner:

a. Into the bucket or bag (for instilling castor oil, a bucket is much preferable to the bag since it is easier to clean), place 4 tbsp of castor oil.
b. Add ¼ tsp of ox bile powder.

c. Take a cake of regular soap (not detergent) into your hand and rub it for a few moments into a regular coffee enema at body temperature.

d. Take this soapy coffee and mix it into the castor oil with ox bile powder, stirring constantly. (Some people find it best to use an electric mixer.)

When mixed, the castor oil still tends to rise to the top; therefore, you need to stir constantly while you allow it to flow into your rectum (quite a trick; if you can't manage it, have somebody do the stirring for you as you take the mixture). This enema along with the castor oil by mouth is virtually impossible to hold. Do not work too hard at holding the mixture. Rather, release when necessary.

Some patients report that when they release the castor oil enema, it burns the anus. Burning can occur, but the circumstance to remember is that *castor oil does not burn*. Instead it's the release of highly toxic material coming out of the body's tissues that burns! This is one more indication of how important it is to take these castor oil enemas. Indeed, after two or three castor oil treatments, the burning is reduced and disappears. Such a disappearance indicates that the toxic level in the system is lower and no longer irritates the rectum and anus. If irritation exists, use a little petroleum jelly to soothe the area. You may also use a little zinc oxide ointment (*not* suppositories, which contain painkillers).

A number of patients, if they previously suffered from hemorrhoids, have a flare-up of this situation. It can be uncomfortable for a few days; but the patient should definitely *not* stop the enemas. Zinc oxide ointment may be applied locally. But please keep in mind that hemorrhoids are usually caused by toxic pressure; therefore, detoxifying is extra-important, and stopping the enemas is entirely wrong. It has also been observed in those patients that the hemorrhoids shortly disappear and do not recur. It just takes a little waiting time and patience.

PHYSICAL FLARE-UPS FROM THE ENEMA TREATMENTS

The frequency of taking coffee enemas as well as castor oil treatments is reduced after a period of time. Some patients are so toxic that reduction of enema frequencies do not apply to them. If they reduce the detoxification too soon and then feel ill, toxic, or headachy, they should go back to the more intensive level for a period of time. Later, they can try to reduce the frequency again. Each patient needs to adjust the frequency of detoxifying to his own needs. At times, when the patient does well upon receiving less-frequent enemas, flare-ups still could occur. These may include new toxic releases, increased swellings or pain, headaches, or lack of appetite. At such times, an extra coffee enema or a castor oil treatment has been known to work wonders.

Occasionally, flare-ups are accompanied by diarrhea. At such times, the patient should only take perhaps two chamomile tea enemas daily to gently cleanse the colon. When the diarrhea lets up, the patient could instill one chamomile tea enema, followed four to six hours later with one coffee enema, and another one of chamomile tea at night. When the colon is calmed, the regular schedule may be resumed, but some of the coffee enemas can still be mixed with chamomile tea.

Some flare-ups are extremely intensive and cause a great deal of bile to be released by the liver. This bile could flow over into the stomach. Bile is highly alkaline, but the stomach cannot hold anything that is not maintained in an acid medium. The alkaline bile will therefore bring on immediate severe nausea, almost always accompanied by vomiting. At such times, the patient should omit the coffee enemas, since they simply stimulate more bile flow and more vomiting! Drink a lot of peppermint tea and eat oatmeal gruel. Use only chamomile tea enemas. When the flare-up is overcome and nausea or vomiting has stopped completely, then resume the coffee enemas.

Some patients have problems with a great deal of gas. When there is much pressure from gas, it is difficult to infuse the coffee. At such times, it will probably be necessary to lower the bucket to the patient's body height while prone or even below the patient's body (if he is in bed or on a bench) to allow the fluid to flow back into the bucket while also allowing the gas to bubble out of the rectum. However, if the gas is too high up in the intestinal tract, this approach will not work.

In A *Cancer Therapy* (chapter 27, p. 201), Dr. Gerson discusses some of the problems of flare-ups, including difficulties with the coffee enemas. We already mentioned (see above) that during these unpleasant flaring reactions, patients occasionally have a problem with infusing the enema although previously this procedure went smoothly. The other problem which occurs is that the patient takes an enema, holds it for the optimum twelve minutes, and then goes to release it. But the infused fluid won't release! Such an uncooperative bowel comes from intestinal spasming or cramping, which may not necessarily be accompanied by pain or discomfort. There are several actions the patient can take for a spasming colon:

1. Lie down on the bed, on the right side, legs pulled up, possibly with a warm water bottle on the abdomen.
2. Don't panic.
3. If after a little while, the coffee still cannot be released, take another coffee enema, adding 3 tsp of a 3 percent solution of hydrogen peroxide to the solution.
4. If the spasm still won't release, take castor oil by mouth.
5. For the next few days, put 3 or 4 tsp of the regular potassium compound into each coffee enema. *Do not continue the potassium in the enema for more than a week; otherwise, the colon becomes irritated.*

During the course of this bowel spasming, at no time is there any danger to the patient even if she or he is not able to release the coffee. The entire enema solution is easily absorbed through the colon and excreted through the kidneys and urine if it is not normally released.

There are still other ways to use the Gerson technique of enema therapy. These are not really cleansing enemas, but rather rectal implants. In a few cases, patients during a healing reaction vomit almost everything they take in. They become dehydrated and hypoglycemic. At such times, it is easy to warm the regular carrot or green juices (including the medications) to body temperature and put the 8 ounces of juice into the bucket or bag and let it run into the rectum. (Use only carrot/apple and green juices, *not* orange juice. *Do not add water to the juice.*) This implant should *not* be expelled. Consisting of only 8 ounces, it can easily be held until it is fully absorbed. And instilling with a juice enema may be repeated every hour as the juices are ready. As soon as the patient is able, he or she should start to drink the juices again normally.

Somewhat in the same area, Dr. Gerson also suggested in cases of severe ulcerations of the uterus or cervix to use a douche made up of green juice. This is gently cleansing as well as detoxifying, and the procedure stimulates healing.

Dr. Gerson suggested that enough coffee for a full day's needs can be prepared at one time. In that case, you can prepare a concentrated coffee solution.

HOW TO MAKE COFFEE CONCENTRATE

To concentrate coffee for later use as a dilution, use a fairly large pot and perhaps 2½ to 3 quarts of water. Here is how to make coffee concentrate:

1. When the water boils, add 15 rounded tbsp of organic drip-grind coffee. Since each enema should contain the equivalent of 3 tbsp of coffee, using 15 tbsp will give you enough coffee concentrate for five enemas.
2. Bring the solution back to a boil for a few minutes, then let it simmer for about fifteen minutes and then strain.
3. Divide the resulting concentrate into five equal portions. (You can put equal amounts into five equal 1-quart glass bottles.)
4. Then fill the bottle to the full quart with distilled water for use.
5. If you need to modify the coffee enema with chamomile tea as we have already explained, you can add a pint of tea to the coffee concentrate.
6. Finally, fill up the container with enough water to make a full quart. Before using this mixture, heat it to body temperature.

Reference for Chapter Thirteen

1. Gerson, M. A *Cancer Therapy: Results of Fifty Cases and The Cure of Advanced Cancer by Diet Therapy*, 6th ed. Bonita, Calif.: The Gerson Institute, 1999, p. 190.

Part Three

ADAPTING THE THERAPY FOR VARIOUS DISEASES

Chapter Fourteen

STANDARD GERSON THERAPY FOR MOST CANCERS

In 1984, Alexandra Lennox of Sacramento, California, aged forty-four, divorced and raising three teenagers, was rediagnosed with invasive, intraductal carcinoma of the right breast after a previous lumpectomy. The patient's initial diagnosis leading to the initial lumpectomy had been simpler and less dangerous than it was this second time.

Immediately following her repeat operation for lump removal, the breast surgeon saw that the margins in her cancerous breast tissues were not "clean," meaning that the lumpectomy had not cut away all the cancer. The surgeon therefore suggested that her lymph nodes needed to be examined and proposed to remove her right breast altogether (mastectomy).

A close friend of Mrs. Lennox was able to secure an appointment for her with the chief of the oncology department at Stanford University School of Medicine. After his examination, the oncologist stated in an unemotional and factual manner, "Undoubtedly this condition of yours is a typical two- to ten-year illness. But I don't think that you'll be alive in two years because the disease is so extensive. Get your affairs in order and have the best time you can. And don't worry; we have powerful medications for you when your pain begins."

The doctor's devastating statement about the potential end of her life was not easy to take, for Mrs. Lennox had been facing numerous complications simply living each day. Prior to her diagnosis, for instance, she had been suffering from severe depression, chronic low blood sugar (hypo-

glycemia), severe constant headaches, black floaters in her eyes that disrupted vision, innumerable allergies, candidiasis (numerous symptoms related to the yeast syndrome), kidney stones, and a great deal of emotional
upset—mainly anger after her divorce from an alcoholic husband following seventeen years of marriage. And she worried about her three teenage
children who were using alcohol and drugs—seemingly learned by association with her ex-husband. Unquestionably, there was tremendous mental and emotional stress for this unfortunate woman.

After the breast reexamination and confirmed cancer diagnosis she
made an appointment with another specialist, a radiation oncologist.
While sitting in his office, she was repelled by being in the company of so
many weak, bandaged, severely sick patients who had been pushed along
and were waiting in wheelchairs. The woman couldn't abide the idea of
existing in the same state of ill health, and she walked out of the doctor's
office without actually seeing him.

As she drove home filled with terror, the distraught woman began to
notice that some of the lawns of her neighborhood were of a lively green
color, while others looked brown and sick. It struck her that if the right
lawn food could improve the growth of grass, why should the human body
not also respond in the same way? Mrs. Lennox figured that with excellent
nutrition, she could at least keep going for, perhaps, another five years or
until a cure for cancer might be found. Then, inside her head, she heard a
clear voice that said: "You can feed and nourish your mind and body and
become well again!"

At that point, she sped right past her house to a health food store for
the purpose of becoming educated about nutrition and cancer by the
store proprietor or in any other way available. Noting on the shop's shelves
that there were lots of books on dieting for weight loss, the patient asked
specifically about cancer treatment information. In considering Mrs.
Lennox's situation, the store owner directed her to Dr. Gerson's book *A
Cancer Therapy: Results of Fifty Cases.*

"The Gerson cancer protocol is the hardest therapy to follow but the
best," this natural food store proprietor said. Consequently, this desperate
victim of cancer purchased the book.

The dietary program in Dr. Gerson's text frightened her at first, but
Mrs. Lennox telephoned the Gerson Institute in Bonita, California, and
four days later arrived at a Tijuana, Mexico, hospital that offered medically supervised Gerson Therapy.

She came alone, accompanied by a great deal of negativity voiced in letters and telephone calls from her family. Still, the woman persisted. Over time, laboratory tests showed her steady improvement and eventually she returned to Sacramento to treat herself.

After two years on the Gerson Therapy, Alexandra Lennox finally could consider herself as having succeeded against breast cancer. She had saved both of her breasts and was flourishing. Sexual relationships with men began again. Her girlfriends described her to others as vivacious, verbal, intelligent, and looking "really fabulous." After some two years more, she felt at the peak of her abilities.

SUMMARIZING THE STANDARD GERSON THERAPY FOR DEGENERATIVE DISEASES

What did Mrs. Alexandra Lennox do to restore her health and eliminate cancer as well as her other health problems? Following is a summary of the standard Gerson Therapy for degenerative diseases.

This chapter presents the standard Gerson Therapy protocol being followed by those degenerative disease patients not attempting to cope with treatment complications. The chapter discusses:

- *Why avoid drinking water* when following the Gerson Therapy for eliminating serious health problems;
- *Why take thyroid extract* on a regular basis five times per day;
- *Why take Lugol (potassium iodide, half-strength)* at the rate of eighteen drops per day as cancer therapy;
- *Why drink liquid potassium compound solution*, 4 teaspoonfuls (tsp), ten times per day, representing 2 grams or 50 mEq each of potassium acetate, potassium gluconate, and potassium monophosphate (but not for certain cancer patients);
- *Why consume cold-pressed flaxseed oil*, 1 tablespoonful (tbs) twice daily (with a reduction of this food oil after four weeks to 1 tbs per day);
- *Why follow the juicing procedure* which requires the daily drinking of thirteen 8-ounce glasses of apple/carrot, carrot alone, green leaf, and/or orange juices;
- *Why ingest niacin* in a dose of 50 mg six times per day;
- *Why supplement with porcine pancreatin*, three 325-mg enzyme tablets four times per day;

- *Why receive a crude liver/B$_{12}$ intramuscular injection of 100 mcg B$_{12}$ with 3 cc of crude liver extract each day;*
- *Why take Acidol® (betaine hydrochloride and pepsin), two capsules three times per day before meals;*
- *Why take coenzyme Q$_{10}$, with its variable dosage;*
- *Why take laetrile (amygdalin), useful for all primary cancers but specifically indicated for bone cancer metastases;*
- *Why use Wobe-Mugos® or Megazyme Forte®, the enzymes for counteracting gastrointestinal gas and for reducing tumor masses;*
- *Why take brewer's yeast with both its positive and negative effects (for instance, it's contraindicated for cancer patients);*
- *Why receive five 32-ounce coffee enemas administered daily for a variable period of up to two years;*
- *Why ingest castor oil (orally and rectally) every other day as a treatment;*
- *Why undergo changes in medications within the first year.*

Considered the foundation for the Gerson Therapy, brief sketches of the topics we provide in this chapter only slightly duplicate treatment instructions which have gone before (or may come after). Indeed, this chapter could be considered the pivot for our entire book and likely will be referred to often by readers attempting to help themselves or loved ones conquer degenerative diseases of all types, but most especially the various cancers and leukemias.

THE REASONS FOR AVOIDING WATER AS A BEVERAGE

Usually, the public is told that, in order to maintain body functions at optimum levels, people should drink about eight 8-ounce glasses (64 ounces or 2 quarts) of water daily. On the Gerson Therapy the rules are different. We must study water from a number of angles to understand why this rule changes.

First, when people eat a salty diet, they are naturally thirsty, for our human physiology forces them to drink enough water to hold excess sodium in solution. If it is too concentrated, sodium buildup causes problems in the blood serum as well as in the cells.

The sodium in salt can kill. As reported worldwide, on July 27, 1999,

Leroy Elders, a three-month-old baby boy in Great Britain, died of a salt overdose after his young parents fed him adult food. London newspapers explained that the child's parents fed him oat breakfast cereal and mashed potato with gravy because they found infant food too expensive. After an autopsy, the baby's pediatrician said, "Leroy's body contained nine grams of salt, compared with a recommended daily maximum of seven grams for adult males. The amount of sodium was too high for the baby's kidneys to process, and it poisoned him to death."[1]

Second, another cause of thirst is eating a diet high in animal proteins and fats. The intermediate or end-products of protein and fat digestion are disturbing to the system and cause the person consuming them to feel thirsty. Nutritionists have observed that fruitarians (people who eat only fruit) don't usually become thirsty. Fruit contains natural distilled water and is easily digested without causing any toxic residue; therefore, the body does not require additional liquids.

Dr. Max Gerson prohibited patients on the Gerson Therapy from drinking water for several reasons. First, Gerson patients consume thirteen 8-ounce glasses (225 cc) of freshly squeezed juices each day—a lot of liquid. Second, Gerson patients also eat unsalted soup twice a day, giving them additional liquids. These two particular components of the Gerson Therapy diet add up to about 4 liters of fluid intake daily, which is more than adequate for human needs.

Some patients on the Gerson program, however, still request additional liquids, or they awaken during some nights with the need to drink more fluids. Since ill persons such as these are not allowed to drink water, they should be provided with herbal teas, such as peppermint, orange blossom, linden blossom, and/or tahebo (lapacho or pau d'arco). A quantity of such teas should be stored in a thermos bottle on a night table, right next to the bed. Also, if the patient has difficulty falling to sleep, certain herbs such as valerian make sleep-inducing teas.

Third, Dr. Gerson did not allow patients to drink water because it tends to dilute stomach acid and the gastrointestinal tract's own digestive juices. It is well known that patients suffering from chronic diseases generally are low in gastric acid, which makes it unwise to allow them to drink water. Dr. Gerson observed that if his patients drank water, their digestion suffered, creating gas and other intestinal discomforts. In contrast, if someone already in intestinal distress drinks peppermint tea, it stimulates digestion and relieves gas or other digestive problems.

Please note: All black and/or green teas containing caffeine (similar to coffee) should be considered drugs, and their consumption on the Gerson Therapy is forbidden.

Fourth, the quality of tap water in the United States is often toxic. In fact, fluoridated or chlorinated tap water in more than 60 percent of American cities or larger communities is responsible for illnesses. Chlorine and especially fluorine are highly detrimental substances; both are in the chemical family of the halogens and have similar properties. Fluorine, second in toxicity only to arsenic, is extremely active and can displace the less active elements in the halogen family, chlorine and iodine. Fluorine is a carcinogen and deadly poison foisted on United States residents with support from the American Dental Association.[2,3,4,5]

Fluoride was originally a highly toxic by-product of the aluminum industry. When it was released into the regular sewer system, it killed millions of fish downstream, which eventually led to the prohibition of this practice. From then on, fluoride had to be specially disposed of, a *very* expensive process. The aluminum industry figured out a way to sell the fluoride in large amounts, rather than having to dispose of it, and hit on the idea of adding it to the drinking water. They, in turn, enlisted the American Dental Association to support the idea (this was not the original idea of the ADA).

How Drinking Fluoridated Water Can Damage the Thyroid

Because iodine is an essential element in the body, it's needed by the thyroid gland to produce the hormone thyroxine. This hormone is extremely important since it controls metabolism, the rate at which food is burned. It is also an essential part of the immune system. Thyroxine controls, through body temperature variations, an individual's normal temperature or fever if needed to overcome infection.

When the thyroid gland's function is lowered by the consumption of fluorine (or chlorine) in drinking water, iodine is displaced from the gland. This weakens the immune system. Then a person's physiology is beset by three types of pathology: (1) it's unable to produce fever, (2) allergies and infections result, and (3) food fails to be burned adequately. These three pathologies result in a lack of energy and the storage of calories as excessive fat. As shown, fluoridated and/or chlorinated drinking water becomes the source of such thyroid gland pathology.

Another problem of low thyroid function is the development and de-posit of plaque in the arteries, called arteriosclerosis or hardening of the arteries. This leads to poor blood supply to the heart, the brain, and the extremities. Too often, heart attacks and strokes are the result of arte-riosclerosis. Endocrinologist Broda Barnes, M.D., demonstrated that low thyroid function and heart attacks are directly related. By administering thyroid extract to his affected patients, Dr. Barnes was able to reverse the formation of arteriosclerosis and overcome their difficulties with heart disease.

With similar kinds of disease reversal occurring from the ingestion of thyroid, it becomes obvious why Gerson Therapy patients take thyroid ex-tract on a regular basis five times per day

In the presence of low thyroid function, moreover, cancer rates go up. Many years ago, in certain areas of the United States, it was noted that an unusually high number of people suffered from goiters (Graves' disease). An affected person's body enlarges the thyroid gland in its attempt to help that gland produce more thyroxine.

The reason this problem exists is lack of iodine in the soil and in the diet of people living in those areas. If adequate iodine is supplied, most enlarged glands usually go back to their normal size. It was noted that in these "goiter belts" around the United States there was also a higher can-cer incidence. In an effort to furnish the population in such goiter belt areas with iodine, the U.S. government introduced "iodized salt." Since it is assumed that everybody consumes salt, the bureaucrats' thinking was that this iodine addition to salt would supply the necessary mineral to the entire population. They were right—goiters almost disappeared after the iodizing of salt.

WHY LUGOL'S SOLUTION IS REQUIRED IN THE GERSON THERAPY

But iodized salt presents a new problem: as illustrated earlier by the death of the three-month-old British baby, salt is a damaging and deadly chemical. Dr. Gerson found that the beginning of all chronic disease is marked by the loss of potassium from the cell and the invasion of sodium chloride, the flavoring chemical compound that comprises salt. Salt in-hibits enzyme production at the cellular level. Furthermore, salt promotes excessive cellular mitosis (cell division). In other words, it promotes cancer. Obviously, we must avoid taking in salt, and must obtain the body's needed iodine from other sources.

In order to restore the thyroid and basal metabolism as well as the most important physiological functioning of his patients, the immune system, Dr. Gerson used Lugol's solution, half-strength. Lugol's is a 5 percent solution of potassium iodide, iodine, and water. This enables patients as well as healthy people to obtain iodine without ingesting harmful sodium.

TAKING LIQUID POTASSIUM COMPOUND SOLUTION

Until their blood tests have been analyzed, patients with any history of cardiac insufficiency, episodes of myocardial infarction, transient ischemic attack, or other types of cardiovascular complications should not receive potassium medicinal ingredients. Otherwise, potassium compound solution (a liquid) is recommended for use in the Gerson therapeutic program in an amount of 4 teaspoonfuls (tsp), ten times per day. This dosage represents approximately 3 1/2 grams or 50 mEq each of potassium acetate, gluconate, and monophosphate (a total of 14 grams or 150 mEq/day).

Gerson patients presenting themselves with a history of kidney (renal) insufficiency or dysfunction, gastritis, nausea, significant bone metastasis, or any indication of bleeding problems should be started with just 1 tsp of potassium compound solution ten times a day. Dosages may be slowly increased with the patient maintained under observation by the Gerson Therapy medical adviser.

RIDDING YOUR DRINKING WATER OF FLUORINE AND CHLORINE

In order to maintain the normal thyroid function, it is imperative that healthy persons, and particularly any Gerson Therapy patients, avoid chlorine and fluorine, which damage the thyroid gland. If tap water is chlorinated, the chlorine pollutant can be destroyed by boiling it.

But boiling one's drinking water does not get rid of fluorine's toxic effects. On the contrary, since fluoride is added to water in the form of sodium fluoride, a salt, boiling the water concentrates the fluoride. Some of the water evaporates and less water volume is left to dilute the fluoride salts.

Also, various filter systems are commercially distributed for people who are aware of water pollution or contamination. Unfortunately, the filters remove much, *but not all* of the fluorides. Even a small amount left in the water is harmful and cannot be tolerated by a seriously ill person. Therefore, if tap water is fluoridated, it should be distilled to remove all the fluoride salts and make it acceptable for the Gerson patient. It is also important to use a carbon filter in the water purifier, since certain volatile fractions, such as commercially manufactured benzenes and other solvents, pass through the distillation process.

A number of articles have been published in magazines about the possible danger of drinking distilled water. It is claimed that distilled water "leaches" minerals from the body. Such leaching, if it really does occur, is not a problem. First of all, minerals contained in some spring waters are inorganic minerals and are poorly absorbed (that's why we need to eat plants: they have enzymes that convert the inorganic minerals to an organic form that the human body can easily assimilate). Furthermore, these inorganic minerals are not in good balance; often they contain too much sodium and calcium, along with frankly harmful nitrates and nitrites. In some cases, well-meaning distributors of mineral drinking water and bottled water even add fluorides to their product. That's the wrong thing to do!

It must be emphasized that the body's requirement for minerals should *not* come from drinking water but from fresh fruit, salads, and vegetable juices. These are amply supplied by the Gerson Therapy diet plan.

Now readers may well ask: If Gerson Therapy patients cannot drink water, why worry about its purity? Here are our answers:

1. While it is true that Gerson patients are not allowed to drink water, they are still going to eat soup made with water, drink teas made with water, and cook some vegetables with a minimal amount of water.

2. More important, patients have three to five coffee enemas daily, made with water, of course. These healing enemas are extremely important to help detoxify the liver. But the colon is a highly absorptive organ. Not only is caffeine absorbed from the coffee enemas, but chemical additives in the water are easily absorbed, as well. Water used for enemas should be the purest available.

3. The fluoride molecule is a very small and active molecule and is

passed rapidly not only through the colon into the bloodstream, but also through the skin. The water used for all the needs of the patient, including soup, teas, cooking, internal enemas, and external washing, must be free of chlorine and fluorine as well as other pollutants.

4.   The water must be purified for any internal purpose. Each time the American Dental Association and its members recommend that people ingest fluorine, almost all of us who follow such an erroneous endorsement become poisoned. Water purification can help eliminate this.

WHY COLD-PRESSED FLAXSEED OIL IS INGESTED

Dr. Gerson, in his earlier work with tuberculosis patients and with persons suffering from many other chronic diseases, was very much aware that these people required some essential fatty acids in their diet. Until he discovered that cancer patients could not tolerate any fats, he used raw egg yolks and a little salt-free butter for noncancerous patients. Yet when tumors in his cancer patients disappeared and he wanted to add some oil, egg yolks, or butter to the individuals' nutrition, he found that their cancer returned.

Since other doctors and researchers were not able to observe cured cancer patients, he had no guidance in regard to this cancer regrowth. Dr. Gerson, therefore, had to experiment on his own patients. He selected those ill people who were affected with external cancers (skin malignancies such as inflammatory breast disease), those lesions which were easily observed. Then, cautiously, after tumors had already disappeared, he added one or another nutritional oil to the patient's diet. Invariably, in a relatively short time (a week or two) the already closed or healed lesion would recur, and tumors grew back. As soon as he omitted the food grade oil or fat, the tumors disappeared again.

Dr. Gerson tried every kind of polyunsaturated oil, all of the many monounsaturated oils such as olive oil, plus nut and seed oils, and others. He found none that were safe for the cancer patients during the process of healing and restoring one's body. For this reason he specified in his famous book, A *Cancer Therapy: Results of Fifty Cases*, that "No Fats, No Oils" be used in all the directions for the patient's therapy.[6]

He finally discovered that it took up to eighteen months, well after the patients' essential organs and digestive system were restored, before he could give these patients a little salt-free butter or vegetable oil. Yet he continued to search, since he was well aware of the importance of the essential fatty acids.

Finally, in 1958, after his book was in print, during the last year of his practice and life, Dr. Max Gerson ran across the work of Johanna Budwig, Ph.D., who had also studied essential fatty acids. Dr. Budwig (still living in Germany and a candidate for the Nobel prize in medicine) had found that flaxseed oil (linseed oil) is different from any other dietary fat or oil and is beneficial for the cancer patient without causing any new problems.

By a strange twist of fate, Dr. Gerson remembered that his father's business consisted of pressing flaxseeds. Yet he had never thought of this product for application in his practice. Dr. Gerson then proceeded to try it immediately on his own patients, and he found that, indeed, the flaxseed oil did improve the results of his cancer treatment. Apparently, the fatty acids helped to carry vitamin A (beta carotene) through the bloodstream to increase the patient's immune response. Aside from this, since flaxseed oil is high in linoleic and linolenic acids, these two omega-3 essential fatty acids helped to dissolve atherosclerotic plaque, thus improving blood circulation. In that way, ingesting flaxseed oil provides the sick (or normal) individual with another benefit.

We are fortunate that we are now able to obtain flaxseed oil from organically grown flaxseed, pressed under cooled conditions (since heat damages the oil), bottled in black plastic so that light cannot oxidize the oil, and carefully refrigerated by health food (natural food) store proprietors. Obviously, it is imperative for this oil to be protected from air, light, and heat to keep it from becoming rancid.

This oil is tasty, with a nutlike flavor, in salad dressings, replacing other oils. When freshly produced and promptly shipped, flaxseed oil will keep in the freezer for about six months and in the refrigerator unopened for three months. But once the bottle is opened, even when kept refrigerated, flaxseed oil should be consumed within three weeks. It should *never* be heated, never be used to cook, bake, or fry anything. It is also unwise to use flaxseed oil in hot soup, or on baked potatoes just removed from the oven and steaming hot. A baked potato should be allowed to cool to a comfortable eating temperature before adding the oil. Do not eat flaxseeds themselves, either whole or crushed, but take only the oil, for it is a medication. Compliance by the patient to prescribed dosages (avoiding over- or underuse) is vital for the best healing.[7]

Since Dr. Gerson didn't mention flaxseed oil in his book for the reason given above, there were no other directions for amounts to be used. Fortunately, we found a letter by Dr. Gerson to his great friend, Nobel laureate Albert Schweitzer, in which he describes not only the good results obtained since he applied the flaxseed oil, but the amounts used. Gerson writes that during the first four weeks on the treatment, his patients are alotted 2 tablespoonfuls a day (1 tbs at lunch and 1 at dinner). Then for succeeding months, the amount is reduced to 1 tbs a day. The Gerson Institute still uses this same prescription with good success. In a few patients, the amounts of flaxseed oil have to be adjusted depending on several factors: serum electrolyte tests, HDL and LDL cholesterol levels, and triglyceride levels.

SUPPLEMENTATION WITH NIACIN/NICOTINIC ACID (VITAMIN B₃)

For cancer patients with little or no history of chemotherapy, who have gone through no ostomy or other surgical interventions, supplementation with niacin/nicotinic acid (vitamin B₃) is appropriate. Niacin is an integral part of the Gerson Therapy protocol. Its standard dosage is 50 mg six times per day.

Patients for which this vitamin is absolutely contraindicated are those with a history of bleeding, ulcers, gastritis, and those concurrently receiving prednisone, other steroids, or Coumadin.

Alternatively, patients with liver (hepatic) insufficiency, primary or metastatic tumor activity in the liver, hepatitis of any type (A, B, C, D, or E), or cirrhosis of the liver may receive a maximum of 100 mg to 150 mg of niacin daily.

SUPPLEMENTATION WITH PANCREATIN

Dr. Gerson wrote: "I found pancreatin [pure pancreatic enzyme derived from crude pork pancreas extract from New Zealand] in many cases a valuable help in the therapy. A few patients cannot stand pancreatin; the majority are satisfied to have less digestive trouble with gas spasms and less difficulty in regaining weight and strength. We use the tablets after the detoxification; each contains five grains and is uncoated. The patient takes three or four tablets three times after meals, and later less."[8]

As Dr. Gerson did, complementary and alternative medicine (CAM) physician Michael B. Schachter, M.D., of Suffern, New York, often prescribes oral pancreatic enzymes to be taken with meals to help break down proteins, fats, and carbohydrates.

They also serve a more cancer-specific function. When taken between meals, some of these enzymes are absorbed intact and can have systemic effects that are beneficial to the cancer patient. The actions include an anti-inflammatory effect and a tendency to dissolve the protective coating around cancer cells.[9]

The pancreatic enzymes in pancreatin "digest away the protein coating which protects cancer cells from being destroyed by our immune system," explains CAM physician Robert C. Atkins, M.D., of New York City. In effect, pancreatic enzymes remove the "shield" that otherwise enables cancer cells to protect themselves. "It's fascinating how many of the successful cancer programs that I have studied incorporate pancreatic enzymes," says Dr. Atkins.[10]

TAKING CRUDE LIVER/B$_{12}$ INJECTIONS

It's advantageous for patients with degenerative disease to receive a once-daily intramuscular injection of 100 mcg vitamin B$_{12}$ (cyanocobalamin) with 3 cc of crude liver extract. Unless a patient exhibits excessive blood levels of vitamin B$_{12}$ or has an allergic reaction to B$_{12}$, there is no known contraindication for its use.

SWALLOWING ACIDOL CAPSULES BEFORE MEALS

For patients without complications, two capsules of the combination betaine hydrochloride and pepsin product named Acidol are swallowed three times per day before meals. However, people experiencing gastric ulcers, gastritis, severe nausea, intestinal bleeding, or esophageal problems should not receive Acidol. Patients taking Coumadin concurrently with the Gerson Therapy also should avoid this product.

COENZYME Q_{10} SUPPLEMENTATION

Almost classified as a vitamin, coenzyme Q_{10} is essential for generating energy in the form of adenosine triphosphate (ATP) in living organisms that use oxygen. It's not considered a vitamin, however, because the body produces its own CoQ_{10}.

CoQ_{10} plays a vital role in the physiology's antioxidant system. When combined with vitamin E, selenium, and beta carotene, CoQ_{10} can significantly reduce free radical damage in the liver, kidney, and heart tissues.[11]

The Gerson Institute recommends initially dosing with 90 mg of coenzyme Q_{10} once per day. If no side effects are experienced (primarily tachycardia or arrhythmia), the patient may increase the dosage to 300 mg on the second day and then 600 mg on the third day and thereafter.

THE LEGITIMACY OF SUPPLEMENTING WITH LAETRILE

"After years of observing patients using amygdalin [laetrile], I can say with complete assurance that it is neither toxic nor worthless," says Douglas Brodie, M.D., of Reno, Nevada. "Nor do I find it to be a cure or panacea for cancer. The experience of my clinic, like that of many clinics worldwide, is that amygdalin has the ability to improve the patient's sense of wellbeing, relieve the pain of cancer, and reduce the requirement for pain medication."[12]

Cancer specialist Etienne Callebout, M.D., of London, England, says: "Amygdalin deserves to have a regular place in cancer therapy. It is nontoxic and water-soluble, and there is considerable evidence that it works against cancer."[13]

Laetrile has strong cancer-fighting potential with regard to secondary cancers, including a 60 percent reduction in lung metastases; other research indicates it can extend the lives of both breast and bone cancer patients.[14,15]

The legitimacy of supplementing with laetrile is assured by the success of its ongoing use for cancer these past forty years. Although pain reduction success takes a minimum of ten days to two weeks of daily administration, laetrile is indicated for bone metastases. Dr. Brodie prefers a dosage of 9 grams per intravenous (IV) application. Those not taking IV laetrile who want it may supplement with 500 mg of oral amygdalin three times a day, continuing with this dosage even after the physical evidence of cancer has disappeared.

TAKING WOBE-MUGOS® OR MEGAZYME FORTE®

The two imported German enzymes Wobe-Mugos® and Megazyme Forte® are derived from both vegetable and animal sources. Both of them are protein-digesting (proteolytic) enzymes used defensively against tumors. They contain the enzymatic substances pancreatin, papain, bromelain, trypsin, chymotrypsin, lipase, amylase, and rutin (a bioflavonoid), which are indicated primarily when the sick person suffers from severe, excessive gas.

Some reports advise that these two enzymes are helpful in shrinking malignant masses. Their administration is in the form of injections, tablets, or suppositories. These supplements offer the degenerative diseased patient an enhancement of whole-body metabolism.

CAUTION IN TAKING BREWER'S YEAST

Originally Dr. Max Gerson had made brewer's yeast a part of his therapeutic program, but that was long before the advent of *Candida albicans* infection, which brings about the yeast syndrome. And it had been introduced by him as treatment for cancer patients prior to his use of liver juice.

Under most circumstances today, brewer's yeast is seldom recommended any longer for cancer therapy owing to an ever-increasing risk of candidiasis, which brings on extreme abdominal distension and gas. Little clinical benefit has been observed from taking brewer's yeast.

In cancer patients, negative responses have been noted after ingestion of brewer's yeast, and it is speculated that the substance is no longer as effective as in Dr. Gerson's day. That's because cancer patients have undergone an increase in their acidity; thus, brewer's yeast is not for them. They seem to have a much greater presence of the pathological candida organisms in their bodies because of dietary changes and other environmental factors.

COFFEE ENEMAS ARE HIGHLY RECOMMENDED

As advised in chapters 12 and 13, five 32-ounce enemas made with coffee beverge are highly recommended for patients suffering from degenerative diseases. They should be taken each day in slowly diminishing numbers for a variable period of up to two years. Each coffee enema helps to purge the colon and liver of accumulated toxins, dead cells, and waste products.

The coffee enema is prepared by brewing organic caffeinated beans and letting the brew cool to body temperature, then delivering it via an enema bag. Coffee contains choleretics, substances that increase the flow of toxin-rich bile from the gallbladder. The coffee enema is probably the only pharmaceutically effective choleretic noted in the medical literature that can be safely used many times daily without toxic effects.[16]

Dr. Gerson recognized early in his therapeutic approach that the coffee enema is effective in stimulating a complex enzyme system involved in liver detoxification, which we described in some of our prior chapters as the *glutathione S-transferase enzyme system*. The increased activity of these enzymes ensures that free radical activity is greatly diminished and that the pathology-producing actions of carcinogens are blocked.[17]

Caffeine additionally stimulates dilation of blood vessels and relaxation of smooth muscles, which further increases bile flow; this effect does not happen when the coffee is consumed daily. In fact, the only beneficial way to ingest coffee is through the rectum.

ROUTINE CASTOR OIL TREATMENT

In following the Gerson Therapy, the application of castor oil treatment is routine. Dr. Gerson recommended its use by mouth and by enema for the elimination of toxic diarrhea, vomiting of bile, and other strong reactions. He wrote, "These strong reactions are actually indications of the beginning of improvement, with increased bile production, greater activity of the liver and elimination of toxins and poisons. After a period of one or two days, patients feel greatly relieved, show better circulation, complexion and color, and have more appetite."[18]

Tumors and cysts of all sizes may also be reduced in volume or eliminated altogether with the application of castor oil packs. In an examination of the immune-stimulating properties of castor oil packs conducted on thirty-six people, those receiving the packs showed significant improvement in the total production of lymphocytes and other immune cells.[19]

Changing Medications within the First Year of Treatment

Approximately one month after discharge from inpatient treatment (about six to nine weeks after admission to a Gerson hospital and start of therapy), thyroid, potassium, and Lugol medications are reduced. Other supplements are generally kept at initial levels. Potassium is typically dropped from 40 tsp per day to 20 tsp per day. Thyroid is lowered to between 2 and 3 grains per day. Lugol is reduced to six drops per day.

Often these medication levels are maintained for nine to fourteen months, and other supplemental adjustments will be based on diagnostic blood work and other means of diagnosis. This is a change in protocol from Dr. Gerson's original presentation in his book as produced more than forty years ago. Instead, patients must now be kept on higher dosages of the three main medications for longer periods than in Dr. Gerson's day. When medications are reduced too rapidly, sick people often experience difficulties and a slowing of recovery or a recurrence of disease.

The standard Gerson Therapy is strictly for uncomplicated cancer or other degenerative disease patients. Modifications from the program occur when chemotherapy is used before this natural and nontoxic protocol is instituted. Unfortunately, it becomes more difficult to treat the patient, as is explained in chapter 15.

References for Chapter Fourteen

1. Nordwall, S.P. "Salt poisoning." *USA Today*. July 28, 1999, p. 6A.
2. Cousins, G. "Health today." *New Frontier*. May 1994.
3. Valerian, V. "On the toxic nature of fluorides, part 2: fluorides and cancer." *Perceptions*. September/October 1995, pp. 30–37.
4. Glasser, G. "Dental fluorosis: a legal time bomb." *Health Freedom News*. July 1995, pp. 40–45.
5. Yiamouyiannis, J. *Fluoride: The Aging Factor*. Delaware, Ohio: Health Action Press, 1993, p. 61.

6. Gerson, M. A *Cancer Therapy: Results of Fifty Cases and The Cure of Advanced Cancer by Diet Therapy: A Summary of Thirty Years of Clinical Experimentation*, 5th ed. Bonita, Calif.: The Gerson Institute, 1990, p. 242.

7. *The Gerson Therapy Physician's Training Manual*. Bonita, Calif.: The Gerson Institute, 1996, p. 114.

8. *Op. cit.*, Gerson, M., pp. 211, 212.

9. Diamond, W.J.; Cowden, W.L.; Goldberg, B. *An Alternative Medicine Definitive Guide to Cancer*. Tiburon, California: Future Medicine Publishing, Inc., 1997, p. 375.

10. *Ibid.*, pp. 35, 36.

11. Leibovitz, B., et al. "Dietary supplements of vitamin E, beta carotene, coenzyme Q_{10}, and selenium protect tissues against lipid peroxidation in rat tissue slices." *Journal of Applied Nutrition*. 120:97–104, 1990.

12. *Op. cit.*, Diamond, W.J.; Cowden, W.L.; Goldberg, B., pp. 78, 79.

13. *Ibid.*, p. 110.

14. Nowicky, J.W. "New immunostimulating anticancer preparation: Ukrain." *Proceedings of the 13th International Congress of Chemotherapy*. Vienna, Austria, August 28–September 2, 1983.

15. Nowicky, J.W., et al. "Ukrain as both an anticancer and immunoregulatory agent." *Drugs under Experimental and Clinical Research*. XVIII: Supplement, pp. 51–54, 1992.

16. Lam, L.K.T., et al. "Isolation and identification of kahweol palmitate and cafestol palmitate as active constituents of green coffee beans that enhance glutathione-S-transferase activity in the mouse." *Cancer Research*. 42:1193–1198, 1982.

17. Hildenbrand, G. "How the Gerson therapy heals." *Gerson® Healing Newsletter*. 6:3/4, 1990.

18. *Op. cit.*, Gerson, M., p. 81.

19. Biser, L. "Study indicates castor oil improves immune system." *The Layman's Course on Killing Cancer*. Charlottesville, Va.: University of Natural Healing, 1992, p. 6.

Chapter Fifteen

MODIFIED THERAPY DURING CHEMOTHERAPY

In 1996, forty-six-year-old F.C., a housewife and piano teacher, underwent a mammogram followed by an ultrasound diagnostic procedure in her hometown of Stockport. To complete her evaluation for breast cancer, she had a needle biopsy, which showed an infiltrating carcinoma measuring 2.5 centimeters (cm). In the course of the subsequent mastectomy, fifteen lymph nodes were removed, fourteen of which proved to be malignant. X-ray examination also showed that the cancer had spread to her lungs.

Her doctors ordered chemotherapy, and a twelve-treatment protocol was initiated and scheduled to last a complete year. The cytotoxic agents planned for her are known to be exceedingly aggressive and tend to accumulate in the patient's body tissues.

In the course of each month's series of chemo treatments, Mrs. C. became so ill, with unbearable nausea and vomiting lasting over multiple days and nights, that she seldom slept and hardly ate. The woman dropped pounds of lean muscle mass steadily. She says, "I couldn't tell you the horror of it." Of course, she also became totally bald.

The chemotherapy seriously reduced her white blood count too, causing an extreme depletion of white blood cells (neutropenia), indicating that her immune system had been devastated. Since neutrophils are an important part of the immune system, their complete suppression caused the patient to suffer multiple types of severe infections. Pneumonia, cold sores, and other illnesses immediately followed each one of the separate monthly chemotherapy courses.

In order to preserve her life by controlling the infections, Mrs. C. had to be admitted to the hospital after each set of treatments. This situation became critical and the doctors were forced to stop the chemotherapies after F.C. had received only nine courses of the proposed twelve. Her lungs were not improved. Cancer remained as before and she was sent home classified as "terminal" with no further treatment available.

From a local naturopath, this dying cancer patient, whose severe illness had been complicated by the cytotoxic agents, learned that the Gerson Therapy had won cancer battles. In March 1997, Mrs. C. arrived at the Gerson treatment facility in Tijuana, Mexico. She writes, "I felt immediately that this Gerson Hospital was a place of healing."

But for this particular ill woman, detoxification was not easy. She had ongoing severe reactions to the prior chemotherapy with a lot of nausea and continuing vomiting. Gradually, however, the Gerson Therapy did work and pulled the accumulated poisons out of her body.

It took Mrs. C. several months to overcome the damage done by her chemo treatment, experiencing about six months of attacks or flare-ups of symptoms from chemicals lingering in the body. Such healing reactions are commonly observed in most patients who have received the cumulative poisons of cytotoxic agents.

About eight months into her Gerson Therapy regimen at home, the patient finally felt much better. At that time, her friends said she looked much healthier, and her demeanor actually became cheerful and vivacious. She still struggled with occasional rushes of nausea, yet she marveled at the transformation in her health.

Previously, upon her discharge from the Gerson Hospital, Mrs. C.'s X-ray films, after she had been on her new dietary program for three weeks, had shown such vast improvement that there was no further lung and breast tumor growth. The cancers remained static in size. Also, the woman remarked then that "spiritually and emotionally I am doing the right thing."

With the passage of a year on the Gerson Therapy, the patient's healing reactions were still coming occasionally from the prior chemotherapy. She writes, "Many times my sense was that I was going through an internal storm, with periods of calm coming on." But it's all turning out right for F.C. She reports that "now, my skin is glowing, my memory is improved, my hair has grown back thick, and it shows beautiful texture without conditioner."

One of the infections that had struck during the courses of chemotherapy was a fungal growth of her toenails, especially of the big toes. Over a period of months on the Gerson Therapy, those fungal areas grew out and she has normal toenails once again. She says, "Seeing the new and clean toenails, I believe they indicate that my immune system is improving. Also, the varicose veins in my left leg are coming down and no longer stick out."

During the six-month healing reaction she went through in late 1997, her skin did show shades of gray coloring and she was again vomiting violently with nausea so severe it kept her from sleeping. Mrs. C. explained, "This was a situation very similar to what I experienced immediately after receiving chemotherapy when I was so sick." Now the stored chemicals were leaving her body, but their poisoning effects continued to make her ill as they emptied out.

Mrs. C. also describes that six-month flare-up as seeming as if flu had invaded, but she found that this healing reaction marked the turning point in her conquering of cancer. The woman's outlook became much more positive. "The Gerson Therapy not only heals mankind, but heals the environment," she told us.

F.C. is not yet fully recovered from the chemotherapy she had received. This former cancer patient who has beaten back the tumors is more than twenty-six months into the treatment and still experiences occasional healing reactions. We are reporting her story because the Gerson Institute is frequently asked if there are recovered cancer patients who had been treated with chemotherapy. We do tell such patients that it takes longer to come back to good health after chemo—but with perseverance, it is entirely possible. Mrs. C. may be considered typical of how one can overcome breast cancer with metastases to the lungs even in the face of having undergone exceedingly aggressive cytotoxic chemotherapy. This chapter is dedicated to just such immune-compromised patients who have undergone chemotherapy.

What Chemotherapy Is and What It Does

The *chemo* part of *chemotherapy* means that chemicals are involved with some process or procedure, and *-therapy* indicates that the procedure is being applied as "treatment." Therefore, the *chemotherapy* term simply advises that the cancer treatment being applied employs chemicals (drugs).

Such chemicals administered as drugs destroy the cancer cells that they reach, either by interfering with cellular growth or by preventing them from reproducing. The various drugs work in different ways to interrupt each cancer cell's life cycle. Some affect the malignant cell during one or more of its phases of growth and offer no adverse effect on the cell during the other phases; other drugs affect the cell throughout its whole cycle of life.[1]

The oncologist's idea is to use chemotherapy as a main means for lowering the multiplication of cancer cells or to destroy them altogether. It would be ideal if a drug being administered spared healthy cells while destroying the deadly ones; however, nearly every cancer chemotherapeutic agent destroys tissue cells—pathological or physiological, sick or well, mutagenic or homeostatic. Almost all of the chemotherapeutic agents in an oncologist's armamentarium are cytotoxic, with *cyto* referring to any cell and *toxic* pointing to poison.

These cytotoxic drugs go back to the 1940s when an observation at the Yale University School of Medicine recognized that the potent World War I gas nitrogen mustard had produced selective damage to the lymphatic system and bone marrow of soldiers. This property, it was surmised, could be useful as treatment against malignancies. Consequently, the first successful application of chemotherapy took place at Yale in the mid-1940s with personnel of that university adapting mustard gas as a method of cancer management. From this practice, alkylating agents were created as cytotoxic therapy. The primary traits of alkylating agents, such as cyclophosphamide, melphalan, and chlorambucil, are that they link up with and destroy normal components of all cells, mainly their DNA (deoxyribonucleic acid) genetic material.[2]

As with all tissue cells in plants and animals, human cancer cells possess DNA. In fact, "cancer" is what happens when a part of one's body grows in an uncontrollable fashion and damages other healthy parts simply because a single group of cells grows and multiplies in a disorderly and uncontrolled manner. So cancer is a condition in which an abnormal body cell mutates and multiplies uncontrollably.[3]

The reason that cellular growth irregularity occurs is that the DNA of one type of cell becomes able to disobey or escape from the control mechanisms that usually keep it growing in a normal, orderly way. The key to understanding the nature of cancer is to find out what normally keeps the

DNA in order and how some cells' DNA are able to escape from regimentation. If medical scientists possessed such knowledge, they would understand what causes cancer, which might help all of us work out how to prevent it.[4]

Not fully knowing the real reason for malignant disease to develop, any of us experiencing tumor growth would benefit by personally applying the standard Gerson Therapy. This will be the case unless a person's immune system has been compromised by pretreatment with the cytotoxic agents of chemotherapy. Then, a lessened or reduced Gerson protocol has to be followed.

THE REDUCED GERSON PROTOCOL FOR CYTOTOXIN-PRETREATED PATIENTS

As we are about to discuss in detail the Gerson Therapy as it relates to cancer patients who have gone through extensive chemotherapy, this chapter is another pivotal portion of our book. Numbers of people who suffer from cancer do expose themselves to chemotherapy as a first resort when it probably should be among the last treatment procedures followed. Be aware that chemotherapy further degrades an already impaired immune system. Note: all cytotoxic drugs are carcinogens: they will *cause* future cancer.

In self-administering the Gerson Therapy, its medication protocol for any chemotreated patients is different from the standard protocol. For instance, the medication quantity varies considerably, and no absolute guidelines may be given. Yet general information can be offered here about a reduced or less intensive cancer protocol. The number of courses of cytotoxic treatment, their dosages, and the specific drugs received must be considered. That's because use of the full, unmodified Gerson protocol can be extremely dangerous for cancer patients who have gone through extensive pretreatment with cytotoxic agents.

The following discussion of the reduced Gerson Therapy protocol is specific for chemotherapy-exposed patients. Acting on such knowledge will help them to respond more quickly and experience better long-term recoveries from their cancers. Otherwise, a few uninformed cancer patients could self-medicate with the more aggressive Gerson protocol we described in chapter 14, which could inhibit their long-term recovery.

For someone ill with cancer, increasing the odds for survival and eventual wellness will occur more quickly and efficiently by following certain admonitions put forth by the Gerson Institute. These particular rules and recommendations are the result of more than fifty years of experience and patient feedback with its use.

Damaged Physical Conditioning After Chemotherapy

Everyone must realize that any form of chemotherapy is a precursor to damaging the physical conditioning of all individuals who take in cytotoxic agents of any kind. That's because the chemotherapeutic drugs enter the bloodstream either directly by intravenous injection or indirectly by absorption through the stomach or intestinal mucosa, after which the drugs are supposedly transported to wherever tumor cells may be thriving. Administering chemical treatment certainly is different from surgery and radiotherapy, which concentrate their effects on some specific part or region of the body. Chemotherapy is used when there is the possibility that cancer cells may be deposited in other places besides the primary tumor, or may be circulating throughout the body via the bloodstream.[5]

As we showed in earlier chapters, chemotherapy seldom allows a five-year survival of ("cures") cancer—less than 15 percent of the time for all malignancies. It may temporarily stop irregular cellular growth, or the drug given may relieve pain and allow life to continue somewhat longer.[6] But, in our opinion chemotherapy as a first recourse is a mistake. Rather, it should be employed as a last resort if other, more gentle treatments have failed.

Over sixty-five commercially available cytotoxic drugs are employed in cancer chemotherapy, and an equal number are being tested right now in clinical trials. Some chemotherapeutic agents produce minor difficulties in the form of adverse side effects such as sleepiness, general fatigue, diarrhea, hair loss, sore mouth, low blood counts, nausea, and vomiting. These are the immediate side effects most often known because a cancer patient experiences them openly and obviously.

What's rarely discussed between oncologist and patient, however, are the other, more serious extra effects which are residual, long-lasting, and have deeper ramifications for one's deteriorated quality of life.

The pretreated chemicalized patient is frequently left in a severely weakened physical condition. Such a weakness arises from causing (1) depressed numbers of blood components which carry oxygen and other nourishment to the cells, (2) various cell mutations, which may finally produce the secondary cancers which are common occurrences, (3) the acceleration of tumor growth rather than shrinkage, (4) deep-seated poisonings of vital tissues unlikely to recover unless the anticancer chemicals are detoxified from the cells of those damaged tissues.

These manifestations of physical weakness are major side effects rarely discussed, but are the chief reasons to avoid taking chemotherapy with cytotoxic drugs.

Even if the patient remains in good physical condition after undergoing chemotherapy, here is a brief discussion of those adverse side effects mentioned:

1. Low Blood Counts

Prolonged depressed numbers of blood components arising from chemotherapy lead to physical weakness, mental lethargy, chronic fatigue, spiritual lassitude, emotional depression, and outright prostration. For instance, a reduced number of white blood cells leaves the individual who has undergone chemotherapy with a vulnerability to infection. The avoidance of anyone suffering from a cold or flu therefore becomes absolutely mandatory. Also, the resulting low platelet count from chemotherapy leads to easy bruising and bleeding. Subsequently, the patient must take care to avoid cuts, burns, or injuries and should steer clear of aspirin, alcohol, and other blood thinners. Sometimes, if the person's platelet numbers drop exceedingly low, transfusions may become necessary.[7]

2. Cell Mutations

Some years after chemotherapy has been received, patients may develop secondary cancers such as acute leukemia. The International Agency for Research on Cancer (IARC) has identified twenty different commonly used anticancer agents which actually are powerful carcinogens in their own right.[8,9] Such cancer-causing occurrences are frequently associated with two particular popular commercial alkylating agents, Cytoxan™ and Alkeran™, as well as almost all of the hormonelike anticancer chemicals. Combinations of these deadly drugs given to patients as a "cocktail" are even worse in their residual cancer aftereffects.

In his respected medical text *Cancer: Principles and Practice of On-*

cology, the staunch chemotherapy advocate Leonard DeVita, M.D., admits to the cancer-promoting properties of cytotoxic drugs. Dr. DeVita states: "Chemotherapy combinations can significantly raise the risk of secondary tumors, especially nonlymphocytic leukemias. The combination of cyclophosphamide, lomustine, and vincristine [three cytotoxins] lead to a leukemia incidence of 14 percent over four years after treatment. Nitrogen mustard, vincristine, prednisone, and procarbazine for the treatment of Hodgkin's disease yield leukemia rates up to 17 percent.... Radiation further increases the risk of leukemia."

3. Acceleration of Tumor Growth

As a direct result of coming in contact with the very chemotherapeutic agents which supposedly will shrink malignant tumors, sometimes the tumors are accelerated in their growth. The cells which make up their structures become seemingly drug-resistant and, in a paradox of purpose, are enhanced in their ability to expand and metastasize. Clinical studies on patients and laboratory investigations on animals have proven this paradox.[10,11]

4. Deep-seated Toxicity

Chemotherapy causes the tissues to undergo complex reactions from the body's attempt to detoxify itself. Cytotoxic agents are the ultimate pollutants, regarded as waste materials by the body, and the metabolism wants to release such waste from its internal environment. During the course of this process, both subclinical and obvious health problems develop internally.

The body organs protest the presence of medical poisons in several ways: (1) by compromised functioning of the liver; (2) by development of an ongoing diarrhea to flush out irritrating bile; (3) by cramping pain in the lower abdomen; (4) by flatulence and gas; and (5) by other general systemic symptoms manifested as periodic flulike feelings of headaches, perspiration, strong body odor, weakness, dizziness, fainting spells, intestinal spasms, and muscular aches and pains.

These discomforts are indications of deep-seated poisons lodged within the tissues from cytotoxics. They are poisonous reactions that show up subtly but repeatedly. Once the cytotoxins are cleaned out by use of the Gerson Therapy, these poisonings flare up as what the Gerson Institute personnel describe as "healing reactions," similar to those described earlier by F.C.

CHEMOTHERAPY PRETREATMENT WITHOUT EXPERIENCING WEAKNESS

We have stated that all chemotherapy is toxic; however, symptoms and signs of resulting physical weakness do not necessarily show up in all cases. Subclinical dysfunctions will likely be present from a patient's receiving toxic chemicals, but obvious signs of such dysfunctions may remain unrecognized. And this set of circumstances brings us to a situation of chemotherapy pretreatment without the patient's experiencing any weakness.

A patient who accepts the Gerson Therapy after having undergone pretreatment with synthetic chemicals and drugs may have avoided experiencing physical weakness. This chapter therefore advises how he or she can proceed in the Gerson Therapy. The drug-treated person blessed with an absence of outward adverse effects will have retained a normal appetite, remained ambulatory, and resisted extreme weight loss. We're describing a truly lucky individual.

Even so, anyone fitting such a description should be receiving the reduced Gerson protocol discussed in the balance of this chapter. The number of courses of chemotherapy, dosages, and specific toxic drugs received must be considered by the patient and any health professional advising on the Gerson Therapy. Pursuing the full, unmodified Gerson protocol for any patient who has undergone chemotherapy, regardless of the time elapsed since the last treatment, can be extremely dangerous.

From the experiences of Gerson Institute personnel, we know that chemotherapy pretreated patients respond more quickly and go through much better long-term recovery when they follow the "reduced" or modified Gerson protocol. Medicating with any aspect of the usual, more aggressive protocol will be done at the expense of safety and long-term recovery. Consequently, we warn that those patients having cancers complicated by chemotherapy should follow the reduced Gerson Therapy program described below.

THE REDUCED GERSON PROTOCOL FOR CHEMICALLY TREATED PATIENTS

Any person suffering from one or more degenerative diseases (with cancer definitely among them) with a medical history of chemotherapy should follow the following modified Gerson Therapy protocol.[12] For example, as described in A *Cancer Therapy: Results of Fifty Cases*, by Max Gerson, M.D., drinking fresh-squeezed organic juices is a potent source of nourishment and an exceedingly powerful detoxifying tool.[13] Consuming juice is therefore done in a different way for the cancer patient pretreated with chemicals.

Juice Consumption

For a cancer patient who has been chemicalized with toxic drugs, it's advisable to start the juicing regimen with only 2 to 4 ounces of fresh-squeezed vegetable or fruit juice. At the beginning of the juicing procedure, because of its strong efficacy, temporarily eliminate the three recommended carrot-only juices.

And the dosage for any of the juices will vary depending on the patient's condition, the ability to tolerate such juices, and any potential side effects which result. If the patient can tolerate the smaller amount of juice, the juice quantities are increased after two or three days. Typically, from 2 to 4 ounces, or four to six ounces at a time, will be imbibed, and eventually, after seven to ten days, progress will be made toward acceptance of the full 8-ounce portions. Finally, the three carrot juices each day may be reintroduced to the chemicalized patient.

Care must be taken to ensure that the patient continues to tolerate all juices without significant nausea or other side effects. If side effects do appear, cut back on the doses of juice.

We recommend that patients should stay with the schedule of juice drinking as follows: Each day it is best to ingest (a) one orange juice, (b) four green leaf juices, (c) five apple/carrot juices, and (d) three carrot juices. To reduce nausea and increase juice-drinking tolerance, add gruel to the juice up to a 50 percent volume.

Potassium Compound Solution (Liquid)

The suggested starting dosage for potassium compound solution is 1 tsp ten times per day, which represents approximately 500 mg or 12.5 mEq each of potassium (K) acetate, gluconate, and monophosphate. This is a total K combination of 1.5 grams or 37.5 mEq/day.

In patients experiencing good condition despite chemotherapy, the normal dosage of 4 tsp ten times per day may be cautiously achieved in several steps over seven to ten days' treatment, if no adverse side effects are observed. Those patients in less than ideal condition should have the dosage increased to 2 tsp ten times daily, then carefully observed, very slowly increasing the dosage to 3, and then 4, tsp ten times per day, as the patient is able to tolerate it.

There are contraindications to K compound solution: Patients presenting themselves with a history of renal insufficiency or generalized kidney dysfunction, gastritis, nausea, significant bone metastases, or any indication of bleeding problems should be started with 1 tsp ten times per day. Dosage may be slowly increased with observation of the compound's effects. Anyone with a history of cardiac insufficiency, myocardial infarction, or congestive heart failure should *not* receive potassium until blood laboratory work has been analyzed by a physician.

Lugol (Potassium Iodide, KI, Half-Strength

The recommended dose of Lugol is six drops per day. However, there are contraindications to taking Lugol for chemo-pretreated patients. Futhermore, if the individual has a history of allergy to iodine, Lugol is also not indicated, at least initially; it can be cautiously added after three to five days, one drop to start, then increasing as tolerance allows.

Patients with hepatic (liver) insufficiency, primary or metastatic tumor activity in the liver, hepatitis, or hepatic cirrhosis should be started on one to two drops of Lugol per day, to avoid bleeding or a decrease in blood platelets. Those patients with bone metastases should also receive reduced Lugol to avoid excessive bone deterioration and pain. Any patients known to be affected by heavy metal toxicity should additionally receive doses of one to two drops per day initially.

Thyroid

Thyroid hormone is taken in a 1-grain dosage once or twice per day, but there are contraindications to thyroid usage similar to those for Lugol. Watch for signs of hyperthyroidism, including tachycardia, anxiety, insomnia, and tremors. Reduce dosage levels if any of these signs and symptoms are present. Also note that transient tachycardia alone can be a toxic or flare-up reaction. Patients with a history of cardiac insufficiency or other cardiac problems should be started on a maximum of 2 grains of thyroid daily.

Niacin

This vitamin B_3 nutrient has a dosage of 50 mg six times per day. Some contraindications do exist, such as for patients who present with hepatic insufficiency, primal or metastatic tumor activity in the liver, hepatitis, or hepatic cirrhosis. These patients should receive a maximum of 100 to 150 mg of niacin daily. Those with a medical history of bleeding, ulcers, or gastritis, or who are concurrently receiving prednisone, other steroids, or coumadin should not receive niacin.

Pancreatin

This pancreatic enzyme from the pig allows for a dosage of three 325-mg tablets taken four times a day. It is contraindicated for sarcoma patients.

Crude Liver/B_{12} Injection

This is taken once daily as an intramuscular injection in a dose of 100 mcg of vitamin B_{12} with 3 cc of crude liver extract. Other than producing excessive levels of vitamin B_{12}, and occasional allergic reactions, there is no known contraindication for the crude liver/B_{12} injection.

Acidol

The gastrointestinal enzyme product known as Acidol (betaine hydrochloride and pepsin) is taken in a dose of two capsules daily, three times a day before meals. There are contraindications to this digestive aid consisting of gastric ulcers, gastritis, severe nausea, intestinal bleeding, or esophageal problems. Patients with these difficulties and those taking Coumadin should not receive Acidol.

Coenzyme Q_{10}

While not a vitamin, coenzyme Q_{10} has vitaminlike properties. The initial dosage is 90 mg once per day. If no side effects in the form of tachycardia or arrhythmia arise, on the second day increase the dosage to 300 mg daily, and on the third day increase the dose to 600 mg. Remain at that higher dosage thereafter.

Wobe-Mugos and Megazyme Forte

These gastrointestinal enzymes are indicated primarily when the patient suffers from severe, excessive gas. Some reports also indicate that the enzymes may be helpful in reducing tumor masses.

Laetrile

Laetrile, known generically as amygdalin, is indicated for the treatment of bone metastases, and it may be useful in the treatment of lung cancers. When laetrile is available, it is primarily used to reduce pain levels, generally effective ten days to two weeks after initial daily administration. The dosage is 3 grams (5 cc) intravenously once per day.

Brewer's Yeast

This type of food yeast derived from the brewing of beer is not recommended under most circumstances because of the risk of the yeast syndrome (candidiasis) developing or worsening. Also, many people taking brewer's yeast report extreme abdominal distension and gas.

Castor Oil Treatment

This plant oil is contraindicated in patients who have undergone chemotherapy. Even so, castor oil treatment may be applicable to chemo patients after six to nine months on the Gerson Therapy. Yet it should be taken with great caution inasmuch as extremely toxic side effects can occur from the body's resulting elimination of chemotherapy residues. Castor oil is a powerful detoxifier, and long-buried cytotoxicity can come out of the tissues. Such a release may produce severe healing reactions.

Coffee Enemas

As we have described in detail, coffee enemas are taken by chemo-pretreated patients in the amount of a 32-ounce enema two to three times per day. In some people, this dosage will be reduced to half strength by mixing 16 ounces of chamomile tea with 16 ounces of coffee. The enema dosage may gradually be increased as needed, but care must be taken not to overstimulate the liver and cause extremely toxic side effects from elimination of the chemotherapy residues lodged within the body.

FOLLOW-UP THERAPY FOR THE CHEMO-PRETREATED CANCER PATIENT

Follow-up therapy is required on this reduced Gerson protocol. Changes in the medications will be made during the first year of treatment. For instance, approximately one month after discharge from the inpatient treatment center (probably six to nine weeks after admission to the Gerson hospital and start of the Gerson Therapy), thyroid, potassium, and Lugol medications are adjusted. If the patient has been on extremely reduced levels, these medications may be increased by 25 to 50 percent. Other supplements are generally kept at initial levels.

If the patient was receiving normal levels of the Gerson protocol (e.g., 40 tsp of potassium and eighteen drops of Lugol), these medication levels are reduced by approximately 50 percent. The adjusted medication levels are generally maintained for nine to fourteen months. Supplemental adjustments are often made based on the diagnostic blood work and other diagnostic means.

Note that this follow-up protocol differs significantly from the information in Dr. Gerson's original book "A Cancer Therapy." Patients must now be kept on higher dosages of the three main medications for longer periods than in Dr. Gerson's day. When medications are reduced too rapidly (such as scheduled in A *Cancer Therapy*), patients often have difficulties and experience a slowing of recovery or a recurrence of disease.

For those special patients who have undergone chemotherapy before undertaking the Gerson Therapy, following the instructions in this chapter will ensure health improvement and potential recovery from disease.

References for Chapter Fifteen

1. Morra, M.; Potts, E. *Choices: Realistic Alternatives in Cancer Treatment.* New York: Avon Books, 1980, pp. 174, 175.

2. Moss, R.W. *Questioning Chemotherapy.* Brooklyn, N.Y.: Equinox Press, 1995, p. 173.

3. Bognar, D. *Cancer: Increasing Your Odds for Survival.* Alameda, Calif.: Hunter House, 1998, p. 10.

4. Buckman, R. *What You Really Need to Know about Cancer.* Baltimore: The Johns Hopkins University Press, 1997, p. 9.

5. *Op. cit.*, Morra, M.; Potts., E., p. 176.

6. *Ibid.*

7. Dollinger, M.; Rosenbaum, E.H.; Cable, G. *Everyone's Guide to Cancer Therapy*, rev. 3rd ed. Kansas City, Mo.: Andrews McMeel Publishing, 1997, p. 67.

8. Ludlum, D.B. "Therapeutic agents as potential carcinogens." In *Chemical Carcinogenesis and Mutagenesis*, ed. by P.L. Grover; C.S. Cooper, Berlin, Germany: Springer-Verlag, 1990, pp. 153–175.

9. Marselos, M.; Vainio, H. "Carcinogenic properties of pharmaceutical agents evaluated in the IARC monographs programme." *Carcinogenesis*. 12:1751–1766, 1991.

10. Houston, S.J., et al. "The influence of adjuvant chemotherapy on outcome after relapse in patients with breast cancer." *Proceedings of the Annual Meeting of the American Society of Cancer Oncologists*. 11:A108, 1992.

11. "Side glance: laboratory-bred mice." *Journal of the National Cancer Institute*. 87:248, 1995.

12. *Gerson™ Therapy Practitioner's Training Seminar Workbook*. Bonita, Calif.: The Gerson Institute, 1996.

13. Gerson, M. A *Cancer Therapy: Results of Fifty Cases and The Cure of Advanced Cancer by Diet Therapy: A summary of thirty years of Clinical Experimentation*. Bonita, Calif.: The Gerson Institute, 1999.

Chapter Sixteen

MODIFIED THERAPY FOR SEVERELY WEAKENED CANCER PATIENTS

From Montreal, Quebec, Canada, Joergon van Zsidy, M.D., N.D., wants people to know that he is a recovered liver cancer survivor. Dr. van Zsidy entered the Gerson therapeutic program on his own when he was in the most weakened state of his former degenerative illness. He's in great shape now, but during that terrible time for him, Dr. van Zsidy affirms, "I was just short of death and sicker than anyone could ever imagine experiencing. Unquestionably, the Gerson Therapy saved my life and it's still working for me today."

In 1988, Dr. van Zsidy, a former practicing psychiatrist in the Netherlands, but currently a naturopathic physician and university professor working in Montreal, Quebec, Canada, noticed his prolonged, extreme tiredness and energy lack—what is now recognized and referred to as *chronic fatigue syndrome*. Simultaneously and close on the heels of his fatigue, Dr. van Zsidy developed the additional discomforts of itchy spots over the length of his body, depression, severe headaches, and nausea. At first, he tried treating himself. "Even so," he now admits, "I had a fool for a doctor and a second fool for a patient."

For the next several weeks, Dr. van Zsidy felt no improvement from his personal ministrations. And then chronic constipation came upon him and lingered for an overly long period. The constipation became so severe that, at times, he didn't move his bowels for five days. As a complication to his constipation, chronic joint pain was always with him as a result of a long-standing osteoarthritis, especially in both of his knees.

To offset the ongoing knee pain, Dr. van Zsidy took aspirin and other painkillers. However, with no letup to any of his symptoms, he began to query health practioners he knew personally. Medical doctors whom he finally consulted professionally for his diverse discomforts offered some treatment suggestions from nebulous to insulting. Consequently, he decided to merely live with his health problems and treat them as best he could.

A year later, the naturopathic physician turned patient had to cope with a different set of signs and symptoms. His new difficulties involved fatty lumps (lipomas) that appeared under the skin, which, upon his undergoing biopsies at several skin sites, proved negative for malignancy. But blood tests which were part of his full diagnostic workup suggested hepatitis had come upon him, and he proceeded to turn yellow with jaundice. Then weight loss began for Dr. van Zsidy, and it became serious. After six months, by the time he had dropped 50 pounds, he had been hospitalized seven times to stop his vomiting, extreme weakness, and swollen lymph nodes. Of course, the patient had long since stopped treating himself and a bevy of medical specialists were tending to his diverse needs. But nothing helped, and the vast number of signs and symptoms remained.

Even under repeated examinations, no cancer was found until an internist who took a computerized tomographic (CT) scan uncovered three lymph nodes which did appear positive for malignancy. From undergoing many additional laboratory and clinical tests, finally it was discovered that the right lobe of Dr. van Zsidy's liver had a number of small malignant tumors growing on it; in addition, the liver's left lobe showed a larger neoplasm 2 cm by 3 cm in size. If the original diagnosis of hepatitis had been correct, it now had turned into a verified hepatic cancer.

Fate still was not finished with the unfortunate man, for further disabilities struck. The patient's feet swelled; his abdomen filled with fluid (ascites); the cancerous liver greatly enlarged; food nauseated him; and pain in his knees grew to be excruciating. Moreover, Dr. van Zsidy's abdomen ached and cramped continuously from what could be described as "chronic indigestion." The man felt absolutely miserable, weak and worn out, and he longed to be put out of his misery.

However, chemotherapy was rejected by both his attending internist and the consulting oncologist because they agreed that their patient was too far gone for the cytotoxic agents to do any good; prednisone was ruled out owing to his having had a prior bout with tuberculosis as a child. (Giving corticosteroids is contraindicated when old and walled-off tubercular lesions are present.)

When Dr. van Zsidy's weight dropped to just 97 pounds, and he was so weak he couldn't leave his bed to eliminate body wastes, the patient and his doctors were convinced that he would not survive more than a couple of days. The man told his brother that he wanted to die at home in the mountains surrounding Montreal, where he could view the river and hills. So the brother immediately arranged for him to be taken there by ambulance. At his request, the next-door neighbor, whom he considered a close friend, dug a grave in the private family cemetery on the van Zsidy property. It was a sad undertaking.

Since he was incontinent and could no longer bear the loss of his personal dignity, Dr. van Zsidy impatiently waited to die and seriously contemplated speeding the event along by committing suicide. He tried this, but his complete physical weakness prevented him from actually carrying out the act. So the patient waited and suffered through his private hell on earth.

Despite his ingesting large numbers of painkilling drugs, bouts of gnawing, aching, and sticking pain constantly interrupted the man's sleep. Observing his condition, one would be hard put to find any person more frail, miserable, and weak than Joergon van Zsidy, M.D., N.D.

Then something happened which dramatically changed all aspects of his situation. Dr. van Zsidy's brother brought him a dog-eared copy of the third revised edition of Dr. Max Gerson's book to read, and it was an eye-opener for him. This patient became determined to try the dietary therapy—a final attempt that he would make to survive.

Dr. van Zsidy set about following the Gerson program. People around him, family, friends, and neighbors, helped him to accomplish the Gerson approach to cancer therapy. Among other procedures for this near-dead individual, he regularly undertook detoxification by means of coffee enemas. In fact, Dr. van Zsidy went overboard with the enemas by increasing their number to one every hour (perhaps eight to ten more per day than he should have taken). His loved ones helped him perform the procedures, and results from these enemas were amazing to the patient and those who gave them to him. The patient has reported to us that he saw massive numbers of parasites in his stools and smelled awful odors coming from them.

Also the man embarked on drinking huge amounts of fresh-squeezed, raw, organic vegetable and fruit juices, eating organically grown vegetables as much as he could hold, and taking the prescribed medications. Subsequently, Dr. Joergon van Zsidy gained weight at the rate of up to 1½ pounds per week. Soon his weakness left and energy returned. After eight months, the arthritis in his knees disappeared entirely and, from walking miles along the mountain paths, he switched to jogging them. Dr. van Zsidy faithfully remained on the Gerson Therapy in this manner for two years, during which he states for publication here, "I felt better than ever I had before."

That beginning experience with the Gerson Therapy for Dr. Joergon van Zsidy took place over seven years ago. Today he continues with most of the program and eats only organic vegetables and fruits. No animal protein and no grains are included in his diet. He drinks lots of fresh, organic vegetable and fruit juices and keeps up with taking coffee enemas, sometimes regularly but mostly irregularly.

To complete his case record Dr. van Zsidy says, "For the past seven years, I have not felt the resumption of weakness of any kind, and I never come down with colds, flu, headaches, arthritis, or any other pains. My liver cancer is gone. Thanks to the Gerson Therapy, I don't experience the symptoms of illness or even vague discomforts anymore. Thanks to God and Dr. Max Gerson I've become a healthy person once again."

THE GERSON PROTOCOL FOR A CANCER PATIENT WHO IS WEAKENED

Dr. Gerson's nutrient, diet, and medication protocol for the treatment of a cancer patient existing in a severely weakened state, whether or not chemical pretreatment has been taken, generally is ultraconservative. Modified Gerson Therapy involves particular guidelines that we give in this chapter. Self-treatment precautions regarding the Gerson Therapy procedures for this class of enfeebled patient are announced in the paragraphs that follow. Furthermore, extra care should be taken by the attending physician to monitor regularly for electrolyte imbalance, bleeding, dehydration, or other complications related to cancer, no matter the type of malignancy. A weakened physical condition for the cancer patient about to engage in Gerson therapeutics is a perilous position to be in. As repeated below, there are risks directly related to the deprivation of strength.

Anyone participating in the Gerson Therapy—patient, caregiver, physician, or other health care professional—must recognize that the detoxification and salt/water management aspects of the Gerson protocol are extremely powerful. No overstimulation of the body systems is allowed because the seriously impaired patient will not be able to mount an appropriate healing if the process is brought about too quickly or intensely. The patient's variables will include the body's overall condition, symptomatology, blood work results, age, diagnosis, and several other factors.

Please note: All patients with a history of chemical pretreatment should receive the reduced Gerson protocol, and those in a weakened physical condition with or without having taken chemotherapy should be given this less intense protocol as well.

This chapter presents the appropriate reduced Gerson protocol for the described type of weakened cancer patients. The program offered is a modification of the standard Gerson Therapy that was described in chapter 14 and varies somewhat from the modified treatment plan discussed in chapter 15. For each of the medications, their dosages, time intervals, contraindications, dietary considerations, and follow-up after the first year of therapy are discussed below beginning with the consumption of juices.

Juice Drinking by the Patient Lingering in a Weakened State

We must emphasize that juice drinking on the Gerson Therapy is a critical aspect of the regimen. The juices provide most of the vitamins, minerals, enzymes, phytochemicals, and other nutrients essential to healing, along with adequate fluid intake. Drinking fresh-squeezed, organically grown vegetable and fruit juices allows for greater absorption and utilization of all of the nutrients found in foods from which the juices are made. Patients who are victimized by degenerative diseases almost always experience difficulty digesting and absorbing food. This can be a result of toxicity, malfunction of the digestive system, a decrease in stomach acid production, or a variety of other causes. Gastrointestinal debilitation like this is the same reason that many patients have difficulty digesting and absorbing vitamin and mineral pills or capsules.

After Dr. Gerson treated a weakened patient—frequently somebody in a terminal state—it became his goal to find ways of increasing the absorption of nutrients. He did this in order to bring about steadily increasing physiological healing and to produce remissions or cures in the otherwise terminal patients. His clinical experimentation showed that fresh juice from organically grown raw foods provided the easiest and most effective means of furnishing high-quality nutrition, and such fresh juice drinking produced the best clinical results.

The Gerson Institute personnel continue to evaluate the effects of the recommended juices. They have considered the addition of other juices and juice products too, and they look for ways to both enhance the healing process and minimize hardship in the practice of the Gerson Therapy. No one says the Gerson approach is easy. As yet, the staff members have not found any means of reducing, substituting, or eliminating any of the juices that have already been recommended.

Additionally, it must be emphasized that preparing the juices fresh *at the time of consumption* is mandatory. This procedure works, which is why the Gerson Institute is reluctant to make changes. It's difficult for the Gerson staff members to justify risking lives for the sake of experimentation when there already exists a proven protocol for treating and healing degenerative diseases.

QUESTIONS ABOUT JUICE-DRINKING GUIDELINES

What are the functions of juice in the healing process? Why have certain juices been chosen? Why are they used in specific ways? For what reasons must the juices be made fresh? These are only a few of the questions asked of us by Gerson patients. We answer them in the following manner:

During the course of Dr. Max Gerson's thirty years of clinical practice (1928 to 1958) his anti-degenerative-disease therapy changed considerably. The variation occurred in the quantity, volume, and type of juices prescribed. Over the years, many patients have successfully used nothing more than the single table of juices and medications published in the sixth edition of Dr. Gerson's book, *A Cancer Therapy: Results of Fifty Cases*, as a road map to healing (see his "Tables" and "Combined Dietary Regime").[1]

While most treatment protocols prescribed by Gerson Therapy physicians will follow the revised guidelines in this book, patients under the care of experienced Gerson physicians may see their "juice prescription" changed in response to their blood test results, healing reaction responses, or other signs and symptoms. Severely damaged or weakened patients often require alterations or modifications of their medications and juices almost daily during the first weeks of the treatment.

Those health professionals who advise about the Gerson approach admit that they do not clearly understand how those very special organic, fresh-squeezed juices enhance healing, except for the obvious vitamin, mineral, enzyme, and trace mineral supplementation that they provide. The nutrient supplementation alone is probably not enough to explain why there is a difference between juices consumed immediately after preparation and those consumed several hours later. Surely, oxidation of a quantity of juice that's been sitting for an interval of time causes loss of certain vitamins and enzymes. Oxygen will do that.

There has been much discussion of the enzyme activity in the juices when they are fresh. The importance of these enzymes in numerous biochemical functions is well accepted. Yet, as any biology student knows, enzymes are immediately destroyed on contact with stomach acid. What makes the difference in healing response between the fresh juice and the hours-old juice? One possibility is that some of the enzymes present in the fresh juice are absorbed directly through the mucous membranes in the mouth and esophagus, before reaching the stomach. This theory is borne out by the observation that patients fed through a nasogastric or stomach tube do not respond favorably to the Gerson Therapy.

Another possibility, from the esoteric medical literature which deals with human and plant energies, is that there is a form of plant "vital force," "qi," or "prana" present in the juices when freshly made. Some believe that this "vital force" benefits the patient's vital force. Such juice promotes healing at the energetic or psychic level rather than at the cellular or biochemical level.

The Gerson Institute possesses little evidence to support any of the assumptions stated above, but its personnel do not wish to rule out any possibility that gives all of us greater understanding. In addition to the nutritional supplementation, the juices also serve to flush the kidneys by virtue of their high liquid content.

So, however the healing process occurs from drinking juice as recommended by the Gerson Therapy advocates, it is vital to recognize that true physiological restoration comes as a result of the intake of fresh juices. Doing so must be consistent. The process has been validated by long-term positive outcomes. All this gives the Gerson Insitute personnel reason enough to follow Dr. Max Gerson's original directives regarding the drinking of juices to overcome cancer and other degenerative diseases.

THE MANNER OF JUICE DRINKING BY WEAKENED CANCER PATIENTS

In most situations, it is advisable to start the juice-drinking regimen of a weakened cancer patient with 4 ounces per dose. Temporarily eliminate the three carrot-only juices. The juice dosage will depend on the condition of the patient and his or her ability to tolerate the juices, and the potential side effects which may result. If the patient can tolerate the smaller amount of juice, juices may be increased after four to seven days, which typically entails raising the quantity from 4 ounces to 5 or 6 ounces per dose. Increases must be carefully monitored, and care must be taken to ensure that the patient continues to tolerate all juices, without significant nausea or other side effects.

The schedule of juice drinking should follow the guideline offered here. Each day drink:

1 orange juice
4 green leaf juices
5 apple/carrot juices
3 carrot juices alone

Gruel may be added to any of the juices—up to 50 percent by volume—to reduce nausea and increase tolerance.

MEDICATION AND OTHER PROTOCOL CHANGES FOR THE WEAKENED CANCER PATIENT

A frustrating factor for someone with a growing malignancy is that the same food calories that support the healthy metabolism of normal cells can be used by malignant cells hungry for energy. Such a situation tends to lead to weakness, debilitating weight loss, lack of energy, early fatigue, and absence of any strength to accomplish even personal tasks such as combing the hair, cooking a meal, or shopping for food. This is known as *cachexia*, a general bodily decline associated with almost any chronic disease. It goes together with weakness for the cancer patient whether or not chemotherapy or immunotherapy or radiation therapy has entered the treatment picture.

Why does weakness associated with cachexia occur? One hypothesis is that the patient, simultaneously with his or her malignancy, additionally suffers from "hypermetabolism," a state in which the immune-impaired body burns up its stores of energy too quickly. A second theory is that the chronically ill patient cannot manufacture lean body mass normally, although fat tissue is readily created. The weight gain that such persons might experience is probably only fat and water weight, not muscle and lean tissue substance.

However, keep in mind that both of these theories have failed their various testings by leading oncologists even in face of repeated clinical and laboratory investigations.[2]

A third likely cause is that the digestive system of the cancer patient is unable to break down fats and animal proteins ("standard foods") to their end product that can be used to feed normal tissues. These foods, partially digested, cannot nourish the normal body cells. However, tumor tissue thrives on these "intermediate" products. Thus, the patient loses weight while the tumor is fed and grows. On the other hand, foods supplied by the Gerson Therapy are rich in nutrients and enzymes that are not only easily digested even by the damaged digestive system of the chronic disease patient, but the enzymes in fresh raw foods and juices help to destroy tumor tissue. That is why patients not only maintain (or gain) weight, but are able to break down tumor tissue.

Staff members and patients who follow the guidelines laid down by the Gerson Therapy know that the patient's weakness, with or without having undergone chemotherapy, requires a special altered protocol. For the sick individual deprived of strength and unnerved by such an experience, listed below are some alterations from the standard Gerson protocol. Note that instructions in this chapter, except for some exclusions or dosage deviations, are quite similar to those directions provided in chapter 15.

Potassium Compound Solution (Liquid)

The recommended starting dosage for potassium compound solution suggested is 1 tsp ten times per day, which represents approximately 500 mg or 12.5 mEq each of potassium (K) acetate, gluconate, and monophosphate. This is a total K combination of 1.5 grams or 37.5 mEq/day.

In patients experiencing extreme weakening, no potassium supplementation should be received for three to five days, or until conditioning improves and stabilizes. The normal dosage of 10 tsp per day may be cautiously increased to 2 tsp ten times per day after five to seven days. If no adverse side effects are observed, increase the dosage to 3 and then 4 tsp ten times per day, as the patient is able to tolerate.

There are contraindications to K compound solution: Patients with a history of renal insufficiency or generalized kidney dysfunction, gastritis, nausea, significant bone metastases, or any indication of bleeding problems should be started with 1 tsp of K ten times per day. Dosage may be slowly increased after observation of the compound's effects. Anyone with a history of cardiac insufficiency, myocardial infarction, or congestive heart failure should *not* receive potassium until blood laboratory work has been analyzed by a physician.

Lugol (Potassium Iodide, KI, Half-Strength)

The KI in Lugol is ingested at the rate of one to two drops per day. There are contraindications to taking Lugol for weakened patients. If the individual has a history of allergy to iodine, Lugol is not indicated, at least initially; however, it can be cautiously added after three to five days, one drop to start, then increasing as tolerance allows.

Weakened patients presenting with hepatic (liver) insufficiency, primary or metastatic tumor activity in the liver, hepatitis, or hepatic cirrhosis should be started on one to two drops of Lugol per day, to avoid bleeding or a decrease in blood platelets. Those patients with bone metastases should also receive reduced Lugol to avoid excessive bone deterioration and pain. Any patients known to be affected by heavy metal toxicity should additionally receive doses of one to two drops per day initially.

Thyroid Hormone

Thyroid hormone is taken in zero to 1½-grain doses once per day. But there are contraindications to thyroid usage similar to those for Lugol. Watch for signs of hyperthyroidism, including tachycardia, anxiety, insomnia, tremors, and other complications. Reduce dosage levels if any of these signs and symptoms are present. Also note that transient tachycardia alone is often indicative for a toxic or flare-up reaction. Patients presenting with a history of cardiac insufficiency or other cardiac incidents should be started on the lowest dosage possible of thyroid daily.

Niacin (Nicotinic Acid), or Vitamin B$_3$

This vitamin B$_3$ nutrient has a dosage of 50 mg three times per day. Some contraindications do exist such as for patients who present with hepatic insufficiency, primary or metastatic tumor activity in the liver, hepatitis, or hepatic cirrhosis. They should receive a maximum of 100 to 150 mg of niacin daily. Patients with a medical history of bleeding, ulcers, or gastritis and those concurrently receiving prednisone, other steroids, or Coumadin should not receive niacin.

Pancreatin

This pancreatic enzyme from the pig allows for a dosage of three 325-mg tablets taken four times a day. It's contraindicated for sarcoma patients.

Crude Liver/Vitamin B$_{12}$ (Cobalamin) Injection

This combination is taken once daily as an intramuscular injection in a dose of 100 mcg of vitamin B$_{12}$ with 3 cc of crude liver extract. Other than the patient attaining excessive levels of vitamin B$_{12}$ and occasional allergic reactions, there is no known contraindication for the crude liver/B$_{12}$ injection.

Acidol

The gastrointestinal enzyme product known as *Acidol* (betaine hydrochloride and pepsin) is taken in a dose of two capsules daily, three times a day with meals. There are contraindications to taking this digestive aid consisting of gastric ulcers, gastritis, severe nausea, intestinal bleeding, or esophageal problems. Patients with these difficulties and those taking Coumadin concurrently with Gerson treatment should not receive Acidol.

Coenzyme Q$_{10}$

While not a vitamin, coenzyme Q$_{10}$ has vitaminlike properties. It provides for an initial dose of 90 mg once per day. If no side effects in the form of tachycardia or arrhythmia arises, on the second day of taking it increase CoQ$_{10}$ to 300 mg daily, and on the third day increase the dose to 600 mg. Remain at that higher dosage thereafter.

Wobe-Mugos and Megazyme Forte

These gastrointestinal enzymes are used primarily when the patient suffers from severe, excessive gas. Some reports also indicate that the enzymes may be helpful in reducing tumor masses.

Laetrile

Laetrile, known generically as amygdalin, is indicated for the treatment of bone metastases, and it may be useful in the treatment of lung cancers as well. When laetrile is available, it is used primarily to reduce pain levels, although this effect requires ten days to two weeks of daily administration for optimum results. The dosage is 2 grams (5 cc) intravenously once per day. It may be useful for severely weakened cancer patients who have or have not undergone chemotherapy. A physician must make that determination.

Brewer's Yeast

This type of food yeast derived from the brewing of beer is not recommended under most circumstances because of the potentially increased risk of the yeast syndrome (candidiasis) developing or worsening. Also, many people taking brewer's yeast report extreme abdominal distension and gas.

Castor Oil Treatment

This plant oil is contraindicated in patients who have undergone chemotherapy pretreatment. In nonchemotreated patients who are much weakened, castor oil treatment may be applicable after six to nine months on the Gerson Therapy. Yet it should be taken with great caution, as extremely toxic side effects can occur from the body's resulting elimination of prior chemotherapy residues. Castor oil is a powerful detoxifier, and long-buried cytotoxicity can come out of the tissues. Such a release may produce severe healing reactions.

Coffee Enemas

Coffee enemas are standard for cancer patients who are sapped of strength. The dosage is a 32-ounce enema once or twice per day. In some people, this dosage will be reduced to half strength by mixing 16 ounces of chamomile tea with 16 ounces of coffee. The coffee enema dosage may gradually be increased as needed, but care must be taken not to overstimulate the liver and cause extremely toxic side effects from the elimination of noxious chemotherapy residues lodged within the body.

First-Year Follow-Up Therapy for the Debilitated Cancer Patient

Follow-up therapy is required on this reduced Gerson protocol for the debilitated cancer patient. Changes in the medications will be made during the first year of Gerson treatment. For instance, approximately one month after discharge from the inpatient treatment center (probably six to nine weeks after admission to the Gerson hospital and start of the Gerson Therapy), thyroid, potassium, and Lugol medications are adjusted. If the patient has been on extremely reduced levels, these medications may be increased by 25 to 50 percent. Other supplements are generally kept at initial levels.

If the patient was receiving normal levels of the Gerson protocol (e.g., 40 tsp of potassium and eighteen drops of Lugol), these medication levels are reduced by approximately 50 percent, assuming the patient is making satisfactory progress and gaining in strength. If the patient has been receiving normal levels of medications such as 40 tsp of K and eighteen drops of Lugol, such medication levels are reduced by approximately 50 percent. The adjusted medication levels are generally maintained for nine to fourteen months. Supplemental adjustments are often made based on the diagnostic blood work and other diagnostic means.

Note that this follow-up protocol differs significantly from the information in Dr. Gerson's original book "A Cancer Therapy." Patients must now be kept on higher dosages of the three main medications for longer periods than in Dr. Gerson's day. When medications are reduced too rapidly (such as according to the schedule in A *Cancer Therapy*), patients often have difficulties and experience a slowing of recovery or a recurrence of disease.

For prostrate, vulnerable, or exhausted patients who have or have not undergone chemotherapy before undertaking the Gerson Therapy, following the instructions in this chapter will ensure health improvement and potential recovery from disease. The weakened state for almost any individual can be overcome by accepting the recommendations originally put forth by Max Gerson, M.D.

References for Chapter Sixteen

1. Gerson, M. A *Cancer Therapy: Results of Fifty Cases: A Summary of 30 Years of Clinical Experimentation and The Cure of Advanced Cancer by Diet Therapy*, 6th edition. Bonita, Calif.: The Gerson Institute, 1999, pp. 223–248.

2. Nixon, D.W.; Zanca, J.A. *The Cancer Recovery Eating Plan: The Right Foods to Help Fuel Your Recovery*. New York: Times Books, 1994, pp. 23–26.

Chapter Seventeen

MODIFIED THERAPY FOR NONCANCER PATIENTS

At the beginning of a weekend in February 1995, Pittsburgh, Pennsylvania, resident Pamela Ptak, now thirty-four years old, drove to her parents' home in Springfield, Massachusetts, for their regular visit. When she woke up the next morning in the bed she had occupied as a teenager, she noted that a large gray spot was stuck in the center of the field of vision of her left eye. When she stood in front of the mirror and closed her right eye, she could no longer see her head. It was blocked by the central eye spot, which appeared dark, warped, rippled, and in a shade of gray. Moreover, this spot in Pamela's left eye caused much of her color vision to be lost.

Alarmed, she returned to Pittsburgh, depending on her right eye to see while driving. Once home, she consulted an ophthalmologist who had been recommended to her by the local hospital in her east Pittsburgh area. The eye doctor thought that his new patient's problem was *central serous retinopathy*, a condition that often disappears by itself. *Central serous retinopathy* is marked by acute localized detachment of the neural retina or retinal pigment epithelium in the region of the macula.

Unfortunately for the patient, this specialist was wrong. Rather, her blocking eye spot did not go away and stayed with Pamela Ptak until June 1995. During the ensuing four-month period, the spot's symptomatic effects had worsened.

After revisiting the same physician, she was put through another diagnostic procedure called *fluorescein angiogram,* which showed that multiple spots were now forming layers on the retinas of both the patient's eyes. The ophthalmologist observed that tissue behind the retina was "eaten away" and pitted. From his viewing scope he saw that a kind of "bird's nest" group of blood vessels had formed, which had hemorrhaged in the center. This graphic description caused her great uneasiness and moved her toward consulting another ophthalmologist for a second opinion.

The second eye specialist diagnosed the young woman as suffering from a different condition—*ocular histoplasmosis,* and he urged immediate surgery to remove the nest of blood vessels. But eye surgery for the correction of her ocular histoplasmosis held no attraction for the patient.

Ocular histoplasmosis is an acute degenerative infection of the eye resulting from the inhalation of spores of the fungus *Histoplasma capsulatum.* The infection, which can become chronic, remains asymptomatic until some alteration in the retina occurs. This second doctor traced her eye disease to her work in a highly toxic job at an advertising agency where she was constantly exposed to spray glues, toxic art materials, lots of deadline pressure, and severe emotional stress. Pamela Ptak also regularly sprayed her apartment with roach poison and other pesticides because of infestation by biological pests. One of them may have been the same fungus causing her disability.

While she was debating whether to undergo the eye operation, a friend suggested that Pamela look into the Gerson Therapy as an alternative method of healing. It does work against any degenerative disease, chronic or acute, including those brought about by pathological microorganisms. Since the young woman was familiar with the treatment's concept (she had watched two friends who had been diagnosed with cancer save their own lives by its application), she decided to start on Dr. Max Gerson's healing program herself. She found it to be no hardship, for a health food supermarket located just down the street furnished their clientele with organically grown produce at fair market prices, and it comprised almost all of Pamela's diet.

Thus, for just one month, from the end of June to July 31, 1995, Pamela Ptak faithfully performed the Gerson Therapy at home, including the taking of two coffee enemas, one before she left for work in the morning and a second immediately upon her arriving home in the evening. The juices she made in quantity and took along with her in thermos bottles for drinking regularly throughout her workday. She hoped that the Gerson program was working during the weeks that followed, but, although her vision seemed to become much less blocked by the gray spot, she was not sure.

On August 1, the patient visited the second retinal surgeon once more to discuss his suggested eye operation. When the doctor looked at his patient's left retina, he was truly surprised, but pleased. The spot had shrunk and was so small it was almost invisible. There was no sign of hemorrhaging. The Gerson Therapy had so stimulated the woman's immune system that it had spontaneously killed off *Histoplasma capsulatum* on its own. She needed no antifungal, antibiotic medications and no operation. The spot eventually stopped blocking her vision, and today she sees just fine.

The therapy took slightly over a month. Pamela Ptak happily reports to us for publication: "Here is one more condition healed by the Gerson Therapy."

THE GERSON PROTOCOL FOR NONCANCER PATIENTS WITH DIFFERENT DISEASES

No single diet/medication protocol for nonmalignant illnesses of different types exists on the Gerson program simply because each disease shows diverse dietary origins and variable treatment needs. Still, the standard protocol that had been offered by Dr. Max Gerson's therapy does provide a starting point which this chapter discusses. There are many modifications of diet, juicing, and medications for the different diseases.

Please be assured that the protocol published here does work, although there are variables. Variables prevail simply because of (a) the patient's overall condition, (b) the results of the sick person's laboratory blood work, (c) his or her symptomatology, (d) the patient's age, (e) the medical diagnosis, and (f) numerous other factors. Yet virtually all types of health problems respond to the Gerson Therapy.

Beginning below with "addictions," a few of the more common illnesses which respond well to a modified Gerson Therapy protocol have their variable treatment programs described in this chapter. First, however, we provide you with the general therapeutic program for patients with nonmalignant diseases to follow. This general therapeutic program is the basic format to follow when someone is weighed down by any acute or chronic illness. Please assure yourself or loved ones you are helping that any appropriate modifications required of specific diseases are incorporated into the general protocol that follows.

Please note: The use of a full, unmodified protocol of the Gerson Therapy for noncancerous diseases ordinarily remains inadvisable. While not usually as dangerous as inappropriate application of the therapy to patients with a chemotherapy history, there are still considerable risks to using the intensive protocol in the presence of some illnesses.

Appropriate explanations must be given to anyone using the therapy regarding the reasoning behind application of the reduced protocol. Otherwise, patients will sometimes self-medicate with the more aggressive protocol, at the expense of their safety and long-term recovery outlook.

THE STANDARD PROTOCOL FOR NONCANCEROUS ILLNESSES

Juices

The regimen for treating a noncancerous illness can begin with the daily drinking of ten 8-ounce glasses of the juices, eliminating pure carrot juice. If the patient is in good physical condition, she or he should be able to take the full 8-ounce portions with no difficulty. However, if this person shows any form of debilitation, start with smaller quantities of juice consisting typically of 4 or 6 ounces.

As always with the Gerson Therapy, be sure that the patient can tolerate all juices without significant nausea or other side effects before an increase in the juice quantity is considered.

The schedule of juice drinking to be maintained by a rather ill but noncancerous individual should be:

a. Orange juice
b. Green leaf combination juice
c. Apple/carrot combination juice

Potassium Compound Solution (Liquid)

The recommended starting dosage for potassium compound solution suggested is 2 tsp ten times per day, which represents approximately 1 gram (1,000 mg) or 25 mEq each of potassium (K) acetate, gluconate, and phosphate (monobasic). This is a total K combination of 3 grams or 75 mEq/day. Most of the time patients do not require the full 40 tsp of potassium that cancer patients would require.

There are contraindications to K compound solution: Patients with a history of renal insufficiency or generalized kidney dysfunction, gastritis, nausea, or any indication of bleeding problems should be started with 1 tsp ten times per day. Dosage may be slowly increased with observation of the compound's effects. Anyone with a history of cardiac insufficiency, myocardial infarction, or congestive heart failure should *not* receive potassium until blood laboratory work has been analyzed by a physician who agrees that K ingestion would be beneficial.

Lugol (Potassium Iodide KI, Half-Strength)

The KI in Lugol is ingested at the rate of three to six drops per day. There are contraindications to taking Lugol for certain sick but noncancerous patients. If the individual has a history of allergy to iodine, Lugol is not indicated, at least initially; however, it can be cautiously added after three to five days, one drop to start, then increasing as tolerance allows.

Other ill patients presenting with hepatic (liver) insufficiency, hepatitis, or hepatic cirrhosis should be started on one to two drops of Lugol per day, to avoid bleeding or a decrease in blood platelets. Those patients known to be affected by heavy metal toxicity should additionally receive doses of one to two drops per day initially.

Thyroid Hormone

Thyroid hormone is taken in a dose of 1 grain once or twice per day. Typically, patients with nonmalignant diseases do not possess as serious a thyroid deficiency as cancer patients. In some cases, the Gerson-trained health professionals have found it beneficial for patients to start on up to 5 grains of thyroid hormone for only three to five days, rather than the fourteen days commonly prescribed for those people with malignancies.

Contraindications to thyroid usage are similar to those for Lugol. Watch for signs of hyperthyroidism, including tachycardia, anxiety, insomnia, tremors, and others. Reduce dosage levels if any of these signs and symptoms are present. Also note that transient tachycardia alone is often indicative for a toxic or flare-up reaction. Patients presenting with a history of cardiac insufficiency or other cardiac incidents should be started on a maximum dosage of 2 grains of thyroid daily.

Niacin (Vitamin B$_3$)

This vitamin B$_3$ nutrient has a dosage of 50 mg three times per day. Some contraindications do exist, such as for patients who present with hepatic insufficiency, hepatitis, or hepatic cirrhosis. These liver-impaired people should receive a maximum of only 100 to 150 mg of niacin daily. Patients with a medical history of bleeding, ulcers, or gastritis, and those who are concurrently receiving prednisone, other steroids, or Coumadin should not receive niacin.

Pancreatin

This pancreatic enzyme from the pig allows for a dosage of three 325-mg tablets taken four times a day. According to Dr. Gerson, pancreatin is contraindicated for sarcoma patients.

Crude Liver/B$_{12}$ Injection

Taken once daily as an intramuscular injection of 3 cc of crude liver extract, added to the extract in the same syringe is 0.05 cc of vitamin B$_{12}$ to make up a normal 100-mcg dose. Other than excessive levels of vitamin B$_{12}$, and occasional allergic reactions, there is no known contraindication for the crude liver/B$_{12}$ injection.

Acidol

The gastrointestinal enzyme product known as Acidol (betaine hydrochloride and pepsin), is taken in a dose of two capsules daily, three times a day with meals. There are contraindications to this digestive aid, including gastric ulcers, gastritis, severe nausea, intestinal bleeding, or esophageal problems. Patients with these difficulties and those taking Coumadin concurrently with Gerson treatment should not receive Acidol.

Coenzyme Q$_{10}$

While not a vitamin, coenzyme Q$_{10}$ has vitaminlike properties. It provides for an initial dose of 90 mg once per day. If no side effects in the form of tachycardia or arrhythmia arise, on the second day of taking it increase CoQ$_{10}$ to 300 mg daily, and on the third day increase the dose to 600 mg. Remain at that higher dosage thereafter.

Wobe-Mugos and Megazyme Forte

These two groups of gastrointestinal enzymes are indicated primarily when the patient suffers from severe, excessive gas. Some reports also indicate that the enzymes may be helpful in reducing tumor masses.

Laetrile

Laetrile, known generically as amygdalin, is not indicated for the treatment of conditions other than cancer.

Brewer's Yeast

This type of food yeast, derived from the brewing of beer, is not recommended under most circumstances because of the potentially increased risk of the yeast syndrome (candidiasis) developing or worsening. Also, many people taking brewer's yeast report extreme abdominal distention and gas.

Castor Oil Treatment

This plant oil, if used at all, usually is administered one or two times a week. It should be taken with great caution as castor oil is a powerful detoxifier, and long-buried toxins can come out of the tissues. Such a release may produce severe healing reactions.

Coffee Enemas

Coffee enemas are standardly taken by ill patients who are following the Gerson Therapy in a 32-ounce enema once or twice per day, and the enemas may be increased in number up to five a day. Remember that coffee enemas tend to stimulate the liver and can cause toxic side effects from the elimination of some long-retained noxious residues lodged within the body's cells.

FIRST-YEAR FOLLOW-UP THERAPY FOR THE PATIENT NOT ILL WITH CANCER

Follow-up therapy is required on this reduced Gerson protocol for the person who suffers from an illness other than cancer. Changes in the medications will be made during the first year of Gerson treatment. For instance, approximately one month after discharge from the inpatient treat-ment center (probably six to nine weeks after admission to the Gerson hospital and start of the Gerson Therapy), thyroid hormone, potassium, and Lugol medications, if at normal levels, are adjusted downward. Other supplements are generally kept at initial levels. Supplemental adjust-ments are often made based on diagnostic laboratory blood examinations and other means of diagnosis.

Note that this follow-up protocol differs significantly from the infor-mation in "*A Cancer Therapy: Results of Fifty Cases*." Patients must now be kept on higher dosages of the three main medications for longer peri-ods than in Dr. Gerson's day. When medications are reduced too rapidly (such as according to the schedule published in A *Cancer Therapy: Results of Fifty Cases*), patients often experience difficulties and go through a slowing of recovery or a recurrence of disease.

Nevertheless, almost any nonmalignant health problem will benefit from being treated with the Gerson Therapy. At the beginning of this book we cite at least fifty-two verified diseases that respond exceedingly well to the Gerson treatment program. We have witnessed their improve-ment, reversal, or outright cure.

SOME NONCANCEROUS ILLNESSES REVERSED BY THE GERSON THERAPY

Here are eighteen examples from the vast number of acute or chronic degenerative health problems that almost anyone can eliminate by fol-lowing the modified Gerson approach to healing (discussed above) and by living the pristine lifestyle originally recommended in the book by Max Gerson, M.D.: (1) addictions of almost all types, (2) atherosclerosis, (3) chronic fatigue syndrome, (4) reversible colostomy, (5) diabetes types I and II, (6) a variety of genetic disorders, (7) emphysema, (8) heart disease and vascular disease, (9) hepatitis A, B, and C, (10) kidney disease, (11) heavy metal toxicity, (12) multiple sclerosis, (13) osteoarthritis, (14) os-teoporosis, (15) steroid treatment, (16) systemic lupus erythematosus, (17) rheumatoid arthritis, and (18) ulcerative colitis.

In accordance with the efficacy of the Gerson approach to treatment, we offer below some commentary on a tiny sampling of these ills. All are able to be corrected permanently using modifications of the Gerson pro-tocol.

ADDICTIONS

Addictions may be reversed or eliminated entirely by the habituated individual by adapting the Gerson program. The addictions most readily responding to some change in the standard Gerson approach are:

Codeine, Morphine, Nicotine, Amphetamines, Sedatives/Hypnotics

Those unfortunate people seeking treatment for these enslavements should be regarded as types of chemotherapy patients, and the addictive drugs in question must be curtailed over a three- to ten-day period. Otherwise, if the treatment is too aggressive, extremely heavy reactions such as diarrhea and an inability to eat and drink may result. There will also be the possible complications involving electrolyte imbalance. For those cases in which the addictive drugs were originally prescribed as medical relief for pain control, placebos may be required in the early stages of addiction treatment.

Heroin, Cocaine

Based on a limited number of patients treated with the Gerson Therapy, our experience is that withdrawal symptoms are almost absent by means of applying the full, intensive Gerson treatment plan. No program modifications are required. However, we cannot rule out the risk of the severe reactions warned about in the narcotic/sedative-hypnotic/amphetamine protocol described immediately above, particularly given the likelihood of multiple drug abuse. These addicts must be watched carefully for reactions, and appropriate interventions by supervising health professionals must be given when necessary.

Alcohol

The Gerson Therapy has not often been employed for chronic alcoholism, but we believe that alcoholics could readily be treated with the narcotic/sedative-hypnotic/amphetamine addiction protocol described above. Liver function must be watched carefully, and the warnings that apply regarding hepatic insufficiency or weakness would be appropriately applied to these unhappy people.

Nicotine

No special modification to the Gerson protocol is required for over-coming nicotine addiction. Some smokers may temporarily call for me-chanical props such as something to put into the mouth or hold in the hands. These props may suffice to replace the physical activity associated with smoking. Niacin is a good adjunctive nutrient to take as a food sup-plement if there are no contraindicating factors to its use. Some patients report that niacin provides a similar effect to nicotine. (Niacin's actual chemical component is, afterall, nicotinic acid.) In most cases, nicotine addiction may be eliminated without any withdrawal symptoms appear-ing for the smoker engaging in the Gerson Therapy.

This treatment for a smoker's habituation or other addictions does work, although some more generalized explanation might be offered for further clarification.

Further General Information about Drug Addiction

Unquestionably, the first thought that comes to mind when we think about drug addiction is what happens on the street, especially in the inner cities. Surely in the last two decades, the use of street or illegal drugs has reached frightening levels; but there are other, possibly even more serious drug addictions for which we have a suggested treatment already.

To clarify: an extremely common addiction is that to alcohol—a legal drug. Some 12 million Americans are known to be confirmed alcoholics and an untold number of undeclared ones exist as well.

Another publicly shared and accepted addiction is the use of another legal drug: coffee drinking. Starbucks Coffee Shops have built themselves into a multi-billion-dollar business, a major franchise operation based on this addiction to coffee. Worldwide, the public has been fooled into be-lieving that drinking this muddy, dark-colored beverage is diversional, nu-tritional, pleasurable, harmless, and socially acceptable, while in reality it has none of these attributes. Rather, coffee drinking is a temporary brain excitant which brings on early fatigue; a hypoglycemic producer, it forces excesses of insulin into the bloodstream; a deteriorator of arteries, espe-cially those already advanced toward blood vessel hardening from athero-sclerosis, it blocks blood flow; a potential producer of birth defects, one can only conjecture as to the number of babies who have paid the price of their mothers' addiction. As for the mothers, coffee drinking is believed by many in the holistic medical movement to be the possible source of breast cancer.

Numerous drugs are used for stimulants; others are considered to be *recreational*. In view of the terrible damage they do, the *recreational* term is unquestionably criminally misleading.

Drugs are also used extensively in medical practice for pain relief. And here we encounter a delicate line of demarcation between use and becoming addicted to opioids (morphine is common). The prescribed opioids are taken for two reasons: painkilling and as an offshoot, psychological addiction. At this point, therefore, we need some definitions when speaking of prescribed drugs.

Tolerance indicates that increasingly heavier dosages have to be used since the body systems do become accustomed to the drug. And *tolerance* is a contrasting term to *physical dependence*, which indicates that withdrawal symptoms occur if the drug substance is suddenly withdrawn. But addiction is considered present when, in addition to tolerance and dependence, *psychological dependence* is also present, or the product is compulsively used for nonmedical purposes.[1]

We believe that a number of addictions, including alcohol and cigarettes, stem from a basic deficiency. The habituated person is aware that he is craving something, often actually nutrients, and is not really functioning at his best level. When he consumes alcohol, cigarettes, or coffee, he feels either calmer or stimulated to increased physical or mental achievement. When such a person then experiments with heavier drugs, street drugs, amphetamines, marijuana, and many more, he is easily "hooked" and cannot stop.

One of the main reasons for this situation of becoming hooked is that the underlying deficiency has not been solved and the nutrient intake of live enzymes, vitamins, and minerals remains inadequate. Worse, an alcoholic may stop eating in favor of drinking and become severely deficient in nutrients. A person addicted to cigarettes will smoke instead of eating a nutritious meal, especially when under stress.

The Gerson Therapy and Drug Addiction

In addition to the protocol we furnished earlier for specific forms of drug addiction, we have some other thoughts about Dr. Max Gerson's procedures. The Gerson Therapy has produced some remarkable results in overcoming addictions, even to cocaine and heroin. When an addicted patient is given thirteen glasses of freshly pressed vegetable and fruit juices to drink, his basic craving is satisfied with optimum nutrition, and to his own surprise, he no longer craves the drug.

Yes, withdrawal may occur. When the withdrawal symptoms set in, at a time when the body tissues begin to release the accumulated drugs from the cells into the bloodstream, a coffee enema clears the toxicity. The nights remain the only problem for the first few days. At night, no juices are served and the patient coming off his or her drug addiction sleeps so that no detoxifying enemas are taking place.

During those first nights of coming off their addictions, the patients tend to suffer from heavy nightmares and wake up around 1:00 or 2:00 A.M. They should then swallow some fruit or juice and get up to take an enema. This relieves the toxicity and possible craving so that the patient can go back to sleep. The nighttime problem also clears after less than a week. We have seen excellent results in overcoming addictions, even the heaviest ones involving not one but multiple drugs.

One young man (see the story of Rob in chapter 7) had been into various heavy drugs and on a particular day he was showing the symptoms. In his middle thirties, he was lying on the floor, too weak to get up, having lost some 45 pounds and feeling ready to die. His mother saved him by providing the foods and juices as well as the enemas of the Gerson Therapy. In a few months, the son gained back 35 pounds and felt like his former self. He had suffered virtually no withdrawal problems even at the start of the treatment, and returned to normal life and activity.

We see that the Gerson Therapy can also achieve prompt and dramatic results in smokers and alcoholics. (See Beata Bishop's book A *Time to Heal.*)[2] One of the Gerson Therapy patients, another young man who is now thirty-four years old and addicted to cocaine (supposedly the most difficult drug addiction to overcome), came to a Gerson hospital for treatment. He reported that *all* of his close friends had died from cocaine use.

This fellow admitted that he was having lung troubles as a result of street drug use and would surely die within two months if the Gerson Therapy was unable to help him. He was also a heavy smoker. After becoming a Gerson patient, the man went through nightmares similar to those we had observed in others. These were relieved with a nighttime coffee enema; thus, he was off the need for drugs, and smoking cigarettes, within a week.

Studies have been completed suggesting that many people are addicted to simple foods to which they are actually allergic. In his book *Diet, Crime and Delinquency*, Alexander Schauss, Ph.D., points out that violent young criminals between ages eighteen and twenty-one are often addicted to sugar and/or heavy milk consumption to which they are actually allergic. Dr. Schauss reported that when the offending substances were withdrawn and vitamins and minerals along with an appropriate diet were substituted, these violent criminals became calm and reasonable.[3]

Of course the Gerson Therapy is intentionally devoid of foods that tend to cause allergies in some people. The organic vegetarian diet, free of pesticides and chemical additives, achieves the purpose of overcoming allergies and allergic reactions.

ATHEROSCLEROSIS

Atherosclerosis (arteriosclerosis), or hardening of the arteries, usually responds exceedingly well to the Gerson protocol. This condition is eliminated by the antiblocking nutrition present in pure, whole vegetarian foods and the detoxification procedures originating in the standard Gerson protocol.

CHRONIC FATIGUE SYNDROME

People suffering from the series of symptoms identified as chronic fatigue and immune dysfunction syndrome (CFIDS) or chronic fatigue syndrome (CFS) get along just fine on the Gerson program, but they should see significant improvement after a short time, with recovery after about nine months. These Gerson treatment participants are allowed to have the full thirteen glasses of juice daily if desired.

CFS patients commonly feel worse after taking enemas in the early stages of treatment because of toxicity escaping from their body cells. Two enemas daily are normally suggested initially, working up to four.

Too many enemas can trigger strong adverse reactions. And patients with chronic fatigue syndrome tend to experience extremely strong emotional responses, such as depression and crying, during and between reaction periods. From a psychological perspective, they often present difficulties in management.

REVERSIBLE COLOSTOMY

Patients with colostomies that are reversible typically receive two combined coffee and chamomile tea enemas per day by use of an irrigation kit. Gerson personnel give instructions for using this kit.

For the colostomy patient, coffee enemas can be mixed 50/50 with chamomile tea, to reduce the potential of cramping and spasms. The volume of juices, particularly the green juice, is often lowered to just 4 ounces. Green juices are not absorbed well and will pass through the gastrointestinal tract rather quickly.

DIABETES, TYPES 1 AND 2

The term diabetes refers to a set of metabolic disorders that cause hyperglycemia, or high blood sugar. The two primary reasons for blood sugar to elevate correspond to the two main kinds of diabetes: juvenile, or type 1, diabetes, and adult-onset, or type 2, diabetes. The body puts insulin into service in several ways; one of them involves converting sugars into energy individual cells can utilize to control their blood sugar levels. The absence or impairment of insulin release brings about serious health problems.

Type 1 diabetes is caused by an insulin absence or deficiency, usually coming from damage to the islets of Langerhans, which are the cells located on the pancreas for producing insulin. While the cause of type 1 diabetes is not fully understood, many factors, such as genetic predisposition and viral infection, may play roles. One theory is that, combined with other factors, childhood bouts with pancreatitis are responsible for damaging those islet cells of the pancreas responsible for insulin production. Immune system malfunction seems to also play a role due to islet cell antibodies that are universally found in type 1 diabetic patients. Again, this may be tied to a present or past viral infection. Patients are usually diagnosed with the disease, enter a short remission period, but then lose islet cell function for life.

Type 1 diabetes generally occurs in children and usually has no relation to a patient's weight. Roughly 8 percent of diabetes cases in the United States are of this kind, with somewhat increased percentages occurring in Europe. Symptoms of type 1 diabetes include increased urination and thirst due to dehydration. Blurred vision and weight loss (despite normal appetite) are also common. Symptoms due to acute insulin deficiency include the above health difficulties as well as nausea, vomiting, and insulin shock.[4]

Type 2 diabetes, in contrast to type 1, is not primarily a result of insulin deficiency, but rather the body's inability to properly use the insulin produced. In such patients, the islet cells function adequately, but only a small amount of insulin actually is used by the cells to produce energy. Again, the cause of this problem is unclear; one theory that seems to be supported by clinically observing the Gerson Therapy working in diabetic patients is that insulin receptors on individual cells can often become obstructed by cholesterol. Other possible causes include genetic predisposition.[5]

Type 2 diabetic patients are quite frequently forty years of age or older and overweight. Often accompanying this diabetic type are high blood pressure and high blood cholesterol, symptoms found frequently with obesity. The disease's symptoms are often more difficult to spot with type 2 patients, although increased thirst and urine output are sometimes noted. Chronic skin infections and reduced circulation to the extremities can also be present.[6]

Conventional Treatment and Potential Complications of Diabetes

Management depends on the type of diabetes affecting an individual. Type 1 diabetes is always managed by a combination of diet and insulin injection. Insulin regimens, designed to supply a continuous though fluctuating supply of insulin to the body, are self-administered by the patient. Diet management, as recommended by the American Diabetes Association, usually suggests that protein intake constitute 10 to 20 percent of caloric intake, with fat no more than that same percentage for fats and oils. The remaining percentage is to be balanced among complex carbohydrates and other products, corresponding to the insulin intake of the patient.

This same diet regimen applies for type 2 patients, although weight loss also becomes a frequent goal. There are a series of noninsulin drugs on the market as well. Their functions range from increasing insulin production in the islet cells to slowing carbohydrate absorption. Type 2 patients will, on some occasions, also self-administer insulin injections.

Diabetes management is almost always geared toward long-term symptom control. Frequently, diet control is a difficult balancing act as the patient has to factor activity levels, different food products, metabolic needs, potential insulin needs, and other health factors into day-to-day treatment.

Despite conventional medical treatment methods, a number of complications still result, which include eye and vision problems such as cataract development, retinal damage, and glaucoma. Kidney problems also strike diabetics frequently; the risk of kidney disease in some form is 15 to 20 percent in type 2 patients and is double that percentage in type 1 diabetics.[7]

Diabetes and the Gerson Therapy

Type 1 diabetic patients, when treated with the Gerson Therapy, often notice a great reduction in their insulin requirements, though many will remain permanently dependent on insulin. When islet of Langerhans cells are destroyed, the body, even in the best of health, cannot regenerate them. If the cells are only damaged, there is some chance that the body, aided by the Gerson protocol, can heal and restore their function.

Additionally, in patients presenting diabetes-associated degenerative changes such as reduced vision, kidney damage, or circulation problems, the therapy is often effective in reversing deterioration. Type 1 diabetes patients do, however, need to indefinitely continue a menu plan very close to the Gerson diet to maintain the best health.

Type 2 diabetes is far more easily corrected. Patients treated with the Gerson protocol are often able to eliminate the need for insulin management. As mentioned previously, one potential cause of type 2 diabetes is a clogging effect on the insulin receptors due to cholesterol deposits. Because the Gerson diet is very low in fat and contains no cholesterol, it is highly effective in rapidly reducing cholesterol. We hold that Dr. Gerson's diet is able to quickly reverse this clogging problem, allowing cell receptors to use insulin. Many Gerson Insitute personnel have observed patients that are able to reduce their insulin dependence almost immediately when following the Gerson protocol.

Diabetic patients pursuing the Gerson Therapy in an inpatient setting will receive an altered version of the Gerson diet with a reduction in sugar intake. Patients frequently work their way back toward the standard Gerson protocol as their bodies respond to the therapy and begin to heal. After several weeks, we have observed cases of type 2 diabetes that are able to resume the full Gerson protocol, including full amounts of the apple/carrot juices that would otherwise have caused severe problems in a diabetic.

Diabetes can be further complicated by many of the other problems it brings to the body, most notably kidney damage. While the Gerson Therapy is able to reverse a good deal of such damage, when the kidneys are past a certain point—generally 20 percent or less of normal function—this treatment program is no longer effective. The same holds true for those people who are undergoing or about to start dialysis, or for those who have already undergone kidney transplant surgery.

A Summary of the Gerson Therapy Application for Diabetics

Type 2 diabetes can often be dramatically improved, and in some cases overcome, using the Gerson Therapy. Type 1 diabetes patients will often see a stabilizing effect in some cases with reversal of kidney damage and retinal damage. Hypertension is often eliminated. Type 1 patients are sometimes able to discontinue insulin completely, but this is not a common outcome. Glucose levels in the blood do require careful monitoring.

In consuming juices and following the diet, certain modifications are made to the Gerson program. Apple juice is eliminated; grapefruit juice replaces orange; the apple/carrot juice is partly replaced with green juice, depending on insulin intake. Raw vegetables replace fruits for snacking. All honey, maple syrup, brown sugar, and other sweeteners are eliminated. If glucose can be stabilized, one or two pieces of fruit per day may be added to the diet. Melons are preferred.

In taking the Gerson-recommended medications, thyroid hormone is reduced to 1 or 1 1/2 grains per day. Lugol is reduced to three drops daily. Potassium (K) is limited to 1 tsp per glass, except in cases of severe edema where K may be increased to 2 tsp per glass. During healing reactions, the individual's need for insulin may temporarily increase. Over time, the requirement for insulin supplementation is usually completely eliminated in type 2 diabetes. Type 1 patients often continue to need some supplementation, but other degenerative processes are usually arrested.

GENETIC DISORDERS

Genetic disorders generally do not respond to the Gerson Therapy, but symptoms of genetic weakness can be improved. One case of cystic fibrosis showed significant improvement while the patient followed the Gerson program.

Emphysema

Positive responses by emphysema patients have been observed when they faithfully adhered to the Gerson protocol. Lung capacity can be increased and related symptoms controlled.

Heart Disease and Vascular Disease

High blood pressure responds exceptionally well to the Gerson Therapy. In fact, improvements are so great that the companions accompanying a heart patient should be screened for antihypertensive effects, since we have observed hypotension in both patients and companions following administration of the Gerson diet alone. Antihypertensive drugs should be slowly decreased starting the third to fifth day of treatment. Malignant high blood pressure can take longer to respond to the treatment.

Heart disease does respond well to the Gerson program, and here is an illustration: In October 1990, a man whom we'll identify as Frank Winslow checked into the Gerson Therapy hospital in Tijuana, Mexico, with a multitude of health problems. He was extremely obese, weighing 303 pounds. Now forty-six years of age, Frank had already suffered a massive heart attack at age thirty-eight, and it had left him not only with heart damage, but with high blood pressure.

Frank Winslow also suffered from gout and was taking standard antigout medication. If he stopped taking it for only one day, he would have a severe gouty attack. He also had intractable diabetes. Even with his taking medication and insulin, his blood sugar ran between 240 and 400 mg/dL (where normal is below 120).

So Frank was given the Gerson Therapy, modified somewhat because of his high blood pressure and diabetes. Usually, as you may know by now, the Gerson juicing program includes thirteen glasses of fruit and vegetable juices: one 8-ounce glass (225 grams) of orange juice, about five glasses containing apples and carrots in approximately a 35 to 65 percent proportion, 1/3 apples to 2/3 carrots), three glasses of carrot juice given with two capsules of liver powder each, and four glasses of juice made with various salad greens, also containing one small apple each. In order to decrease his glucose intake somewhat, he was given not orange juice but grapefruit juice. And Frank's other juices contained fewer apples. He was also given more green juices in the place of some of the carrot juice.

Making an additional dietary adjustment which is usually done for diabetics, this patient was not furnished with a fruit plate to eat in his room, as the other patients ordinarily receive. Instead, Frank was served a plate of raw vegetables: cut-up carrot sticks, green pepper strips, celery sticks, little cauliflower heads, tomatoes—so that he would have something to "nibble" in case he was hungry. Outside of that, he could eat three full Gerson Therapy meals at regular mealtimes. They included all organic vegetarian foods, freshly prepared without any salt or fats, no frozen or canned foods, and very limited herbal spices.

Between his three meals and thirteen glasses of juice, plus his raw vegetable plate daily, Frank was never hungry even for one moment. But he did get rid of a pound a day for over two and a half months! Of course the man was also administered the other components of the Gerson Therapy: 2 tsp of potassium compound in each glass of juice, along with a little thyroid, Lugol's solution (iodine), and digestive enzymes.

Frank was taken off his antigout medication from the first day and never had another gout attack! He was also receiving the regular coffee enemas of the Gerson Therapy and an intramuscular injection of 3 cc of crude liver extract which contained 0.1 cc of vitamin B_{12} daily. Exceptionally (this next medication is not given to nondiabetic patients), he also received three times daily 200 mcg of chromium picolinate, a glucose tolerance factor.

Meantime, Frank's blood pressure came down (without salt and fat, the Gerson Therapy usually produces reduction of blood pressure within a few days); therefore, his blood pressure medication was lowered.

Within five weeks, not only had Frank Winslow lost 35 pounds, but his blood sugar was a normal 105 (from a high of 240) without his receiving any medication or insulin. He continued to lose 1 pound a day until he was a reasonably normal 205 pounds (at a height in his stocking feet of 6 feet 2 inches or 190 cm). All this time, consuming the right foods, the patient was able to eat according to his appetite's needs without being hungry at any time.

One very important aspect of Dr. Max Gerson's therapy is the coffee enema. When a patient of this diabetic type with other complications of illness is losing weight rapidly, he is also metabolizing many of the toxins that are stored in the fatty tissue. In other words, when the fat dissolves, the chemicals contained in the fatty tissue go into the general blood circulation and poison the patient if one does not intensively detoxify. The coffee enemas help to open the bile ducts in the liver and allow the toxins to be eliminated through the bowel. (See full details of the Gerson Therapy procedure in our separate chapters about the juices, food preparation, and coffee enemas.)

There are several interesting facts in this case that deserve attention. On the one hand, it became obvious to the Tijuana hospital's staff of physicians that Frank was a typical case of low thyroid function, in addition to his other problems. He was extremely overweight and had already suffered one severe heart attack plus diabetes, all of which relate to his having a low thyroid function. Also, both of his sons, aged fourteen and seventeen, suffered from allergies and asthma, respectively. These are also signs of low thyroid function (often hereditary) and immune deficiency. The boys had them too.

Still more astonishing in this family situation is the fact that Frank's father, now about seventy-six years old, had been a patient on the Gerson Therapy some seven years earlier, suffering from advanced pancreatic cancer. His doctors had given him a "hopeless" prognosis, saying that he had perhaps three to six months to live. He came to the Gerson Therapy hospital facility in Tijuana, stayed faithfully on the Gerson Therapy, and recovered completely. It is now over eight years since the senior Mr. Winslow's recovery, and the man remains well today. He too had already suffered three heart attacks prior to his diagnosis of pancreatic cancer. Today, as well, he remains free of heart disease, is active and enjoying life.

There is something to be learned by studying this unique family situation. We see here another member of the Winslow family with low thyroid function, suffering heart attacks and eventually cancer. Even though the son watched this dramatic recovery in his father, he allowed himself to become so seriously ill that he was close to death before presenting himself for the treatment which had already saved his father's life!

An important factor in the Gerson Therapy for heart disease is the use of thyroid medication to increase metabolism, burn off fats, and use up cholesterol. Obviously, thyroid hormone must be started at a low level in order not to overtax the damaged heart. Second, food supplementation with flaxseed oil helps to dissolve fat and cholesterol deposits in the arteries and increase the ability of the blood to carry oxygen. Also of great importance is the use of potassium, which helps in enzyme function (also to dissolve plaque) and keeps the blood from coagulating excessively; thus, potassium reduces the danger of clots forming and causing heart attacks and/or strokes.

Dr. Gerson was aware early in the development of his therapy of the extreme importance of potassium in treating all chronic disease. He stated that, in his opinion, the beginning of all chronic degenerative disease is the loss of potassium from the cell and the invasion of sodium (which we have referred to as *tissue damage syndrome*). In the area of heart disease, this opinion about tissue damage syndrome was later stated by Professor Demetrio Sodi-Pallares of the Mexico City University Medical School. He wrote more than twelve books and over 300 articles on his treatment of heart disease.

Dr. Sodi-Pallares also states that, in his opinion, heart disease is not a disorder of the heart but a disease of the body—particularly the loss of potassium and excess sodium. He too, in his treatment of heart disease patients, gives only a low-sodium and high-potassium diet. It was much after his original work with heart disease and many publications that he became aware of Dr. Gerson's work and similar philosophy. Only Dr. Gerson applied his low-sodium, high-potassium diet to all chronic diseases, with the same excellent results. Low sodium and high potassium work well in combination against all kinds of illnesses.

Of course, the Gerson Therapy also includes many other items and procedures, such as intensive nutritional therapy with many freshly prepared juices, digestive enzymes, flax oil, and the detoxifying coffee enemas. In arteriosclerosis and heart disease, Dr. Gerson achieved not only improvement but long-term survival. Contrary to the belief and teaching of orthodox medicine, in the Gerson patient arterial plaque and invasion is reversible so that the artery walls become clear of plaque again.

One other patient is Dr. Gerson's longtime friend, Professor Henry Schaefer-Simmern of New York City. This patient, in his mid-forties, a heavy smoker, had suffered several heart attacks within a few days of each other. He was barely alive with little blood circulation, as evidenced by his blue lips. Professor Schaefer-Simmern was put on the Gerson Therapy in the late 1940s and remained alive and active into his middle eighties.

Nearly all additional acute or chronic degenerative diseases may find permanent correction by the patient's application of a modified Gerson Therapy.

HEPATITIS A, B, AND C

We have observed apparent full remission and restoration of liver function using the Gerson protocol. Treatment is identical to that of almost any cancer chemotherapy patient. Liver enzymes should be carefully watched.

KIDNEY DISEASE

Owing to the low-protein diet offered in the Gerson protocol, kidney disease can be controlled and any remaining kidney function of not less than 15 percent can be maximized. Once patients have been started on dialysis, they cannot be accepted for treatment with the Gerson Therapy. Since kidneys won't be fully restored in most cases, kidney patients must remain for the rest of their lives on the Gerson Therapy.

METALLIC TOXICITY

Lugol's solution should be reduced to one or two drops per day when metallic toxicity is being conquered. The detoxification process should be allowed to occur slowly. The modified Gerson regimen for chemotherapy patients in fair physical condition is normally used to overcome metallic toxicity.

MULTIPLE SCLEROSIS

The Gerson Therapy has obtained excellent results in cases of MS. With the proper nutrition and detoxification, the body is able to clear the damaged myelin sheaths, which insulate the nerves so that they can carry electrical messages to the brain and back. Clearing the damaged "insulation" may cause a temporary worsening of the symptoms, frightening the Gerson patient. However, if one persists and stays with the treatment, the body will restore and heal these sheaths, resulting in ultimate full recovery.

Warning: MS is "assumed" to be an "auto-immune" disease. Namely, it is felt that the body's own immune system is destroying the myelin sheaths. With that assumption and with no other treatment choice, orthodox medicine often treats victims of MS with immune-suppressants, such as cancer chemotherapy. After such treatments, the Gerson Therapy is not easily effective. Also, such patients are often treated for long periods of time with prednisone. This, too, holds back recovery by the Gerson Therapy.

Osteoarthritis

More commonly occurring and less quickly debilitating than rheumatoid arthritis, osteoarthritis is usually found in older people. It's due to a
slowly deteriorating process in the joints, and it arises from the same underlying damage caused by excess proteins which the body is unable to assimilate and the kidneys cannot excrete. However, osteoarthritis is not
accompanied by the inflammatory process, so it's slow to cause joint damage and destruction. The disease is fairly common to observe as hard,
bony lumps in the index finger, the little finger, or in almost any of the
joints in the hands and toes. Osteoarthritis eventually lodges in the larger
joints as well.

Both types of arthritis—osteo- and rheumatoid—are theorized to be
genetically related. There is good reason to support this theory, since in either case we have to remember that the body is unable to handle the overload of animal proteins. This would presume a weakened pancreas, unable
to generate the necessary proteolytic enzymes. The tendency to a weak
pancreas could well be inherited.

But there is another point to consider. When a disease runs in the family, we have to remember that the family members are likely to eat the
same foods. Not only that, but the daughters will again eat the foods they
have learned to prepare from their mothers. In this way, the same type of
diet will be carried on through the family and into the next generation.

At the Gerson Institute, we had an interesting illustration of this situation. A vivacious woman named Lillian Stomatis, aged about fifty-five, arrived at the Gerson Therapy hospital to find relief for her rheumatoid
arthritis. Her right knee was very swollen and so painful that she was unable to help herself. In order to manage at the hospital, she brought her
daughter Rosalie along to help her walk to the bathroom, dress, and perform other personal tasks.

The daughter, an attractive young woman, was twenty-eight years old
and already clearly showed the beginning symptoms of arthritis. Still
more unfortunate, Rosalie had brought along her own daughter, a pretty
little girl in pigtails, aged five, who already had the first symptoms of
arthritis! So we see that the degenerative changes of arthritis set in earlier
and earlier in each generation.

The older people still have somewhat better reserves and are less damaged by the toxins in the air, water, soil, and daily food and newer drugs.
The younger people are getting more and more used to taking drugs for

pain, discomfort, sleeplessness, low energy, and worse. This drug taking causes more rapid deterioration. Moreover, in very young children, there is always the additional problem of vaccination.

There has been a great deal of evidence, as described by Robert A. Mendelsohn, M.D., former head of the American Pediatric Society and chief of a large pediatric hospital in Chicago before his death, that damage to young children has been caused by vaccination. In many children, the introduction of attenuated germs or viruses is sufficient to cause severe damage, brain dysfunction, diabetes, and rheumatoid arthritis. Dr. Mendelsohn's warnings and writings were violently disputed by orthodox medicine, but the fact remains that a large number of children became brain-damaged owing to vaccinations. The other disease effects were more difficult to prove. But we have to ask again about the underlying problem of vaccinating against disease: What does vaccination do to cause disease rather than prevent it? Toxins introduced into the body and not completely excreted can cause enzyme inhibition. When particular enzymes are blocked or inhibited, certain nutrients are improperly digested and excreted. And that is where disease begins.

An eighty-two-year-old physician, H. R. Feinstein, M.D., of Los Angeles, was seen at the Gerson Therapy hospital mainly because he suffered from rather severe osteoarthritis pain in his hip and other doctors had urged him to submit to a hip replacement operation. He refused and came into the Gerson program instead. However, he had other problems. This physician maintained himself on medication for high blood pressure, had a blood cholesterol count of over 300 (up to 200 is normal), and suffered from a severe loss of hearing. Dr. Feinstein brought his wife along, who also suffered from arthritis, but her problem was rheumatoid rather than osteoarthritis. She too was victimized by a high cholesterol count.

The doctor was amazed that his cholesterol count came down by over 100 points in one week. Then he was able to reduce his high blood pressure medication. Toward the end of their second week at the hospital, the Feinstein's son was in a serious auto accident, and the father was, understandably, very anxious and nervous. Just to be sure, he took an extra dose of blood pressure medication and promptly had a fainting episode. The Gerson physicians at the hospital were worried since this man, after all, was eighty-two years old. So the physicians took emergency measures. But they found that Dr. Feinstein's blood pressure was simply too low from his having popped down the medication.

As time passed and the hypertension medication left his bloodstream, he became normal again and was perfectly fine. By the end of the third week at the hospital, the patient's hearing had vastly improved, and his blood pressure remained normal without medication.

The pain in Dr. Feinstein's hip disappeared, and his osteoarthritis stopped bothering him. Of course, his hip did not heal completely, but from an X-ray examination he could see that the healing process had started and the friction was down, eliminating the pain. In his wife's case, her swollen finger, too, was improved, but due to her rushing off to her son's side, Mrs. Feinstein's treatment was interrupted and her results were not as dramatic.

Another patient with osteoarthritis, Mrs. Marion Sands, a librarian aged sixty-one, arrived at the Gerson Tijuana hospital with extremely deformed knuckles and fingers. She wore a leather shaping form to hold her fingers aligned in a normal position. She went through a three-week program and went home with knowledge to help herself. After some two years on the Gerson Therapy, at home, her hands became almost normal. The fingers were straight and her muscles were restored so that she was able to use her hands fairly well thereafter, never again needing any kind of leather brace.

As mentioned before, patients suffering from osteoarthritis have long-term, deep damage, and it takes a good deal of time and ongoing adherence to the Gerson Therapy to slowly restore the bones and muscles. But the important thing is that it can be done if the patient has enough determination and will stay long enough with this demanding and rather restrictive nutritional therapy.

OSTEOPOROSIS

In osteoporosis, patients suffer from decalcification of the bones. The presence of that problem tends to produce a reaction from the average allopathic physician. More often than not, he or she tells the patient to drink plenty of milk (for calcium). Unfortunately, this is a simplistic and incorrect approach to the problem.

First of all, we must remember that excess protein as in milk causes the disease in the first place. Second, we have seen in Pottenger's classic book *Cats, a Study in Nutrition*,[8] that heat-damaged, pasteurized milk or cooked milk products are not absorbed without the live enzymes and do no good at all, only harm. Using calcium supplementation doesn't work, either. Calcium tablets are not well assimilated. Calcium has to enter the body in the proper combination, together with active, live enzymes that we find in carrot juice, juice from green salad leaves, and a great deal of fresh lettuce.

In those fresh organically grown foods, the body receives not pharmaceutical calcium but the complete mineral nutrients aside from calcium: magnesium, manganese, zinc, copper, potassium, iodine, and many more together with the active enzymes to allow the body to assimilate these minerals and lodge them in the bones. In this manner, the Gerson Therapy not only alleviates calcium deficiency but allows one's body to actually rebuild bone.

The Gerson Therapy has been observed to be effective in improving calcification of bone for osteoporosis.

STEROID TREATMENT

When conventionally administered allopathic steroid treatment is received by patients such as those with systemic lupus erythematosus, rheumatoid arthritis, gastrointestinal disorders, brain tumors, and other conditions, such cortisone medication must *not* be discontinued suddenly and the Gerson Therapy substituted in its place. Using appropriate monitoring, the proper procedure is to slowly wean the patient off steroid medications as appropriately as possible. These sick people on steroids, which have terrible side effects, are more likely to experience stomach irritation. Acidol and niacin should be eliminated until five days after steroids have been deleted from the bloodstream, and potassium should be reduced to 10 or 20 tsp per day.

SYSTEMIC LUPUS ERYTHEMATOSUS, RHEUMATOID ARTHRITIS, AND SCLERODERMA

Upon elimination of steroids, systemic lupus erythematosus (SLE), rheumatoid arthritis (RA), scleroderma (all collagen diseases) respond exceptionally well to the Gerson Therapy. However, there will be poor healing even with the Gerson Therapy in those situations where steroids have been taken by the patient for periods over two years, or when the patient has been pretreated with chemotherapy. For SLE and RA, enemas should be limited to two to three per day. Reactions can be severe, and patients must be monitored carefully during the reaction period.

ULCERATIVE COLITIS

People who are the victims of ulcerative colitis, even when bleeding, may respond surprisingly well to the Gerson Therapy. We have observed several people who have gone into full, long-term remissions. Chamomile replaces coffee in enemas at the outset of treatment, and certain raw foods are avoided for a short period. Ulcerative colitis, Crohn's disease, irritable bowel syndrome, leaky gut syndrome, and other intestinal difficulties do show positive reactions when the Gerson Therapy is made the patient's treatment plan.

References for Chapter Seventeen

1. McPhee, S.J.; Schroeder, S.A. "General approach to the patient; health maintenance & disease prevention; & common symptoms." In *Current Medical Diagnosis and Treatment*), 36th ed., ed. by L.M. Tierney, S.J. McPhee, and M.A. Papadakis. Stamford, Conn.: Appleton & Lange, 1997, p. 14.

2. Bishop, B. A *Time to Heal: Triumph over Cancer: The Therapy of the Future.* New York: Penguin Putnam, 1985.

3. Schauss, A. *Diet, Crime and Delinquency.* Seattle, Wash.: Life Sciences Press, 1988.

4. Karam, J.H. "Diabetes mellitus & hypoglycemia." In *Current Medical Diagnosis and Treatment*), 36th ed, ed. by L.M. Tierney, S.J. McPhee, M.A. Papadakis. Stamford, Conn.: Appleton & Lange, 1997, pp. 1069–1109.

5. Kumar, P.; Clark, M. *Clinical Medicine.* London: Balliere Tindall Publishing, 1994, pp. 830–831.

6. *Op. cit.,* Karam, J.H., *p. 1090.*

7. *Ibid.,* Karam, J.H., p. 1096.

8. Pottenger, F. *Cats, a Study in Nutrition.* San Diego, Calif.: Price Pottenger Nutrition Foundation, 1983.

Part Four

USING THE GERSON APPROACH

Chapter Eighteen

PSYCHOLOGICAL APPROACHES OF THE GERSON THERAPY

Gerson patients bear an extra heavy psychological burden. Often, they come to the Gerson Therapy after having run the gauntlet of some difficult-to-accept orthodox treatments. These establishment-type therapies offered in North America are frequently adversely extensive, somewhat unpleasant, uncomfortable, and sometimes life-threatening. The patient usually will have already drained his financial resources, squandered his immunity, and made heavy demands on his emotions. Such a situation happens because of a patient's need to go through frequent diagnostic laboratory procedures, frightening clinical examinations, anxiety-driven biopsies, and numbers of other upsetting medical or psychological experiences.

The cancer patient especially is often traumatized by a widespread belief that nothing much can be done to conquer cancer. And that view may be true in many cases, judging from the high mortality rates accompanying most forms of allopathic chemotherapy and radiation therapy.

Even the newly accepted immunotherapy has its unwelcome pitfalls. From the conventional viewpoint, a patient may be led to believe that in the end, cancer is unbeatable.

The cancer patient and his or her family may arrive at the Gerson treatment facility depressed and, in many instances, taken over by a range of negative feelings, including worry, grief, fear, sadness, anger, irritability, and self-centeredness. Even for these depressed, anxious, and generally unfortunate people, the Gerson Therapy offers healing and hope.

We have observed that other patients who strive to employ the Gerson procedures at an earlier, less-damaged stage often have fewer difficulties overcoming their lack of wellness. Receiving Gerson Therapy sooner rather than later is better for achieving healing and health maintenance.

Either way, the two types of unhappy patients, early attendees and later arrivals, embark on the unfamiliar Gerson treatment outside the bounds of orthodox medicine. Consequently, they do face a long, demanding, monotonous, and lonely labor, with strong hope and determination, but with no guarantee of success at the end. Psychological aspects do play a role in the healing process, and either the standard or the modified Gerson protocol will provide some procedural guidelines.

PSYCHOLOGICAL ASPECTS OF THE GERSON THERAPY

Because of cancer's life-threatening nature, patients beset by malignant neoplasms in particular and those who suffer from other chronic diseases progress faster and more competently toward healing when they receive psychological support. An important factor of the Gerson Therapy is that its several detoxification aspects have excellent effects on the patient's outlook. The inherent toxicity of the standard American diet (SAD) and lifestyle tends to bring toxins into the blood and general systemic circulation. These poisons also reach the brain and tend to affect the mind by increasing anxiety, depression, fear, panic, and more.

Just starting with the detoxification of the Gerson Therapy, in a few days the patients improve considerably, feel more confident, and exhibit greater emotional stability. Nevertheless, we are advocates of additional psychotherapeutic help whenever available.

Dr. Gerson once stated that more human beings die of panic than from cancer. *The body involves but one part of the illness.* When the sickness also produces fear, the combination causes a systemic accumulation of more and more toxins in the body and a quickening of physiological deterioration. A better understanding of fear and the other negative emotions and what they do to someone on the mend is essential.

Inasmuch as our every human thought and emotion equals a biochemical act, the science of psychoneuroimmunology tells us that feelings, moods, and general outlook affect each person's immune system. It is boosted by a hopeful, determined outlook and undermined by a despairing, helpless attitude. If the truth be known, any cancer diagnosis equals mental and emotional trauma with reactions ranging from despair and panic to apathy or rage, all of them powerful negative perturbations of the conscious mind. These emotions hamper the affected individual's immunity to a malignancy's deadly attack.

Since the aim of Gerson personnel is to rebuild the diseased patient's damaged immune system, psychological factors must not be allowed to sabotage physical healing. A holistically oriented therapist dispels mental and emotional (psychic) negativity in order to reinforce the physical (somatic) immunity. If you are working on your own as the patient or as a caregiver for such a patient without the support of a Gerson hospital setting, our advice is to focus your healing procedures on handling negative emotions. They are destructive and must be eliminated. The patient's traumatized negative inner state must be reprogrammed and turned positive.

"No attempt should be made to cure the body without [curing] the soul," wrote Plato nearly 2,400 years ago. Body and mind are inseparable; they sicken together and must be healed together. Otherwise, chances for success in regaining health will be greatly lessened. Neither the Gerson program nor any other therapeutic method will work effectively if something in the patient's consciousness keeps saying no to life.

Indeed, negative emotions have a devastating effect upon the function of the body, and especially the nervous system. The stressful experiences arising from negative emotions cause unhealthy stimulation of the autonomic or involuntary division of the nerves, including both the sympathetic and parasympathetic branches. Blood pressure, heart rate, respiration rate, and oxygen consumption are increased. Glucose is needlessly used up. Kidney filtration, gastrointestinal secretions, and activity are decreased, affecting digestion and the release of body wastes and toxins. Insomnia, fatigue, loss of appetite, listlessness, avoidance, and boredom are observed in the patient.

All of these physical faults manifesting themselves in the autonomic nervous system must be diluted and countered to the point of eliminating them. How may somebody do that for himself or herself? How might a therapist help the patient to neutralize such negative physiological responses? The renowned author Norman Cousins, Ph.D., furnished his readers with substantial healing tools when, in his best-selling *Anatomy of an Illness*, he described how positive emotions are powerful mobilizers for the patient's natural healing resources.

EMPHASIS ON POSITIVE EMOTIONS AS POWERFUL HEALING TOOLS

Positive emotions are powerful weapons in the unwell individual's war against disease. Laughter, courage, tenacity, love and consideration for others, and a connection to the patient's own understanding of spirituality are all positive passions or sentiments. Dr. Cousins wrote:

Increasingly, in the medical press, articles are being published about the high cost of the negative emotions. Cancer, in particular, has been connected to intensive states of grief or anger or fear. It makes little sense to suppose that emotions exact only penalties and confer no benefits. At any rate, long before my own serious illness, I became convinced that creativity, the will to live, hope, faith, and love had biochemical significance and contribute strongly to healing and to well-being. The positive emotions are life-giving experiences.[1]

The French physicist and Nobel laureate Marie Curie, Ph.D., stated, "Nothing in life is to be feared; it is only to be understood. Now is the time to understand more, so that we may fear less." The understanding of a disease process and its cause should be the first step in conquering any sickness. Identifying the underlying reason that an illness exists will enable a distressed patient to comprehend the workings and purpose of the Gerson program and why it's bound to be effective.

Someone critically ill will likely find it difficult to concentrate on thoroughly learning Dr. Gerson's concepts; consequently, the family or accompanying caregiver must assist with this function. Understanding and accepting the Gerson approach to achieving wellness takes away some of the fear by showing that there is hope of reversing the disease process.

Words alone will not obliterate all of the fear, and we acknowledge that a favorable result is really what counts. Early improvement in the diseased state will do more than anything else to resurrect hope. Many patients newly arriving at a Gerson health facility have lost the will to eat and drink.

But that situation soon changes for the better. The Gerson program helps such a person over this difficult period, giving the individual simple foods and juices which the body is able to easily digest. Such an easing of the metabolism is vital, for then we will see a restoration of blood flow, an improvement in the nervous system, and an overall pickup of bodily functions. The patient begins to eat, drink, and sleep much better, and almost immediately he or she starts to feel strengthened. An interest in life is stimulated. Probably for the first time since the patient heard his or her diagnosis and prognosis, there is a prospect of living a long life. There *can* be a future.

SOME FUNCTIONS OF A CAREGIVER (FAMILY MEMBER OR FRIEND)

Still, a drastic change of lifestyle is required by the Gerson Therapy. For the patient, living each day inevitably has its ups and downs with healing crises occurring all too frequently. The healing process offers a severe test for even the most committed patient. It becomes the job of any caregiver to lighten that patient's burden with steady support, empathy, and well-focused counseling. How are these caregiving functions carried out? By the caregiver's achieving full completion of specific beneficial tasks. They include:

- Creating a safe space for the patient to occupy through total listening and offering nonjudgmental attention.
- Building a healing partnership with the patient, turning him or her into an active ally able to share responsibility for the therapeutic process.
- Dispelling the superstitious fear attached to cancer. This is done by reprogramming the patient's consciousness, helping to reframe harmful concepts; and by identifying self-defeating patterns and eliminating them.
- Exploring the patient's belief system and the family dynamics in which he or she is embroiled. If the family dynamics are negative or hostile to the therapy, an attempt must be made to reverse such dynamics. Or, get the patient out of the disruptive environment. Or, take the source of disruption away from the patient's environment.
- Dealing with resentment and unfinished business facing the patient.
- Coping with the drastic mood swings and sometimes antisocial behavior that can accompany the detoxification process.

A caregiver is very necessary to prevent the patient from deciding that the Gerson treatment program is impossible to face at home on one's own. The caregiver assists a patient in almost all aspects of accomplishing the Gerson Therapy. It starts out with shopping for food and moves on to securing deliveries, cooking the foods, checking on helpers, preparing juices, allotting juice portions, establishing the daily routine, keeping on top of the program routine, washing up endlessly, making the enema coffee, offering aid if an enema goes askew, coping with healing reactions and other forms of flare-up, relieving boredom, injecting enthusiasm into the treatment, and above all, causing sanity to prevail for both patient and caregiver.

The caregiver needs to be prepared for alterations in emotions that arise as the patient's body is freed of its residual poisons. Journalist and psychotherapist Beata Bishop of London, England, tells us, "Physical detoxification inevitably brings about psychological detoxification, too. Toxins passing through the central nervous system evoke strange reactions and out-of-character behavior: violent mood swings, snappiness, anger, instability, unfair accusations, and aggression. The patient's normally civilized behavior gives way to drives and emotions that have been denied and repressed for a long time, perhaps since childhood. . . . It is part of the process. In whatever capacity we work with the patient, we remain calm, caring, unchanged, waiting for the inner upheaval to pass."[2]

TOOLS AND METHODS FOR PSYCHOLOGICAL IMPROVEMENT

To offset the negative psychological aspects of serious illness—whether cancer, heart disease, diabetes, arthritis, serious infections, or any other form of degenerating pathology—practitioners of the Gerson Therapy are taught to incorporate certain considerations into their treatment programs. The extracurricular considerations include a number of psychology tools and methods for patient application:

1. Employing relaxation techniques,
2. Creating visualizations linked to self-healing,
3. Engaging in simple meditations,
4. Repeatedly using affirmations,
5. Educating and developing the imaginative power of the right brain that is creative, artistic, and idealistic,

6. Reversing negative family dynamics,
7. Emphasizing positive actions in all situations or relationships,
8. Fully understanding the Gerson program to bring about confidence and a willingness to become involved in such a demanding, rigid, and comprehensive treatment which asks for so much self-discipline,
9. Removing internal physical pain relatively quickly by use of coffee enemas and other sources of detoxification, and
10. Steadily exhibiting symptomatic results the patient sees and feels.

Below, we briefly discuss the first five methods and tools. These five afford a psychological uplift for the person who is ill with cancer or another life-threatening disorder.

Use a Relaxation Technique

For fifteen minutes, three times a day—upon arising, after lunch, and before retiring—relax deeply by use of a progressive relaxation technique. First relax the head, next the neck, then the shoulders, and in progression all of the rest of the body from top to bottom completely down to the toes.

This relaxation is achieved by proceeding with the technique taught by Jose Silva of Silva Mind Control fame. Here is how to proceed:

1. Sit comfortably in a chair or lie on the floor.
2. Close the eyes and relax.
3. Take a deep lung-filling inhalation.
4. During exhalation, relax the body even more.
5. Count slowly backward from 100 to 1.
6. Daydream about some peaceful place you know.
7. Mentally verbalize a strong affirmation such as "I will always maintain a perfectly healthy body and mind."
8. Go into the well-practiced creative visualizations you've developed for yourself which provide the greatest comfort.[3]

Create Visualizations

There is a basic technique of creative visualization which Shakti Gawain, renowned pioneer and teacher of the consciousness movement, offers to her students. It involves the following step-by-step procedure:

1.   Apply your personal method of relaxation, perhaps the same technique suggested by Jose Silva;
2.   Imagine a healthy state of the body that you want very much to possess;
3.   Imagine this healthy body state in your possession, admire it, enjoy it, show it to loved ones and friends;
4.   Make some positive statements (affirmations) about this healthy body state;
5.   End the visualization with firm avowals that you will have this healthy body state permanently.[4]

Once relaxed and able to visualize readily, start the healing process in earnest. Picture the body with its growing tumor, and imagine that tumor stopping its growth. Then see it getting smaller. During each of these relaxation sessions, visualize the tumor shrinking a tiny bit more than the last time. Also imagine the very active immune system, however you may picture it, with that protective system's all-encompassing white blood cells (leukocytes), which consist of the lymphocytes, the phagocytes, the monocytes, and much more.

Engage in Simple Meditations

Meditation, a state of consciousness in which one stops awareness of the surroundings so the mind can focus on a single precept, leads to rest and relief from stress. It takes patience and persistence to develop the power of concentration required in meditation. The mind will naturally wander to other things and images. One's attention must be returned to the subject over and over again. It may be frustrating to discover just how easily the attention wanders. Consider that the subject of a meditation is similar to that of a target; stray thoughts will often prevent hitting the bull's-eye.[5]

A wide variety of meditation techniques are used to clear the mind of stressful outside disturbances. The method that follows below, as taught by Dr. Lawrence LeShan, is just one of many meditation procedures that we could describe.

Meditation is a purposefully directed and harmonious application of the mind. And the Indian Yogi Maharishi's teachings ask: "What is the mind? It is only a bundle of thoughts. Stop thinking and show me then, where is the mind?"

Psychotherapist Lawrence LeShan, Ph.D., another pioneer who explores therapeutic and ethical implications of meditation and visualizations, offers us a means of reaching into the mind by counting breaths. It is a technique used in Zen training, and the object is to be doing just one thing as completely and fully as possible. The single thing, in this case, is counting one's exhalations.

"Strive to be aware of just counting breaths and be as fully aware of it as possible," Dr. LeShan advises. "All your attention is gently and firmly and repeatedly brought to bear on this activity. The goal is to have your whole being involved in the counting. . . . In this exercise one is paying as full and complete attention as possible to the counting itself. Thoughts, feelings, impressions, sensory perceptions, to the degree that they are conscious, are a wandering away from the instructions."

We suggest that you draw in your senses by counting the breaths up to four counts. Then begin the count again. To fill up the time elapsed between counts, add the word "and" after each of the exhalation counts. Thus you would count "one"—"and"—"two"—"and"—"three"—"and"— "four." Then repeat the count. This is a very fine technique for bringing you into a meditative state.[6]

Repeatedly Use Affirmations

Among the most important elements of creative visualization are affirmations, strong and positive statements declaring that something exists or is already so.[7] When an individual states, "I am getting better and better," the mind tells the body. Be assured: *The body believes everything that it hears the mind say.* The stream of thoughts that runs through one's mind are vital to the body's health, for if the ideas and words we use are unknowingly negative, a small amount of this negation attaches itself to one's physical self. Those words get stuck in the mind and seep out to the rest of oneself.

And, if the negative notions are knowingly painful to others, those ideas are *dis*affirmations that come back to destroy you. Remember that old cliché which has proven itself all too true: "What goes around comes around."

The practice of silently verbalizing affirmations (or speaking them aloud) allows the verbalizer to replace negative, stale, worn-out programming from the past with positive or constructive concepts and themes to transform attitudes and expectations about life and health. You can write down the affirmations too or chant them as rhymes or sing them as songs. Repeatedly using affirmations is vital for bringing about healing.

Exponents of the Gerson Therapy encourage the application of tangible health-producing affirmations having to do with acute or chronic illnesses and infectious or degenerative diseases that are causing difficulty. Here we offer just a few samples of affirmations you might create and use for yourself:

- Every day in every way I am getting better, better, and better.
- I am vibrantly healthy and radiantly beautiful!
- I am healthy and whole and complete in myself.
- I give thanks now for my life of perfect health and happiness.
- I am happy to be alive and well, anticipating what the future brings.
- I now recognize and accept the excellence of my healing path.
- I love and appreciate myself just as I am.
- I am conquering illness because the treatment is working.

At this point we have some suggestions about how to use affirmations to create health and happiness:

1. Always phrase affirmations in the present tense, as if what you aim for already exists. See your goal as being reality now and as something to come. That's because everything is created first in the mind before it becomes manifest in the physical.
2. Phrase affirmations in the most constructive manner possible by stating what is definitely wanted, rather than what is *not* wanted. Avoid disaffirmations except when eliminating emotional blocks or bad habits. If it is necessary to say something negative, follow up immediately with another thing that's positive.
3. Use shorter affirmations instead of longer ones so that they remain clear and convey strong feelings.
4. Hold on to the affirmative statement only if it fits you well and feels right for your body and mind.
5. Have the affirmation produce a feeling of belief within you by suspending doubts or hesitations about its practicality.
6. Use affirmations repeatedly whether alone or in combination with creative visualizations. (Affirmations accompany visualizations very well.)

Develop the Imaginative Power of the Right Brain

It's only in the last century and a half that real progress has been made in understanding the mind's workings, and even that progress has shown us how much is yet to be learned. Just when scientists think they have located areas where activities such as thinking, remembering, and speaking are based, a new situation appears which proves that the answer is by no means certain. Yet we are gathering knowledge about the imaginative power of the right brain—at least we know that the mind is infinitely more subtle than was previously thought. Everyone who possesses what has been called a "normal" mind actually owns a much larger ability and potential than had been determined a mere fifty years ago.[8]

The brain of each human being has two sides, the left hemisphere and the right hemisphere. Each side of the brain has different mental functions which scientists refer to as *lateralization*, meaning that various mental abilities are parceled out laterally (to the left or right side).

The left hemisphere functions most effectively for purposes of reading, writing, arithmetic and number skills, calculation, spoken language and language skills, scientific skills, reasoning, linear processing, logical procedures, and right-hand control. The right hemisphere best controls music awareness, spatial construction and artisitic intelligence, holistic thinking, imagination, insight, intuition, three-dimensional and pattern perception, and left-hand control. Added to these, the right brain deals with relaxation, imagination, creativity, visualization, meditation. and affirmations.[9]

As an interesting aside, women have more-developed left hemispheres and thus outperform men on tests of verbal fluency. And women do better on remembering details. In navigating through the world, however, men possess more of a sense of a spatial map in their mind, while women pay attention to and use local landmarks as guides. The mental differences between the sexes may be partly due to hormones.[10,11,12]

Inasmuch as the right hemisphere provides more efficacy with the psychology of surviving cancer, we highly recommend that the person with a degenerative disease develop the imaginative power of the right side of the brain using the methods we have described.

References for Chapter Eighteen

1. Cousins, N. *Anatomy of an Illness.* New York: W.W. Norton & Co., 1979, p. 86.

2. Bishop, B. "Psychological considerations for the Gerson patient." In *Gerson Therapy Physician's Training Manual*. Bonita, Calif.: The Gerson Insititute, 1996, p. 62.

3. Silva, J.; Stone, R.B. *You the Healer*. Tiburon, Calif.: H.J. Kramer, 1989, p. 18.

4. Gawain, S. *Creative Visualization*. Novato, Calif.: Nataraj Publishing, 1995, pp. 27–28.

5. Ozaniec, N. *Meditation for Beginners*. London: Hodder & Stoughton Educational, 1995, p. 2.

6. LeShan, L. *How to Meditate*. Boston: Little, Brown & Co., 1974, pp. 58–59.

7. Gawain, S. *Creative Visualization*. New York: Bantam Books, 1982, pp. 21–26.

8. Buzan, T. *Use Both Sides of Your Brain*. New York: E.P. Dutton, 1974, p. 13.

9. Leviton, R. *Brain Builders!* (West Nyack, N.Y.: Parker Publishing Co., 1995, pp. 330–331.

10. Herlitz, A.; Nilsson, L.G.; Backman, L. "Gender Differences in Episodic Memory." *Memory and Cognition* 25(6):801–811, 1997.

11. Sherwin, B.B. "Estrogen and cognitive functioning in women." *Proceedings of the Society for Experimental Biology and Medicine* 217(1): 17–22, 1998.

12. Fink, G.; Sumner, B.E.; Rosie, R.; Grace, O.; Quinn, J.P. "Estrogen control of central neurotransmission: effect on mood, mental state, and memory." *Cellular and Molecular Neurobiology* 16(3):325–344, 1996.

Chapter Nineteen

HOW TO FOLLOW THE GERSON THERAPY ON YOUR OWN

W hat are the characteristics of a person who survives cancer or another "incurable" disease? We, whose work entails furnishing information for coping with incurables, have observed the traits shown by those who thrive, even against life-threatening odds. To open this chapter, we are sharing such information.

Every day, the incurable disease survivor embarks on a healing journey and:

- asks lots of questions and makes multiple new health discoveries;
- seeks out others knowledgeable about health care;
- questions the practices of conventional oncological medicine (COM);
- examines offerings in complementary and alternative medicine (CAM);
- uncovers and then puts aside the abundant myths perpetuated by both medical disciplines (COM and CAM);
- associates closely with a higher spiritual power;
- keeps faith in, acquires hope for, and expects healing from that higher power;
- abandons self-pity and accepts personal responsibility for homeostatic bodily functions;
- avoids stressors and masters stress; and
- prepares a set of principles for living well and abides by them.

In the October 1999 issue of the *Townsend Letter for Doctors & Patients*, Al Schaefer of Seattle, Washington, discusses the successful cancer survivor. Mr. Schaefer writes: "The survivor questions him/her self and wonders what steps to take for correction—how to recover [and remain in a state of wellness]. He/she asks [informed persons], 'If you were in my shoes, what would you do?' "

The cancer survivor discovers that there is a definite belief system about malignancy programmed into allopathic doctors that trickles down to medical consumers through the journalistic media, which invariably take their material from organized medicine's propaganda mechanisms. This programming states: "Cancer is death; it is tumor; tumor is autonomous; under no circumstances can it be conquered!" If accepted by a cancer patient, these erroneous beliefs severely hinder recovery and are likely to come true. Alternately, when they are not believed their falsity becomes apparent, and the person with cancer survives splendidly.[1]

A second set of falsehoods leveled at the public by a brainwashed North American medical orthodoxy is that (1) surgery, radiation, or chemotherapy is the only effective cancer treatment, and all other therapies should be considered quackery; (2) biopsy, excision of the lump accompanied by a pathology examination, CAT scans, mammograms, X-ray films, and other forms of high technology are the most reliable diagnostic methods; (3) food quality and good nutrition have no effect upon cancer's progress; (4) early detection and treatment increase the odds of survival; and (5) if someone with cancer lives five years, such an interval counts as a cure of the disease.

The above five propaganda pronouncements are unmitigated myths perpetrated by the cancer industry, usually for financial gain. The knowing cancer survivor recognizes statements such as these as coming from allopathic sources. He/she knows that they are sheer fantasies, and subsequently, develops more accurate personal beliefs based on observation and education.

"Identifying these fabrications as altogether wrong and harmful to the ill individual, I know there must be a more effective way to gain healing and health maintenance," says the "incurable disease" survivor who puts the lie to such an inaccurate label. This positive-minded patient seeks out and finds the better way. In doing so, he or she becomes totally confident and self-reliant.

Some survivors discover their inspiration through the actions of an empathetic health professional who has become disenchanted with the various conventional myths of medicine. This doctor radiates love for patients who eventually do push him or her into some form of alternative method of healing—a rare physician who deserves to be cherished. Other patients become inspired by the testimonies of survivors who are proof that cancer or another illness is reversible. Tumor, for instance, turns out to merely be a symptom of some pathology that's treatable, but to which treatment had not yet been applied.

The "incurable disease" survivor becomes anchored in reality. He/she wastes no time searching for "silver bullets" or some anticancer vaccine or another form of "miracle" cure repeatedly being promised but never delivered by the cancer establishment. It's realized by the sophisticated individual that our cancer industry reaps vast profits each time it predicts such a cure if only enough money could be donated.

Instead of a miracle cure, the disease survivor searches for nontoxic alternatives and asks, "How many have been helped by this treatment? Do you know someone who recovered by its use? Can I talk to the recovered person? Does it have detrimental side effects? What are they? Also, what are the product's ingredients or the method's procedures?"

A cancer survivor continues to nourish his/her body with excellent food containing all the essential nutrients and cleanses it internally and externally. One's body is considered a temple for the soul. The patient has become vegan with the ingestion of no animal products, drinking from ten to fourteen glasses of vegetable or fruit juices a day. All drugs, soft drinks, coffee, chocolate, and processed foods are avoided. And only those certain adjunctive practices or medications permitted by the Gerson program are brought home to be introduced into the body.

If engaging in the Gerson Therapy at home, the supposedly "incurable disease" survivor requires self-discipline, determination, and the vigorous pursuit of human body knowledge. He or she becomes a student of organic agriculture, nutritional science, body detoxification, psychology, visualization, meditation, the politics surrounding cancer's medical treatments, and much more general information connected with degenerative diseases. This individual becomes an educator about what's pure, good, and true for the welfare of body and mind. There is much sharing with others. Most of all, although difficult to pursue, complete recovery from illness using the program developed by Dr. Max Gerson continues for the patient at home.

Without any question or doubt, an incurable disease survivor affirms that self-administering the Gerson Therapy at home is the principal means by which one ensures that perfect health remains evermore.

AN INTRODUCTION TO
SELF-ADMINISTERING THE
GERSON THERAPY AT HOME

To understand and apply the Gerson Therapy at home to increase the chances of beating back most of the incurable diseases, the balance of this chapter offers a quick reference format for various aspects of the healing program. It also explains recent developments in adjuvant therapies, too. Practical help for those seeking the required materials and supplies used for the Gerson Therapy, sometimes difficult to obtain, is given. The authors, primarily Charlotte Gerson, who is most conversant with her father's therapy, are drawing on more than forty years of experience in "curing the incurables".

For people who are afflicted, or who have loved ones suffering with all types of life-threatening degenerative diseases, starting immediately below with information about adjuvant therapies we show how patients can become their own healers.

Because the Gerson Therapy is the primary management tool for eliminating illness, any agent, material, technique, or procedure added to it must be characterized as adjuvant, or supportive in nature. No adjuvant agent should be used at the expense of a regular Gerson procedure or medication in the hope of improving that adjuvant's performance. If a Gerson-trained physician makes an alteration in the healing program, however, adjunctive treatment under that doctor's supervision is permissible. Furthermore, always consult your Gerson Therapy physician with regard to any promising new addition to the treatment.

ADJUNCTIVE THERAPIES THAT FIT INTO
THE GERSON PROCEDURE

The procedures and materials listed below are available at all Gerson facilities in a form compatible with the Gerson Therapy. Please be aware that each Gerson Center is separately owned and licensed by the Gerson Institute. At any given facility, certain additional therapies cited below may or may not be available. The Gerson-trained physician in charge may choose to recommend the addition of one or more of such adjunctive therapies.

Laetrile, the purified form of amygdalin, which occurs naturally in the pits of apricots and in some other foods, is a cyanogenic glycoside (containing cyanide). While it is nontoxic, laetrile by itself does not cure. It is used as an analgesic and has other purported anticancer properties. Laetrile is not part of the routine Gerson Therapy.

When a Gerson patient elects to add laetrile to the Gerson program, this supplemental material must in no way replace the central and continuous work of the Gerson Therapy. (Some laetrile therapists have recommended dietary measures counterproductive to natural healing progress with the Gerson Therapy. Do *not* follow those non-Gerson measures.)

Polarizing treatment, described in *Merck's Manual of Standard Medical Procedures*, aids potassium travel through the cell membrane by a transport mechanism. It is an addition to the Gerson protocol pioneered by Dr. Demetrio Sodi-Pallares, a noted Mexico City cardiologist and researcher. The basic polarizing solution, GKI, is necessary to provide a transport mechanism to help potassium (K) travel through the cell membrane for those patients who are deficient in K. It is combined with glucose (G) and insulin (I) together as an intravenous injection.

Polarizing treatment promotes healing in the diseased heart and in tissues damaged by cancer and other degenerative diseases. Patients with edema in the extremities note a rapid reabsorption and release of the fluids from the body.

Oxygen therapies, including hydrogen peroxide (H_2O_2) and ozone (O_3) therapy, boost serum oxygen levels to revitalize normal cells while damaging viruses and other pathogens. It may be absorbed through the skin by bathing in it (4 to 5 pints of 3 percent H_2O_2 in a standard-size bathtub), applied topically, or insufflated rectally. Ambient air ozone generators are used to benefit patients by delivering O_3.

In addition to the usual intensive Gerson Therapy, some adjuvant procedures such as those mentioned and several others are being made available in the Gerson hospital or other Gerson facilities but at an extra charge.

Live cell therapy, the ingestion by injection or orally of fetal tissue cells for the strengthening of specific organs, is more effective after good detoxification has taken place. It should not be tried during the initial stages of Gerson Therapy. It may be available on request from your Gerson Therapy facility.

Pancreatin, highly concentrated pancreatic enzymes for dissolving and digesting tumor tissue, help patients if they carry a heavy tumor load. The additional intensive pancreatin has improved the patient's ability to eliminate many kinds of neoplasms.

Tahebo tea (pau d'arco or lapacho), has been shown repeatedly to have anticancer properties. It is used as a tea by native Indians of the Americas.

Vitamin C, administered orally and rectally, works to offset the free radical pathology connected with chemotherapy and radiation.

Hyperthermia/Hydrotherapy, full-body immersion in a bathtub containing hot water to elevate the body temperature to 104°F for the induction of a mild fever, tends to deteriorate tumor tissue. It's best used after the administration of laetrile. This combination of hot tub fomentation with laetrile is one of the best remedies for overcoming pain. It dulls and calms the discomfort and is a great assist to detoxification by improving the blood flow and lymphatic circulation. Patients with nervous system disease such as MS should not be subjected to high temperature. Cool compresses are more beneficial for them. Important: not to be used with fluoridated water systems.

Clay poultice, a soft composition powder mixed with water and applied as a mud pack to an inflamed body part for purposes of absorbing toxins of arthritis, cancer, insect stings, diarrhea, and poisons, it has an adsorptive effect like that of charcoal. The clay poultice aids detoxification. Clay powder can also be used internally to clear gastrointestinal difficulties and inflammations. The procedure for applying a clay poultice should involve the following steps:

1. Prepare enough warm water to mix the needed amount of clay powder into a paste.
2. Apply the paste quickly to a square of clean muslin to prevent cooling.
3. Place the muslin on an area to be treated.
4. Cover the area with plastic and wool cloth.
5. Pin the covering in place and leave it on overnight or until dry.
6. Remove and gently rub the area with a cold wet cloth.
7. Repeat this procedure as required.
8. Discard used clay pack.

References for Chapter Nineteen

1. Schaefer, A. "Some characteristics of cancer survivors." *Townsend Letter for Doctors & Patients.* 195:70–71, October 1999.

Chapter Twenty

GERSON LAB TESTS EXPLAINED

In this chapter we explain the significance of certain laboratory tests that are necessary for monitoring one's healing progress. Laboratory testing of blood and urine are a standard part of follow-up protocols for Gerson Therapy patients employed by all Gerson-trained health professionals. Among practitioners invited to administer the Gerson program are medical doctors, osteopathic physicians, and naturopathic physicians.

If you are a patient utilizing the Gerson approach to healing but have no access to a trained Gerson health practitioner to act as your ombudsman, it's still possible to have appropriate monitoring performed. Accomplish this by hiring the services of a conventionally praciticing allopathic physician who is willing to order laboratory examinations for you or for ill loved ones (of course, for a fee). Then, using the guidance of this chapter, you probably will be able to interpret the test results. But, you do need a licensed health professional's prescription to have laboratory tests conducted.

Moreover, from observations made over many years of counseling degenerative disease patients, the coauthors know that combining a doctor's interpretation with information offered below will give you an understanding of what is happening physiologically in your healing body. We offer this caution, however: Suggestions by allopathic, non-Gerson-educated practitioners for you to take drugs or make food changes may not be in your best interest and could very well be contraindicated.

Explanations and interpretations are provided here to help our readers feel less intimidated by unfamiliar medical terms, and to acquaint them with current knowledge about the required laboratory tests in the event they must monitor themselves without assistance by any health professional. If you want education about some specific test other than what is furnished here, we recommend that you query the laboratory conducting the particular examination for you. It's your right to know about tissues and other specimens taken from your own body.

THE SERUM CALCIUM LABORATORY TEST

The laboratory test for serum calcium is a measurement of the levels of calcium in the blood. Knowing such levels helps a health professional to interpret the patient's physiological status regarding neuromuscular activity, enzyme activity, skeletal development, and blood coagulation.

Calcium (Ca^+) is a predominantly extracellular ion (a cation) derived from the calcium absorbed in food through the gastrointestinal tract, provided sufficient vitamin D is present in the food eaten. Excess quantities of calcium ions in the blood are excreted in the urine and feces, while insufficient calcium concentrations can move out of the storage areas of bones and teeth to restore low blood levels. Daily ingestion of 1 gram of calcium is necessary for normal calcium balance. For Gerson patients, this should not be given in the form of supplements. Juices and foods contain more than adequate amounts of calcium.

Serum calcium testing aids in diagnosing arrhythmias, blood-clotting deficiencies, acid-base imbalance, and disorders of the neuromuscular, skeletal, and endocrine systems. Normal adult serum calcium levels range from 8.9 to 10.1 mg/dL (atomic absorption is 2.25 to 2.75 mmol/L). Serum calcium levels for children are higher than for adults.

When the level of Ca^+ is too high, a condition of *hypercalcemia* prevails indicating the possibility of one or more of the following pathologies: hyperparathyroidism, Paget's disease of the bone, multiple myeloma, metastatic carcinoma, multiple fractures, and prolonged immobilization. From inadequate excretion of calcium, also shown by elevated serum calcium, kidney disease and adrenal insufficiency may result.

In contrast, low calcium levels (known as *hypocalcemia*) may come from hypoparathyroidism, total parathyroidectomy, or malabsorption. Decreased serum Ca^+ levels may arise from calcium loss in Cushing's syndrome, kidney (renal) failure, acute pancreatitis, and periotonitis.

Hypercalcemia may bring on deep bone pain, flank pain from renal calculi, and muscle hypotonicity. Its beginning symptoms are manifested by nausea, vomiting, and dehydration, leading to stupor and coma, and may end in cardiac arrest.

Hypocalcemia may produce peripheral numbness and tingling, muscle twitching, facial muscle spasm (Chvostek's sign), carpopedal spasm (Trousseau's sign), seizures, and arrhythmias.

THE SERUM PHOSPHATES LABORATORY TEST

The laboratory test for serum phosphates is a measurement of the blood levels of phosphates to tell the state of body energy, carbohydrate metabolism, lipid metabolism, and acid-base balance. Phosphate ion (P^+) is the dominant cellular anion, which is essential for bone formation. Testing for its blood level aids in the diagnosis of acid-base imbalance plus renal, endocrine, skeletal, and calcium disorders.

In a normal adult, serum phosphate levels range from 2.5 to 4.5 mg/dL (0.80 to 1.40 mmol/L) or from 1.8 to 2.6 mEq/L. Children show a higher range that can rise to 7 mg/dL (2.25 mmol/L) during spurts of increased bone growth.

Phosphates are absorbed through the intestines from dietary sources in the presence of vitamin D. Excess quantities of them are excreted through the kidneys, which act as the regulating mechanism. Because calcium and phospate interact in a reciprocal relationship, urinary excretion of phosphates increases or decreases in inverse proportion to serum calcium levels.

Abnormally high concentrations of phosphates in the blood (*hyperphosphatemia*), which can come from drinking an overabundance of carbonated beverages, sets up a pathological process of bone loss, tooth demineralization, poor healing of fractures, hypoparathyroidism, acromegaly, diabetic acidosis, high intestinal obstruction, and renal failure.

Depressed phosphate levels in the blood (*hypophosphatemia*) may result from malnutrition, malabsorption syndromes, hyperparathyroidism, renal tubular acidosis, or treatment of diabetic acidosis. In children, such hypophosphatemia can suppress normal growth.

THE SERUM SODIUM LABORATORY TEST

The laboratory test for serum sodium is a measurement of the blood levels of sodium to determine body water distribution, osmotic pressure of extracellular fluid, neuromuscular function, and acid-base balance. The sodium ion (Na^+) is the major extracelullar cation, and it influences both chloride and potassium blood levels.

Sodium is absorbed by the intestines and is excreted primarily by the kidneys; a small amount is lost through the skin by sweating. This mineral aids the kidneys in regulating body water, for decreased Na^+ promotes water excretion and an increased level promotes water retention (edema).

Testing for Na^+ aids in evaluating fluid electrolytes, acid-base balance, and certain disorders of the kidneys, adrenals, and neuromuscular system. The sodium blood test also determines the effects of drug therapy such as diuretics on the body. For an adult, normally serum sodium levels range from 135 to 145 mEq/L (mmol/L). For Gerson patients, a level of 127 is still acceptable.

Sodium imbalance comes from either a change in water volume intake or variation in how much sodium gets consumed. Elevated serum sodium levels (*hypernatremia*) may be caused by inadequate water intake, diabetes insipidus, impaired renal function, prolonged hyperventilation, severe vomiting, or severe diarrhea. Sodium retention also comes from consuming excessive salt. The signs and symptoms of hypernatremia are thirst, restlessness, dry mouth, sticky mucous membranes, flushed skin, oliguria, diminished reflexes, hypertension, dyspnea, and edema.

Ingesting too little sodium mineral for serum Na^+ (*hyponatremia*) is rare and doesn't even happen on the low-sodium dietary program encouraged by the Gerson Therapy. There is always some sodium coming from food. Still, hyponatremia can occur, and its indications appear as apprehension, lassitude, headache, decreased skin turgor, abdominal cramps, tremors, or convulsions. It can come on from profuse sweating, gastrointestinal suctioning, diuretic therapy, diarrhea, vomiting, adrenal insufficiency, burns, and chronic renal insufficiency with acidosis. If you do have testing for serum sodium performed, make sure to get a urine sodium determination simultaneously.

THE SERUM POTASSIUM LABORATORY TEST

The laboratory test for serum potassium, a quantitative analysis, is the measurement of blood potassium for regulation of homeostasis, osmotic equilibrium, muscle activity, enzyme activity, acid-base balance, and kidney function. Potassium (K^+) is the body's major intracellular ion (a cation); small amounts of it are also found in the extracellular fluid.

Since the kidneys excrete nearly all the ingested potassium, a dietary intake of at least 40 mEq/day (mmol/d) is essential. A normal diet usually includes 60 to 100 mEq/day of this mineral. In the blood, normal K^+ levels range from 3.8 to 5.5 mEq/liter (mmol/L).

Vital to maintaining electrical conduction within the cardiac and skeletal muscles, K^+ is affected by variations in the secretion of adrenal steroid hormones and by fluctuations in pH, serum glucose levels, and serum sodium levels. A reciprocal relationship exists between K^+ and Na^+; the substantial intake of one causes a corresponding decrease in the other. Although the body readily conserves sodium, potassium deficiency may develop rapidly and is quite common, because there is no efficient method for conserving potassium.

The laboratory test for serum potassium is used to evaluate clinical signs of either potassium excess (*hyperkalemia*) or potassium depletion (*hypokalemia*). It also monitors kidney function, acid-base balance, and glucose metabolism, and evaluates arrhythmias, neuromuscular disorders, and endocrine disorders. Hyperkalemia is common in patients with excessive cellular K^+ entering the blood as in cases of burns, crushing injuries, diabetic ketoacidosis, and myocardial infarction. It will also be present where there is reduced sodium excretion from renal failure that causes an abnormal Na^+-K^+ exchange and in Addison's disease caused by the absence of aldosterone, with consequent K^+ buildup and Na^+ depletion.

Note: Although elevated serum potassium is uncommon in Gerson Therapy patients, if it does occur, supplemental potassium should be reduced or temporarily discontinued. Then the consulting Gerson-trained physician should immediately be consulted.

The signs and symptoms of hyperkalemia are weakness, malaise, nausea, diarrhea, colicky pain, muscle irritability progressing to flaccid paralysis, oliguria, and bradycardia. An electrocardiogram (EKG) reveals a prolonged PR interval; wide QRS; tall, tented T wave; and ST depression. Indications of hypokalemia are decreased reflexes; rapid, weak, irregular pulse; mental confusion; hypotension; anorexia; muscle weakness; and paresthesia. The EKG shows a flattened T wave, ST depression, and U wave elevation. In severe cases of hypokalemia, ventricular fibrillation, respiratory paralysis, and cardiac arrest could occur.

THE SERUM CHLORIDE LABORATORY TEST

The laboratory test for serum chloride, another quantitative analysis, is a measurement of blood levels of the chloride ion (Cl^-), the major extracellular fluid anion. Interacting with Na^+, Cl^- helps maintain the osmotic pressure, blood volume, arterial pressure, and acid-base balance. Chloride is absorbed from the intestines and is excreted primarily by the kidneys.

By evaluating the body's fluid status, the serum chloride laboratory test detects two types of fluid imbalances, acid-base (acidosis and alkalosis) and extracellular cation-anion. Normally serum chloride levels range from 100 to 108 mEq/liter (mmol/L). Maintaining a normal amount of chloride in the blood reflects acid-base balance by its inverse relationship to bicarbonate. Excessive loss of gastric juices or other secretions containing chloride may cause hypochloremic metabolic alkalosis or excessive chloride retention. Ingesting it may lead to hyperchloremic metabolic acidosis.

Elevated serum chloride levels (*hyperchloremia*) can come on from severe dehydration, complete renal shutdown, head injury (which produces neurogenic hyperventilation), and primary aldosteroism. Manifestations consist of stupor, rapid and deep breathing, and weakness that leads to coma.

A situation of low chloride levels in the blood (*hypochloremia*) is associated with reduced blood sodium and potassium levels coming from prolonged vomiting, gastric suctioning, intestinal fistula, chronic renal failure, or Addison's disease. Congestive heart failure, or edema resulting in excess extracellular fluid, can cause dilutional hypochloremia. The indications are hypertonicity of muscles, tetany, and depressed respirations.

THE LACTIC DEHYDROGENASE (LDH) LABORATORY TEST

The laboratory test for lactic dehydrogenase (LDH) is a measurement of five specific isoenzymes which catalyze the reversible conversion of pyruvic acid present in all muscles of the body into lactic acid. Many common diseases—myocardial infarction (MI), pulmonary infarction, anemias, liver disease, kidney disease, erythrocytic damage, and others—cause elevations in total lactic dehydrogenase, and the LDH laboratory test is useful for differentiating between them.

The five identified isoenzymes in lactic dehydrogenase are LDH[1] and LDH[2] appearing in the heart, red blood cells, and kidneys; LDH[3] in the lungs; and LDH[4] and LDH[5] in the liver and the skeletal muscles. Testing for these enzymes is especially appropriate for the delayed measurement of creatine phosphokinase (CPK) associated with MI and for monitoring patient response to some forms of chemotherapy. Total LDH levels normally range from 48 to 115 U/L. Normal distribution of the five isoenzymes is as follows:

LDH[1]: 17.5% to 28.3% of total
LDH[2]: 30.4% to 36.4% of total
LDH[3]: 19.2% to 24.8% of total
LDH[4]: 9.6% to 15.6% of total
LDH[5]: 5.5% to 12.7% of total

Since a vast number of illnesses involve the enzymes of LDH, this laboratory test for lactic dehydrogenase is broadly employed for establishing diagnoses.

THE ASPARTATE TRANSAMINASE/SERUM GLUTAMIC-OXALOACETIC TRANSAMINASE (AST/SGOT) LABORATORY TEST

The laboratory blood examination for aspartate transaminase and serum glutamic-oxaloacetic (AST/SGOT) is a measurement of specific amino acid residues left behind by nitrogenous portions of the metabolized amino acids. Aspartate aminotransferase (AST) is found in the cytoplasm and mitochondria of many tissue cells, primarily in the liver, heart, skeletal muscles, kidneys, pancreas, and red blood cells.

AST is released into blood serum in proportion to cellular damage, and its detection (together with creatine phosphokinase and lactate dehydrogenase) indicates myocardial infarction. The test also helps in the diagnosis of acute liver disease. It monitors patient progress in healing. AST adult serum levels range from 8 to 20 U/L. Normal values for infants are four times higher.

Maximum elevations of AST are associated with viral hepatitis, severe skeletal muscle trauma, extensive surgery, drug-induced liver injury, and passive liver congestion. Levels ranging from 10 to 20 times normal may indicate severe MI, severe infectious mononucleosis, and alcoholic cirrhosis. Moderate-to-high levels ranging from 5 to 10 times normal indicate Duchenne muscular dystrophy, dermatomyositis, and chronic hepatitis, along with prodromal and resolving stages of diseases. Low-to-moderate levels of 2 to 5 times normal may show hemolytic anemia, metastatic liver tumors, acute pancreatitis, pulmonary emboli, alcohol withdrawal syndrome, fatty liver, and the first stages of biliary duct obstruction.

THE SERUM BILIRUBIN LABORATORY TEST

The laboratory test for serum bilirubin, the main product of hemoglobin catabolism, is a measurement of bile pigment which indicates the state of health of the liver and gallbladder. After being formed in the reticuloendothelial cells, bilirubin is bound to albumin and then transported to the liver, where it's conjugated with glucuronic acid to form bilirubin glucuronide and bilirubin diglucuronide. These two compounds are then excreted in bile. Measurement of indirect or prehepatic (unconjugated) bilirubin helps to evalute hepatobiliary and erythropoietic functions.

The serum bilirubin laboratory test showing elevated levels often indicates liver damage in which the parenchymal cells can no longer conjugate bilirubin with glucuronide. Then indirect bilirubin reenters the bloodstream. Also, an elevated reading alerts the health professional to the possibility of severe hemolytic anemia. This test aids in the differential diagnosis of jaundice, biliary obstruction, and dangerous levels of unconjugated bilirubin.

Normally in an adult, indirect serum bilirubin measures 11 mg/dL or less; direct serum bilirubin of less than 0.5 mg/dL). Neonates have total serum bilirubin ranging from 1 to 12 mg/dL; if elevated to 20 mg/dL (for them, it indicates neonatal hepatic immaturity or congenital enzyme deficiencies. An exchange blood transfusion may then be required.

If readings of bilirubin are elevated for adults, the test advises about the possibility of autoimmunity or transfusion reaction, hemolytic or pernicious anemia or hemorrhage, and hepatocellular dysfunction perhaps from viral hepatitis. Needless to say, elevated levels of direct conjugated bilirubin usually show biliary obstruction with overflows into the bloodstream. Intrahepatic biliary obstruction may come from viral hepatitis, cirrhosis, or chlorpromazine reaction. Extrahepatic obstruction may come from gallstones, gallbladder cancer, pancreatic cancer, or bile duct disease.

THE SERUM GAMMA-GLUTAMYL TRANSPEPTIDASE (GGT) LABORATORY TEST

The laboratory test for serum gamma-glutamyl transpeptidase (GGT) is a measurement of obstructive jaundice in neoplastic liver disease, and it's also useful for the detection of excessive alcohol consumption. The GGT enzyme is sensitive to drug use and detects alcohol ingestion; therefore, it's used to determine compliance with alcoholism treatment. It also helps in the diagnosis of obstructive jaundice and liver cancer.

The normal range for GGT varies with age in males but not in females. For men ages 18 to 50 it varies between 10 and 39 U/L. Older than that, males show a GGT range from 10 to 48 U/L. The normal range in women is 6 to 29 U/L. Elevation signals a cholestatic liver process.

Note: The immune-stimulating effect of the Gerson Therapy frequently causes a rise in GGT blood levels.

THE ACID PHOSPHATASE LABORATORY TEST

The laboratory test for acid phosphatase is a measurement of the prostatic and erythrocytic isoenzymes to detect cancer. Active at a pH of 5, the two phosphatase enzymes appear in the liver, spleen, red blood cells, bone marrow, platelets, and prostate gland.

Successful treatment for prostate cancer decreases acid phosphatase levels. Its normal values range from 0 to 1.1 Bodansky units/mL; 1 to 4 King Armstrong units/mL; 0.13 to 0.63 Bessey-Lowery-Brock units/mL; and 0 to 6 U/L in SI units. Normal range of radioimmunoassay results is 0 to 4.0 ng/mL.

An elevated prostatic acid phosphatase test indicates Paget's disease, Gaucher's disease, multiple myeloma, and a tumor that has spread beyond the prostatic capsule. If metastasized to bone, the high acid phosphatase level accompanied by a high alkaline phosphatase shows increased osteoblastic activity—metastatic bone cancer.

THE ALKALINE PHOSPHATASE (AP)
LABORATORY TEST

An enzyme that is most active at pH 9.0, alkaline phosphatase (AP) influences bone calcification and the transport of lipids and metabolites. The alkaline phosphatase laboratory test measures combined activities of those AP isoenzymes found in the liver, bones, kidneys, intestinal lining, and placenta. Bone and liver AP are always present in adult blood serum, with liver AP most prominent—except during the third trimester of pregnancy when the placenta originates half of all AP.

The AP laboratory test is particularly sensitive to mild biliary obstruction and indicates liver lesions. Its most specific clinical application is in the diagnosis of metabolic bone disease and detecting skeletal diseases characterized by osteoblastic activity and local liver lesions causing biliary obstruction such as tumor or abscess. It furnishes supplemental information for liver function studies and GI enzyme tests, and it assesses the response to vitamin D treatment in rickets.

The normal range of serum alkaline phosphatase varies in accordance with the laboratory method employed, but the usual total AP levels range from 30 to 120 U/L in adults and from 40 to 200 U/L in children. Since AP concentrations rise during active bone formation and growth, infants, children, and adolescents normally show levels three times higher than adults. Additional normal ranges for AP are 1.5 to 4 Bodansky units/dL; 4 to 13.5 King-Armstrong units/dL; 0.8 to 2.5 Bessey-Lowry units/dL; 30 to 110 U/L by SMA 1260.

High AP blood levels indicate skeletal disease, intrahepatic biliary obstruction causing cholestasis, malignant or infectious infiltrations, fibrosis, Paget's disease, bone metastases, hyperparathyroidism, metastatic bone tumors from pancreatic cancer, and liver diseases before any change in blood serum bilirubin levels.

Moderate rise in AP levels shown by this laboratory test may reflect acute biliary obstruction from liver inflammation in active cirrhosis, mononucleosis, osteomalacia, deficiency-induced rickets, and viral hepatitis.

The Alanine Transaminase, Serum Glutamic-Pyruvic Transaminase (ALT/SGPT) Laboratory Test

Alanine aminotransferase (ALT), one of the two enzymes that catalyze a reversible amino group transfer reaction in the Krebs citric acid (tricarboxylic acid) cycle, is necessary for tissue energy production. (The second enzyme is aspartate aminotransferase.) Elevated serum ALT indicates acute hepatocellular damage before jaundice appears. The ALT/SGPT laboratory test makes use of spectrophotometric or colorimetric methods which detect and evaluate treatment progress for hepatitis, cirrhosis without jaundice, liver toxicity, and acute liver disease. It also distinguishes between myocardial and hepatic tissue damage.

ALT values range from 10 to 32 U/L in men; from 9 to 24 U/L in women; twice those levels in infants. When they are very high—up to 50 times normal—viral or drug-induced hepatitis must be suspected. Or there may be other liver disease with extensive necrosis.

Moderate-to-high levels of ALT may indicate infectious mononucleosis, chronic hepatitis, intrahepatic cholestasis, early or improving acute viral hepatitis, or severe hepatic congestion due to heart failure.

Slight-to-moderate ALT elevations may appear with any condition that produces acute cellular injury in the liver such as active cirrhosis and drug-induced or alcoholic hepatitis.

Marginal elevations possibly show acute myocardial infarction or secondary hepatic congestion.

An interfering factor for the alanine transaminase, serum glutamic-pyruvic transaminase laboratory test is the taking of opiate analgesics such as morphine, codeine, and meperidine.

The Total Serum Cholesterol Laboratory Test

This quantitative serum analysis measures the circulating levels of free cholesterol and cholesterol esters and reflects the amount of cholesterol compound appearing in the body tissues. Both absorbed from the diet and synthesized in the liver and other body tissues, cholesterol is a structural component in cell membranes and plasma lipoproteins. It contributes to the formation of adrenocorticoid steroids, bile salts, androgens, and estrogens. A diet high in saturated fat raises cholesterol levels by stimulating absorption of lipids, including cholesterol, from the intestine; a diet low in saturated fat lowers them. Elevated total serum cholesterol is associated with an increased risk of atherosclerotic cardiovascular disease.

Thus, the total serum cholesterol laboratory test assesses the risk of coronary artery disease (CAD), evaluates fat metabolism, and aids in diagnosing kidney disease, pancreatitis, liver disease, hypothyroidism, and hyperthyroidism. Total cholesterol concentrations vary with age and sex. Its common range is from 150 to 200 mg/dL.

A desirable blood cholesterol is below 200 mg/dL, and levels from 200 to 240 mg/dL are considered borderline or at high risk for CAD. A level in excess of 250 mg/dL (*hypercholesterolemia*) indicates high risk of cardiovascuar disease, incipient hepatitis, lipid disorders, bile duct blockage, nephrotic syndrome, obstructive jaundice, pancreatitis, and hypothyroidism. They require treatment. Hypercholesterolemia from high dietary intake requires modification of eating habits and possibly medication to retard absorption.

Hypercholesterolemia can occur from taking adrenocorticotropic hormone, corticosteroids, androgens, bile salts, epinephrine, chlorpromazine, trifluoperazine, oral contraceptives, salicylates, thiouracils, and trimethadione.

Low serum cholesterol (*hypocholesterolemia*) is associated with malnutrition, cellular necrosis of the liver, and hyperthyroidism. Cholesterol often drops below normal in the Gerson program, because patients are eating an extremely low-fat diet.

THE LIPOPROTEIN/CHOLESTEROL FRACTIONATION LABORATORY TEST

To assess the risk of coronary artery disease, the lipoprotein/cholesterol fractionation laboratory test is conducted. By centrifugation or electrophoresis, it isolates and measures the cholesterol in blood, which appears as low-density lipoproteins (LDL) and high-density lipoproteins (HDL). It's known that a lower HDL level in the population gives rise to a higher incidence of CAD. Conversely, higher HDL levels produce a lesser amount of CAD.

Note: Since the Gerson Therapy offers a minimal amount of fat, it often lowers the risk of coronary artery disease; but it does provide an adequate

*supply of certain polyunsaturated essential fatty acids and fat-soluble vita-
mins that cannot be synthesized in adequate amounts for optimal body
function.*

Normal HDL cholesterol ranges from 29 to 77 mg/100 mL of blood,
and normal LDL cholesterol ranges from 62 to 185 mg/100 mL. Too-high
LDL levels increases the risk of CAD, while elevated HDL generally reflects a healthy state. Or it might indicate chronic hepatitis, early-stage
primary biliary cirrhosis, or too much alcohol consumption.

THE SERUM TRIGLYCERIDES LABORATORY TEST

Triglycerides being the body's main storage form of lipids (constituting
95 percent of fatty tissue), the serum triglycerides laboratory test provides
a quantitative analysis of them. It identifies *hyerlipemia* in kidney disease
and CAD. The triglyceride values vary according to age:

Age	Trigyceride Values	
	mg/dL	nmol/L
0–29	10–140	0.1–1.55
30–39	10–150	0.1–1.65
40–49	10–160	0.1–1.75
50–59	10–190	0.1–2.10

Test abnormality suggests that other measurements are needed. High
triglycerides indicate the risk of atherosclerosis or CAD. Mild-to-moderate
levels advise of biliary obstruction, diabetes, kidney disease, endocrin-
opathies, or too much consumption of alcohol. Decreased levels are rare
but may show malnutrition or a betalipoproteinemia.

*Note: On the Gerson diet, flare-ups and healing reactions are shown by
elevated triglycerides.*

THE SERUM PROTEIN ELECTROPHORESIS LABORATORY TEST

The major blood proteins of the body, albumin and four globulins, are
measured in an electric field by separating them into patterns according
to size, shape, and electric charge at pH 8.6. Comprising more than 50

percent of total serum protein, albumin prevents leakage of capillary plasma by oncotic pressure (the pressure exerted by plasma proteins on the capillary wall), and it transports the many water-insoluble substances such as bilirubin, fatty acids, hormones, and drugs. Of the four globulins, alpha^1, alpha^2, beta, and gamma, the first three act as carrier proteins for transporting lipids, hormones, and metals through the blood, and the fourth, gamma globulin, acts in and upon the immune system.

As indicated by its label, the serum protein electrophoresis laboratory test uses electric current to measure the total serum protein and albumin-globulin ratio to convert them into absolute values. These values help to uncover the presence of liver disease, blood dyscrasias, kidney disorders, gastrointestinal illnesses, neoplastic (benign and malignant) diseases, and/or protein deficiency. Here are the normal blood serum ranges for these proteins:

Total serum protein	6.6 to 7.9 g/dL
Albumin fraction	3.3 to 4.5 g/dL
Alpha^1 globulin fraction	0.1 to 0.4 g/dL
Alpha^2 globulin	0.5 to 1.0 g/dL
Beta globulin	0.7 to 1.2 g/dL
Gamma globulin	0.5 to 1.6 g/dL

The balance between total albumin and total globulin (known in medicine as the A-G ratio) is evaluated in relation to the total protein level. A reversed A-G ratio (decreased albumin and elevated globulins) and low total protein shows chronic liver disease; reversed A-G ratio with normal total protein shows myeloproliferative disease (leukemia and Hodgkin's disease) or certain chronic infectious diseases (tuberculosis and chronic hepatitis).

THE BLOOD UREA NITROGEN (BUN) LABORATORY TEST

Measurement of the blood's nitrogen fraction of urea, the chief product of protein metabolism, is accomplished by the blood urea nitrogen (BUN) laboratory test. Formed in the liver from ammonia and excreted by the kidneys, urea constitutes 40 to 50 percent of the blood's nonprotein nitrogen. The BUN level reflects protein intake and kidney excretory capacity, but it's a less reliable indicator of uremia (urine in the blood) than the serum creatinine level (see the test description which immediately follows).

With normal values ranging from 8 to 20 mg/dL, the BUN test helps to evaluate kidney function, aids in the diagnosis of kidney illness, and assesses the body's hydration. An elevated BUN happens in reduced renal blood flow from dehydration, renal disease, urinary tract obstruction, and increased protein catabolism as in burns. Depressed BUN levels occur in severe liver damage, malnutrition, and overhydration.

Note: Due to initial decreased dietary protein intake, a person following the Gerson Therapy will likely show a slightly reduced level of BUN .

THE SERUM CREATININE LABORATORY TEST

Providing a more sensitive measure of kidney damage than the BUN, the serum creatinine laboratory test is a quantitative analysis of the non-protein end product of metabolism, creatinine. Kidney impairment is virtually the only cause of creatinine elevation in the blood; therefore, creatinine levels are directly related to the glomerular filtration rate. They assess renal glomerular function and screen for kidney damage.

Creatinine concentration in males normally ranges from 0.8 to 1.2 mg/dL; in females it ranges from 0.6 to 0.9 mg/dL. Elevation of serum creatinine means that serious renal disease is present with 50 percent damaged nephrons as in gigantism and acromegaly. Interfering factors are too much absorption of ascorbic acid, barbiturates, diuretics, and sulfobromophthalein. Also, athletes may have above-average creatinine levels, even with normal kidney function.

THE SERUM URIC ACID LABORATORY TEST

Used mainly to detect gout, the serum uric acid laboratory test measures levels of uric acid, a metabolite of purine in the blood. Glomerular filtration and tubular secretion gets rid of uric acid, but it's less soluble at a pH of 7.4 or lower which occurs in certain diseases such as gout, excessive cellular generation and destruction as in leukemia, and kidney dysfunction.

Uric acid concentrations in men range from 4.3 to 8 mg/dL; in women they range from 2.3 to 6 mg/dL. Although elevated levels of serum uric acid don't correlate with severity of disease, they do rise in congestive heart failure, glycogen storage disease, acute infectious diseases such as infectious mononucleosis, hemolytic anemia, sickle cell anemia, hemoglobinopathies, polycythemia, leukemia, lymphoma, metastatic malignancy, and psoriasis. Depressed uric acid levels indicate defective acute hepatic atrophy or tubular absorption as in Wilson's disease and Fanconi's syndrome.

Drug factors interfering in the serum uric acid laboratory test include loop diuretics, ethambutol, vincristine, pyrazinamide, thiazides, and low doses of salicylates which elevate blood levels. Also, starvation, a high-purine diet, stress, and alcohol abuse raise uric acid. When uric acid is measured by the colorimetric method, false elevations come from acetaminophen, ascorbic acid, levodopa, and phenacetin. Decreased uric acid is caused by high doses of aspirin, Coumadin, clofibrate, cinchophen, adrenocorticotropic hormone, and phenothiazines.

THE GLUCOSE, FASTING BLOOD SUGAR (FBS) LABORATORY TEST

Following a 12- to 14-hour fast, the glucose, fasting blood sugar (FBS) laboratory test measures glucose metabolism as required in diabetes mellitus. In the fasting state, blood glucose levels decrease, stimulating release of the hormone glucagon. Glucagon then raises plasma glucose by accelerating glycogenolysis, stimulating glyconeogenesis, and inhibiting glycogen synthesis. Normally, secretion of insulin checks this rise in glucose levels. In diabetes, absence or deficiency of insulin allows persistently high glucose levels.

Normal ranges for fasting blood glucose on the FBS laboratory test after an eight- to twelve-hour fast are:

- fasting serum, 70 to 100 mg/dL;
- fasting whole blood, 60 to 100 mg/dL;
- nonfasting whole blood, 85 to 125 mg/dL in persons over age 50, and 70 to 115 mg/dL in persons under age 50.

These laboratory readings help to screen for diabetes mellitus and other disorders of glucose metabolism. They also monitor drug or dietary therapy for diabetics, insulin requirements for uncontrolled diabetics, and known or suspected hypoglycemics.

Fasting blood glucose levels of 140 to 150 mg/dL or higher obtained on two or more occasions are diagnostic of diabetes mellitus. Nonfasting levels that exceed 200 mg/dL also show diabetes. The elevated blood glucose may come from pancreatitis, hyperthyroidism, pheochromocytoma, chronic hepatic disease, brain trauma, chronic illness, chronic malnutrition, eclampsia, anoxia, and convulsive disorders as well.

Depressed blood glucose occurs from hyperinsulinism, insulinoma, von Gierke's disease, functional or reactive hypoglycemia, hypothyroidism, adrenal insufficiency, congenital adrenal hyperplasia, hypopituitarism, islet cell carcinoma of the pancreas, hepatic necrosis, and glycogen storage disease.

THE SERUM IRON AND TOTAL IRON-BINDING CAPACITY LABORATORY TEST

Two separate blood tests conducted with buffering and coloring reagents measure (1) the amount of iron bound to the glycoprotein transferrin and (2) the plasma's total iron-binding capacity (TIBC) if all the transferrin were saturated with iron. The percentage of saturation is obtained by dividing the serum iron result by the TIBC, which reveals the actual amount of saturated transferrin. Normal transferrin is 30 percent saturated. Thus, the two tests (a) estimate total iron storage, (b) diagnose hemochromatosis, (c) distinguish between iron deficiency anemia and chronic disease anemia, and (d) evaluate a person's nutritional status.

Normal serum iron and TIBC values have been determined to be:

	Serum Iron	TIBC (mcg/dL)	Saturation (mcg/dL)
Men:	70 to 150	300 to 400	20 to 50
Women:	80 to 150	350 to 450	20 to 50

In iron deficiency, serum iron falls and TIBC increases to decrease the saturation. With chronic inflammation as in rheumatoid arthritis, serum iron is low in the presence of adequate body stores, but TIBC remains unchanged or drops to preserve normal saturation. Iron overload does not alter serum levels until relatively late in the pathology, but serum iron increases and TIBC remains the same to increase the saturation.

THE ERYTHROCYTE (RED BLOOD CELL, RBC) COUNT

Traditionally counted by hand with a hemacytometer, red blood cells (RBCs) are now commonly counted with electronic devices, which provide faster, more accurate results. This erythrocyte count does not provide qualitative information about the RBCs' hemoglobin content, but it does tell mean corpuscular volume (MCV) and mean corpuscular hemoglobin (MCH). Thus, the erythrocyte blood count offers indices for RBC size and hemoglobin content and supports other hematologic tests in diagnosing anemia and polycythemia.

Depending on age, sex, sample, and geographic location, normal RBC values in adult males range from 4.5 to 6.2 million/microliter (4.5 to 6.2 x 1,012/L) of venous blood; in adult females from 4.2 to 5.4 million/microliter (4.2 to 5.4 x 1,012/L) of venous blood; in children, 4.6 to 4.8 million/microliter of venous blood; in full-term infants, 4.4 to 5.8 million/microliter (4.4 to 5.8 x 1,012/L). An elevated RBC count indicates polycythemia or dehydration; a depressed count shows anemia, fluid overload, or recent hemorrhage. With total bed rest, RBC counts drop considerably from decreased oxygen requirments.

THE TOTAL HEMOGLOBIN (HGB) LABORATORY TEST

The total hemoglobin (Hgb) concentration in a deciliter (100ml) of whole blood is measured by the total hemoglobin laboratory test. The Hgb-RBC ratio (mean corpuscular hemoglobin or MCH) and free plasma Hgb affect the RBC count. This test, a usual part of the complete blood count, measures the severity of anemia or polycythemia, monitors therapy response, and supplies figures for calculating MCH and mean corpuscular Hgb concentration.

Based on venous blood samples, normal values for different patients are:

Age	Hemoglobin Level (g/dL)
Less than 7 days	17–22
1 week	15–20
1 month	11–15

Age	Hemoglobin Level (g/dL)
Children	11–13
Adult males	14–18
Elderly males	12.4–14.9
Adult females	12–16
Elderly females	11.7–13.8

THE HEMATOCRIT (HCT) LABORATORY TEST

The volume of RBCs packed in a whole blood sample is measured by the hematocrit (Hct) laboratory test. Number and size of the RBCs determine the Hct concentration, and such a readout aids in the diagnosis of abnormal states of hydration, polycythemia, anemia, fluid imbalance, blood loss, blood replacement, and red cell indices. According to a patient's sex, age, laboratory competence, and type of blood sample, the test routinely screens one's blood in a complete blood count.

Hct reference values range from 40 percent to 54 percent (0.4 to 0.54) for men and from 37 percent to 47 percent (0.37 to 0.47) for women. Low Hct indicates anemia or hemodilution; high Hct shows polycythemia or hemoconcentration caused by blood loss. If a hematoma develops at the venipuncture site, ease discomfort by applying ice, followed later by warm soaks.

THE ERYTHROCYTE INDICES LABORATORY TEST

Mean corpuscular volume (MCV), mean corpuscular hemoglobin (MCH), and mean corpuscular hemoglobin concentration (MCHC) are the three measurements accomplished by the erythrocyte indices laboratory test. The MCV expresses the average size of erythrocytes and indicates whether they are undersized (microcytic), oversized (macrocytic), or normal (normocytic). MCH gives the weight of hemoglobin in an average red cell. MCHC defines the concentration of Hgb in 100 mL of packed red cells.

The normal RBC indices are:

MCV   = 84 to 99 cubic microliters/red cell (femtoliters (fl)/red cell)
MCH   = 26 to 32 picograms (pg)/red cell
MCHC = 30% to 36% (300 to 360 g/L)

These indices aid in diagnosing and classifying anemia. Low MCV and MCHC show microcytic hypochromic anemias caused by iron deficiency anemia, pyridoxine-responsive anemia, or thalassemia. High MCV indicates macrocytic anemia caused by megaloblastic anemias coming from folic acid or vitamin B_{12} deficiency, inherited disorders of DNA synthesis, or reticulocytosis.

THE ERYTHROCYTE SEDIMENTATION RATE (ESR)

Measuring the time required for erythrocytes in a whole blood sample to settle to the bottom of a vertical tube, the erythrocyte sedimentation rate (ESR) is a sensitive but nonspecific test that indicates the presence of disease when other chemical or physical signs are normal. It rises in widespread inflammatory disorders caused by infection, autoimmune disease, or malignancy.

Thus, the ESR monitors inflammatory or malignant illness and detects occult disease such as tuberculosis (TB), tissue necrosis, or connective tissue disorders. The normal ESR ranges from 0 to 20 mm/hour. It rises in pregnancy, acute or chronic inflammation, TB, paraproteinemias, rheumatic fever, rheumatoid arthritis, and some cancers. ESR also rises in anemia. ESR drops in polycythemia, sickle cell anemia, hyperviscosity, and low plasma protein.

Note: ESR is frequently raised during and after reactions and fevers induced by the Gerson Therapy.

THE PLATELET COUNT

Platelets, or thrombocytes, are tiny formed elements in the blood which create the hemostatic plug in vascular injury. They promote coagulation by supplying phospholipids to the intrinsic thromboplastin pathway. The platelet count is vital for monitoring chemotherapy, radiation therapy, or severe thrombocytosis and thrombocytopenia. A platelet count that falls below 50,000 brings on spontaneous bleeding; below 5,000, fatal central nervous system bleeding or massive gastrointestinal hemorrhage is possible.

The platelet count evaluates platelet production, assesses effects of cytotoxic therapy, aids the diagnosing of thrombocytopenia and thrombocytosis, and confirms visual estimate of platelet number and morphology from a stained blood film. Normal platelet counts range from 130,000 to 370,000/mm (130 to 370 x 10^{11}/L).

A decreased count comes from aplastic or hypoplastic bone marrow; infiltrative bone marrow diseases like carcinoma, leukemia, or disseminated infection; megakaryocytic hypoplasia; ineffective thrombopoiesis caused by folic acid or vitamin B_1 deficiency; pooling of platelets in an enlarged spleen; increased platelet destruction from drug use or immune disorders; disseminated intravascular coagulation; Bernard-Soulier syndrome; or mechanical injury to platelets.

Medications decreasing the count include acetazolamid, acetohexamide, antimony, antineoplastics, brompheniramine maleate, carbamazepine, chloramphenicol, ethacrynic acid, furosemide, gold salts, hydroxychloroquine, indomethacin, isoniazid, mephenytoin, mefenamic acid, methazolamide, methimazole, methyidopa, oral diaoxide, oxyphenbetazone, penicillamine, penicillin, phenylbutazone, phenytoin, pyrimethamine, quinidine sulfate, quinine, salicylates, streptomycin, sulfonamides, thiazide, thiazidelike diuretics, and tricyclic antidepressants. Heparin causes transient reversible thrombocytopenia.

An increased platelet count results from such diseases as hemorrhage; infectious disorders; malignancies; iron deficiency anemia; myelofibrosis; primary thrombocytosis; polycythemia vera; myelogenous leukemia; recent surgery, pregnancy, or splenectomy; and inflammatory disorders, such as collagen vascular disease.

THE LEUKOCYTE (WHITE BLOOD CELL, WBC) COUNT

Reporting on the number of white blood cells (WBCs) found in a microliter (cubic millimeter) of whole blood by use of a hemacytometer or Coulter counter, the leukocyte count varies with strenuous exercise, stress, or digestion. It's used to detect infection or inflammation, the need for further tests such as the WBC differential or bone marrow biopsy, and the response to chemotherapy or radiation therapy.

The WBC count ranges from 4.1 to 10.9 x 10^{11}. An elevated count signals infection such as an abscess, meningitis, appendicitis, or tonsillitis, and it may indicate leukemia, tissue necrosis from burns, myocardial infarction, or gangrene. A low count shows bone marrow depression from viral infections or from toxic reactions such as those following treatment with antineoplastics, mercury or other heavy metal toxicity, benzene or arsenic exposure, and invasion by the organisms of influenza, typhoid fever, measles, infectious hepatitis, mononucleosis, and rubella.

THE WHITE BLOOD CELL DIFFERENTIAL

Being a relative number of each type of white blood cell, the white blood cell differential test is determined by multiplying the percentage value of each WBC type to give an absolute number of each kind of the 100 or more WBCs. There are granulocytes, agranulocytes, juvenile neutrophils, segmented neutrophils, basophils, eosinophils, large lymphocytes, small lymphoctyes, phagocytes, histiocytes, and so on.

The WBC differential evaluates the body's capacity to resist and overcome infection, various types of leukemia, the stage and severity of infection, allergic reactions, severity of allergic reactions, and parasitic infections. There is a long list of reference values in the WBC differential test, divided into adult and child. For example some of them are:

For Adults—	Relative Value (%)	Absolute Value (mcL)
Neutrophils	47.6–76.8	1950–8,400
Lymphocytes	16.2–43	660–4,600
Monocytes	0.6–9.6	24–960
Eosinophils	0.3–7	12–760
Basophils	0.3–2	12–200

To make an accurate diagnosis, the test examiner must consider both relative and absolute values of the differential counts. For the vast number of variables and illnesses which are diagnosed by them, please see Appendix I of the *Gerson Therapy Handbook: Companion Workbook to A Cancer Therapy: Results of Fifty Cases: Practical Guidance, Resources and Recipes for Gerson Therapy Patients*. To acquire a copy of this handbook/workbook, contact the Gerson Institute, in Bonita, California.

THE ROUTINE URINALYSIS

Elements of routine urinalysis include the measurement evaluations of physical characteristics, specific gravity and pH, protein, glucose, and ketone bodies, plus examination of urine sediment, casts, and blood cell crystals. The analysis of urine is an exceedingly important test that tells a lot about the internal workings of a person. Routine urine test results have a great number of implications for how the physiology is functioning or how it is responding to the diet, nonpathologic conditions, specimen collection time, and other factors.

For the vast number of variables and illnesses which are evaluated by urinalysis, please see Appendix I of the *Gerson Therapy Handbook: Companion Workbook to A Cancer Therapy: Results of Fifty Cases: Practical Guidance, Resources and Recipes for Gerson™ Therapy Patients.* To acquire a copy of this handbook/workbook, contact the Gerson Institute in San Diego, California.

Chapter Twenty-One

SUCCESS STORIES BY PATIENTS

Writing in the *Townsend Letter for Doctors & Patients*, medical anthropologist Tim Batchelder advises that people do not arrive at health care systems for diagnosis and treatments; rather, they come to find wellness and wholeness.[1]

People often feel symptoms and even exhibit signs of illness when they seek the services of a doctor or clinic but return home labeled with a disease. Other medical anthropologists call such a result the "veterinary practice of medicine" since the patient's experience of illness becomes irrelevant except as it reveals an underlying presence of disease. A patient's opinions, beliefs and other aspects of sociocultural identity only cloud the doctor's mind-set.[2] Preferable for some technically oriented and conventionally practicing health professionals is that the patient be passive like a sedated animal in a veterinarian's clinic.

Not so the situations for Gerson patients whose case histories of chronic illnes you're about to read. They have been far from passive or sedated; instead these people actively sought out the Gerson Therapy and practiced it—this despite knowing their selected approach to wellness offers a difficult, highly restrictive, and isolating lifestyle. The goal for each of these folks has been to live as close as possible to the full complement of mankind's allotted years. The Gerson Therapy has been allowing them to reach that goal.

REVERSING LATE-STAGE LUNG CANCER

To his shock and dismay, in November 1989, sixty-year-old John Peters of Pittsburgh was diagnosed with lung cancer—an adenocarcinoma. Although he had eaten a good diet, swam a thousand yards in his swimming pool five days each week, never smoked, and had been given an excellent health report by his doctor just three months before, Mr. Peters still had come down with non-small-cell carcinoma of the lung, staged at level IIIA by his consulting oncologist.

Lung Cancer is the second most common cancer and the number-one cause of death from malignancy in both men and women. Although there has always been a higher incidence in men, lung cancer in women has risen rapidly in recent years. While lung cancer has long been the top cancer killer of men, it has now surpassed breast cancer as the main malignancy killer of women.

In 1997, 178,100 Americans developed lung cancer, and 160,400 died of it. This high incidence of death is true even though lung cancer is the most preventable of malignancies; if every bit of tobacco were removed from the earth, the number of *all* cancer types (not only those affecting the lung) would fall by 17 percent. Of the two general kinds of lung cacner, small-cell and non-small-cell, the latter is more common, accounting for approximately 75 percent of all diagnosed cases.

Conventional oncological treatment of lung cancer, which primarily depends on surgery with chemotherapy, radiation therapy, and sometimes hyperthermia, has offered a poor prognosis for remaining alive over a prolonged period of time.

- The success rate for five-year survival of stage I lung cancer (no spread to lymph nodes) is 30 to 80 percent because the tumor is tiny in size and surgery removes it.
- The success rate for five-year survival of stage II lung cancer (spread to the hilar nodes) is 10 to 35 percent with both surgery and radiation therapy administered. (*Hilar nodes* are those lung indentations where arteries enter and veins and lymphatics leave.)
- The success rate for five-year survival of stage IIIA lung cancer (surgery is possible combined with radiation therapy and occasional chemotherapy) is 10 to 15 percent.
- The success rate for five-year survival of stage IIIB lung cancer (surgery offers no benefit; radiation therapy and experimental

chemotherapy may be attempted) is less than 5 percent because usual orthodox oncological treatments truly fail the patients.

- The success rate for five-year survival of stage IV lung cancer (metastases to distant sites) is considerably less than 5 percent—perhaps only 3 percent—for treatment usually is directed merely toward relieving symptoms.

Non-small-cell lung cancer, spreading by the lymphatic system and through the blood, contains three distinct types: squamous-cell or epidermoid carcinoma of the lung (most related to smoking), large-cell carcinoma (associated with brain metastasis), and adenocarcinoma. For no known reason, adenocarcinoma has steadily increased in frequency (above 30 percent of all lung cancers). Treatment is similar for these three non-small-cell lung cancer types.

Upon an emergency recommendation of his consulting oncologist, John Peters underwent immediate open-chest surgery, followed by twenty-four radiation treatments. Thus, his various symptoms consisting of constant cough, sometimes containing blood, hoarseness and shortness of breath, excessive sputum, recurrent episodes of lung infection, weight loss, and swelling of the face, plus the sense of overwhelming fatigue, lessened to the point of almost disappearing.

A year later, however, the patient's original coughing and some of his other symptoms recurred. Another series of diagnostic tests, including bronchoscopic examination, revealed that he again required chest surgery for excising the non-small-cell lung cancer. "When I refused surgery and chemotherapy, the doctors told me that there was no chance for my survival at all," John Peters explained.

"I had researched lung cancer and realized that the only reason I got cancer was that my body supported it. Thus, if I didn't change the internal environment of my body, the cancer would just come back again. In May 1991, I started on the Gerson Therapy at home," said Mr. Peters. "I was very weak, and this Gerson Therapy was demanding, but I was facing the Grim Reaper, so I was also highly motivated.

"In only three weeks, I knew the Gerson treatment was working—I was getting stronger, coughing less, and feeling much better. Most surprising, I was actually gaining weight on this vegetarian diet. After losing so many pounds the months before, I was finally becoming more than just skin and bones," Mr. Peters wrote in a letter to the Gerson Institute. "I have remained cancer-free and in good health for the past seven years. I am vegan, avoid refined flour, sugar, salt, caffeine and alchohol and still press vegetables and drink their juices, about twenty-four ounces per day. There is no doubt in my mind that I would have been in the cemetery six or seven years ago without the Gerson Therapy.

"Incidentally, before going through my 1989 lung removal surgery, I had obtained a second opinion from the head of the Pittsburgh Cancer Institute. When I returned to him for a follow-up cancer test in 1996, he was shocked to see me surviving. The lung surgeon told me that I'd never know how lucky I was to be alive and that with my disease, there was only about a 3 percent chance of five-year survival. Eating the Gerson vegetarian way has saved my life," John Peters confirmed.

At his latest report to this book's two authors, as a former lung cancer patient who subscribes rather closely to the eating program of the Gerson Therapy, John Peters has gone well beyond doubling the usual cancer patient's five-year survival time for adenocarinoma of the lung. (As you've been informed, five-year survival of any cancer is defined by the American Cancer Society as a "cure.)"

A TWENTY-YEAR CURE OF INOPERABLE STAGE IIIB LUNG CANCER

In mid-January 1979, Jesus Lechuga Valdez of Durango, Mexico, returned from a business trip to Mexico City with a severe cold. A week later it had deteriorated into a persistent cough and lingering hoarseness that made it difficult for him to speak. Senor Lechuga, who, at this writing, is eighty-six years old, in 1971 had retired from his position as general manager and partial owner of a truck and tractor dealership. His travels for business had been successful but hard on the man's body. During the next six months, his chronic cough and hoarse voice were treated by three allopathic physicians and a homeopath, all of whom thought such signs of illness came from adult-onset asthma. At that time he was sixty-six years old.

The doctors' diagnosis and treatment were incorrect, for X-ray films eventually taken of Senor Lechuga's thoracic area showed a 5-centimeter (cm) round spot in the upper region of his right lung. A chest surgeon he consulted confirmed the existence of a lung tumor 2½ inches across.

Since an El Paso, Texas, internist, Walter D. Feinberg, M.D., had been keeping annual records of the patient's physical examinations, on June 18, 1979, Senor Lechuga traveled to Dr. Feinberg's office for comparing previous and current radiographs. It turns out that there had been no sign of the potential for a chest lesion the year before. Within half a dozen months, therefore, his mass had formed spontaneously and quickly.

Pulmonologist E. S. Crossett, M.D., at El Paso's Hotel Dieu (French for "God's house") Hospital performed a bronchioscopy and mediastinoscopy during lung surgery to remove the tumor. But because excision would have left his patient too weak, the surgeon decided not to remove the tumor and only performed a biopsy. The resulting tissue pathology and instrumentation reports indicated that Senor Lechuga was victimized by stage IIIB "large cell undifferentiated carcinoma with metastasis to the bronchial and mediastinal areas."

Staging in cancer terminology is a relative index of how much cancer exists in an individual's body, including its size, location, and containment or metastasis.[3] *Stage III* indicates that metastases have spread the cancer to areas other than the primary site. In lung cancer, stage III is divided into two types, IIIA and IIIB. *Stage IIIB lung cancer* classifies the tumor as not removable because of technical reasons relating to the surgical technique or because there would be no benefit to the patient.[4] The several malignant metastases of Jesus Lechuga Valdez were declared inoperable, and his prognosis became established at only three to six months of life remaining.

High-Dosage Radiation Exposure for Senor Lechuga

Consultation with oncologist Ira A. Horowitz, M.D., medical director of the El Paso Cancer Treatment Center, followed. Dr. Horowitz emphatically recommended radiation therapy, but the machine used for this external radiation failed to be state-of-the-art; its old-fashioned cobalt-60 electron beams would present the patient with some awful side effects. The machine's radioactive source was housed in a lead container, and as the cobalt isotope decayed, it produced a beam in the megavoltage range.[5]

With advice from his family, Senor Lechuga decided instead that he would take radiation therapy in Chester, Pennsylvania, close to the Wilmington, Delaware, home of his daughter, Georgina Lechuga Potter. (Mrs. Potter, who now lives in Vienna, Virginia, acted as translator for her father's Spanish-spoken case history. Besides hospital records, she is a main source of the information you are reading. The patient's wife, Dolores A. Lechuga, signed the permission form to release this story.)

From Wilmington, Mrs. Potter brought her father to consult with oncologist Robert Enck, M.D., located at the Crozer-Chester Medical Center in Chester. He confirmed the need for radiation therapy. Upon Dr. Enck's referral, radiologist Warren Sewall, M.D., from July 10 to August 21, 1979, used a linear accelerator to administer radiation doses of 4,400 rads (the modern dosage term is *centigray* [cGy]) to the right lung and mediastinum for four weeks. The patient also received 1,600 rads to the upper lobe of the right lung plus 5,000 rads simultaneously to cancer-filled "supraclavicular nodules." He took this high-energy therapy five days per week for four weeks. Then the radiologist added another 5,000 rads to those supraclavicular nodules for two additional weeks.

The linear accelerator, one of the most popular machines now being used, was truly state-of-the-art back in 1979. It is available in energies ranging from 4 to 35 megavolts and uses a mixed beam of X rays and electrons. Electrons are accelerated along a wave guide to their high velocity. Penetration into tissue is determined by the energy of the beam selected.[6]

With the object of relieving his symptoms (not curing the cancer), Jesus Lechuga Valdez underwent multiple exposures to the hospital's linear accelerator's high-energy X rays. They were responsible for certain discomforting side effects and may be responsible for cancer to have appeared currently, twenty years later. The massive amount of X rays given then to normal tissue supposedly never exceeded safe doses.

Through a process of "ionization," the radiation is designed to kill some cancer cells by damaging their chromosomes and DNA to stop cell division. Of the centigray dose, one gray equals 100 rads, so that Senor Lechuga each day actually received 44 cGy plus 16 cGy plus 50 cGy for a four-week total of 2,200 cGy, and then he accepted another 1,000 cGy for two weeks more. The 3,200 cGy dosage is enormous and, as you will learn later, such radiation therapy held significance for the man's future health prospects.

The beam's adverse effects caused Senor Lechuga to experience mental depression, loss of appetite, serious weight loss, darkening of the skin in the irradiated chest area, and difficulty swallowing from esophageal scarring that resulted from the radiation burns he sustained. Even today, almost twenty-one years later, he must swallow carefully because he can be choked by an overly large food particle getting stuck at the esophageal scar site.

By means of follow-up diagnostics back at the El Paso Cancer Treatment Center, on August 31, 1979, Dr. Horowitz confirmed that his patient's lung tumor had been reduced by about 80 percent. The coughing fits were less strong and not striking Senor Lechuga as often; his appetite had returned; and the annoying hoarseness improved. Throughout his examinations and treatments, the doctors put no dietary restrictions on him whatsoever, permitting Danish pastries, fatty hamburgers, french fried potatoes, pizza, cola drinks, and other assorted junk. He was told merely to avoid sunlight directly on his irradiated skin areas.

When pressed for a prognosis as the result of radiation therapy received, Dr. Horowitz gave him an estimated 50 percent chance of either having a lung cancer recurrence or living somewhat longer. It was then that the man returned home to Durango and resumed working in his truck and tractor dealership.

Lung Cancer Returns

Less than a month after conclusion of the radiation, his cancer came back. Coughing spells and hoarseness returned worse than ever for Senor Lechuga. It was then that he and Dolores decided to act upon information about the Gerson Therapy provided by their daughter, Georgina Lechuga Potter. Her friend, practicing pharmacist Irwin Rosenberg, Ph.D. (a doctorate in nutrition), acquired information and taught Mrs. Potter about healing cancer using Dr. Max Gerson's dietary/detoxification program. Dr. Rosenberg is owner of the Apothecary Pharmacy on Georgetown Road in Bethesda, Maryland (ironically, located across from the National Institutes of Health).

On October 28, 1979, Senor Lechuga accompanied by his wife arrived at the Gerson Therapy hospital in Tijuana, Mexico. Victor Ortuno, M.D., the hospital's medical director, initially examined the patient and then turned the Lechuga case over to his cousin, Arturo Ortuno, M.D., who took full responsibility for supervising treatment.

Although very uncomfortable from his numerous healing reactions, Senor Lechuga's physical response was rapidly positive. His cancer markers and other laboratory tests improved; however, his state of mind hit bottom—depression set in. Still, from Dr. Arturo Ortuno's efforts and with much encouragement from Dolores Lechuga, Senor Lechuga stayed on the dietary/detoxification program at the Gerson hospital and then later at home.

On his own back in Durango, Senor Lechuga struggled with tolerating the many glasses of Gerson juices, coffee enemas, castor oil treatments, salads, and eating the well-done and unsalted foods. The Gerson diet was contrary to his Mexican cultural background and abhorrent to his psyche.

During healing reactions, appetite left him completely, and such reactions came on frequently for prolonged periods. Sometimes they lasted for a week, but the love and support of Dolores, his companion for life, prevailed over his discouragement. Dolores prepared the foods, juices, enemas, and other healing components; she became his self-contained caregiver and the household's Gerson therapist. In effect, his wife saved the life of Senor Lechuga.

By the week between Christmas and New Years day of 1980, his healing flare-ups diminished, and he began to feel better. However, the man did experience extreme weakness and had to force himself to eat anything at all. He preferred to do nothing more than rest in bed and sleep frequently. In another week he made enough progress to return to work part-time and sporadically. Sitting at his desk gave him a renewed will to fight his cancer with all his might. With an office a mere five minutes by car from home, the patient went home for coffee enema cleansings, to eat his meals, and to drink the green juices. He carried carrot juice in a thermos with him to work for hourly drinking.

By the end of April 1980, the patient traveled to the Gerson hospital once again for his first six-month checkup. (In all, after November 1979, he returned to that hospital for semiannual examinations twelve times.) His cancer markers and blood tests showed a near-normal physiology so that the Gerson diet was modified by Dr. Arturo Ortuna, who after eight weeks had included yogurt, rye bread, raw skimmed milk, infrequent meals of fish, chicken, and a few other items heretofore forbidden. Senor Lechuga was feeling better and better, and his mental outlook became optimistic. He told stories, joked, sang, and became a joy to everyone around him.

Having reported his progress to Charlotte Gerson during the weekend of October 17 and 18, 1981, he accepted her invitation to participate as a speaker in San Diego at a "Gerson Survivors' Conference." In June 1985, Dr. Arturo Ortuno traveled with Senior Lechuga to a San Diego diagnostic center for him to undergo a magnetic resonance imaging (MRI) to confirm that after five years his cancer had completely cleared. It had! Receiving the affirmative MRI report, Dr. A. Ortuno declared his patient officially cured of cancer and asked him to return to the Gerson Hospital in one year for another checkup. Then the doctor suggested that he go back to the very restrictive Gerson Therapy for just one month more as a kind of "insurance" toward his cure. This Senor Lechuga agreed to do along with promising that he would report results of his following the difficult lifestyle for a final month that's demanded by the therapy.

When the patient telephoned Dr. Arturo Ortuno that single month later to report on the experience, he learned that his forty-year-old physician had just died and was being buried. While Dr. A. Ortuno had been playing hard at racquetball with Dr. Victor Ortuno the day before, he suffered a massive heart attack. He succumbed in his cousin's arms.

Shocked by the terrible news, Senor Lechuga never returned to Tijuana. Also, he markedly reduced his adherence to the Gerson Therapy. Although he continued to consume a sensible diet, his juice intake fell to about four glasses daily. During the fourteen years following, Jesus and Dolores Lechuga lived the good life. They traveled extensively to Hawaii, Canada, Washington State, New York City, and other places. They flew, cruised, drove, took train trips, and went places all over North America.

Then, from July 25 to August 5, 1999, he enjoyed a cruise to Alaska to walk on glaciers, hike mountain trails, and eat the multiple massive meals

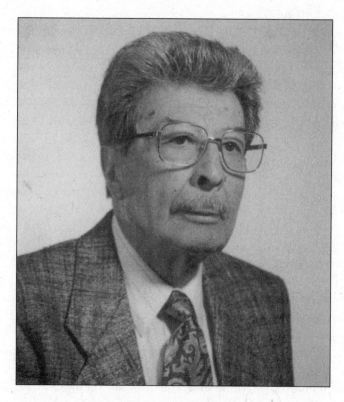

Jesus Lechuga Valdez

served aboard ship. During this Alaskan excursion, the patient felt back pain just below the right shoulder blade. Upon his return home, he was treated in Durango by two medical doctors for a "contracted and knotted muscle" until the lack of relief caused them to request a biopsy. The surgeon who did the biopsy in Durango, J. Roberto Salas Gracia, M.D., reported that this muscle "knot" actually was a tumor. It was diagnosed as a malignant pleomorphic fibrotic hysticytoma in the soft tissue of the right shoulder blade. Because of insufficient viable tissue surrounding the tumor unable to be biopsied, it remains undetermined as to whether Senior Lechuga's cancer is a malignant schwannoma.

The *malignant schwannoma* is a sarcoma, one of the slow-growing tumors that develop in soft tissue surrounding the nerve sheaths of smooth muscles. Some 75 percent of such sarcomas are called *leiomyosarcomas*.

Receiving this diagnosis of malignancy in mid-October 1999, Senor and Senora Lechuga and their daughter Georgina Potter immediately made arrangements to admit him as a patient at the Gerson Therapy facility in Tijuana. On October 25, 1999, he became a resident of the Oasis of Hope Hospital. The attending clinician there, Jaime A. Martinez, M.D., advised that such a cancer cannot be completely excised by surgery because the procedure would negatively affect the use of his right arm. Dr. Martinez conjectured that the new cancer might be a delayed adverse side effect of the original radiation therapy that Senor Lechuga had undergone some twenty years before.

Three weeks after entering the Oasis Hospital, he left to follow the Gerson Therapy at home. While the specific diagnosis of disease remained uncertain, there was no doubt that this eighty-six-year-old man once again needed to fight for his life—but with a different form of cancer. Then, during the last week of November 1999, Senor Jesus Lechuga Valdez died suddenly of heart failure. (See Illustration 21-2 depicting Senor Lechuga).

A FOURTEEN-YEAR RECOVERY FROM OVARIAN CANCER

In November 1999, while taking maintenance care at the Oasis Hospital, the only official Gerson Therapy facility in Tijuana, Mexico, fifty-one-year-old Sandra Whitwell, now of Stuart, Virginia, described her permanent recovery from carcinoma of the ovary. Sandra currently works as a nanny and nutritionist. Fourteen years ago ovarian cancer had threatened her life; today she shares her story about using the Gerson Therapy to cure herself of the most common gynecologic malignancy.

As the fourth most frequent cause of cancer death in American women, ovarian cancer's mortality rate exceeds that for all of the other gynecologic malignancies combined. Every seventieth woman develops it, and 1 in every 100 dies from the tumorous growth at its primary site or from metastases. Arising from cells covering the surface of an ovary (epithelial carcinoma), in 1997 in the United States 26,800 ovarian cancers were diagnosed, which caused 14,200 deaths. Subsequent years have shown even higher incidence. Despite all of the money invested in research by American taxpayers, the incidence of ovarian cancer is rising steadily.

Cancer of the ovary spreads by a shedding of malignant cells into the abdominal cavity and the peritoneum (its covering membrane) and then implanting on the surface of the liver, the large intestine, the omentum, the small intestine, the bladder, the diaphragm, or the stomach's attached fatty tissue. Ovarian cancer cells also metastasize to lymph nodes in the pelvis, aorta, groin, and neck. Talcum powder containing asbestos is suspected as one of the probable causes.[7]

Sandra Whitwell's ovarian cancer came upon her gradually starting with the breakdown of her body when she was seventeen years old. Invariably her menstrual periods were beset with unbearable cramps, and these carried over to her early twenties when she married Lawrence Whitwell, a Nashville, Tennessee, policeman. "My painful menstruation was abnormal and an indication of ovarian problems to come," advises Sandra. "By age twenty-three, cysts had developed on both of my ovaries which were removed by surgery. Next, endometriosis struck, which required more surgery to scrape the endometrium. After each of these two operations I had been asked by the consulting surgeons as to whether I had ever been pregnant, and I had not. They never explained why they wanted to know about pregnancy, but the doctors seemed anxious to perform an ovariectomy or hysterectomy on me.

"I never gave birth to a child. We adopted our son, Aaron, as a baby. But then, when he was three years old his daddy was killed in the line of police duty," she reveals. "Ovarian cysts formed again, one of them the size of a baseball, and these were excised. After recuperating from a third operation for cyst removal, I had begun running for exercise—at least four miles a day. I enjoyed the running and thrived on it. This vigorous daily movement continued for me over an eight-year period. Early in 1985, however, running stopped abruptly for me. I awakened one morning in tremendous pain and with a distended fluid-filled abdomen [ascites]," describes Sandra. "The operation that followed for removal of a grape-fruit-sized cyst also included a hysterectomy, which left me feeling awful pain. Two days later my gynecologist together with the gynecological surgeon told me I was the victim of ovarian cancer. They wanted to go back in and take biopsy tissue from the ovaries and several other organs.

"Since blood transfusions were required as well, and this was during the time when AIDS resulted from such transfusions, I refused the operation and three pints of blood that went with it. Simultaneously, my health insurance carrier did not honor our insurance contract. The insurance company just outright canceled my coverage," Sandra states. "Upon my contacting a lawyer to enforce reimbursement, he informed me that a loophole in the policy allowed such cancelation under terms stating that this ovarian cancer was a 'preexisting condition.' I was just out of luck unless I had lots of money to pay court costs and legal fees for litigation without any guarantee I would win.

"Having no treatment available to me, I left the hospital after resting for seven days diagnosed with ovarian cancer. At age thirty-six, I was alone, a widow, the mother of a seven-year-old son showing diabetic tendencies, and without income. Except that I owned my Nashville house and some small compensation from my husband's death, I could not afford the sophisticated chemotherapy or other toxic modalities being offered by orthodox medicine. But I do have loving parents living in Stuart, Virginia, who would do anything to save my life, and they were the people who did just that.

"My mother, who has nursed cancer patients, did research and helped me in deciding to do nothing rather than take toxic therapy. With assistance from mom and dad in caring for Aaron, I moved in with my parents. Then a friend from Alaska sent me information about the Gerson Therapy," Sandra says. "Sitting with them in their living room, I remember watching videotapes showing lectures by Charlotte Gerson. My mom said, 'This program makes so much sense. Feed the immune system and give it a chance to fight off the cancer itself.' So not having hospital insurance was a benefit, because I couldn't even consider taking any conventional therapy.

"Accompanied by my mother as companion and caregiver, I traveled to Tijuana's Gerson Hospital. My intent was to receive the Gerson Therapy and take instructions in following it at home. The trip occurred in September 1985, exactly one month after my hysterectomy and cancer diagnosis. During that short period before learning the Gerson program, I became what looked like a bag of bones," describes Sandra. "My weight loss was excessive, falling from 120 to 92 pounds. With a height of five feet, six-and-a-half inches, I looked really skinny. I was weak to the point of collapse, and I did remain bedridden for four months. Only the love and devotion of my caregiving parents pulled me through that worst period of my life.

"But first spending ten days at La Gloria Hospital to learn the Gerson Therapy, and then returning to my parents' home to be nursed by them, saved me. I had rented my Nashville house to fellow church members. Then bringing my son, I moved in with my mother and dad," explains Sandra. "At the Gerson hospital, I immediately underwent detoxification reactions—many of them—including emotional depression, many tears, constant nausea, vomiting, headaches, burning sensations from taking castor oil both orally and rectally, loss of appetite, sleeplessness, whole body pain in the joints, muscles, and bones. And I smelled like permanent-waving solution. It was my habit to periodically take hair permanents, perhaps five times a year, and that poisonous liquid had permeated my body organs to poison them. The Gerson Therapy pulled out those accumulated toxins, and I gave off the stinky odor of permanent-waving solution. I reeked of perm."

A lesson learned from Sandra Whitwell is that a person becomes what he or she puts into and onto the body. That is, eat garbagelike foods and you become garbage. Consume carcinogens and you turn into a walking cancer factory. Bathe a body part in poison as Sandra did to her head, and you make the entire body a receptacle for cancer. To stay healthy, you must expose yourself only to good stuff.

"Out of ignorance, I harmed myself with convenience or so-called 'beauty' items. In college, I had my room and the halls of that dormitory smelling really bad from the permanent-waving liquid. Just think of all the contaminated air I inhaled. Also, before I knew better, it had been my habit to drink up to three full, six-cup pots of coffee a day," admits Sandra. "But instruction in the Gerson Therapy taught me how to live correctly. At my parents' home back then, body weight began to come back from my dad and mom making juices for me to drink. They used only fresh, organic vegetables and fruits, which are more expensive than the supermarket variety. Originally, my mother was afraid for my life; she truly thought I was gone, but then she saw that slowly I was improving.

"It took nearly two years of detoxifying and nourishing my body before the immune system kicked in and took over against ovarian cancer. I observed it do this when one day my temperature rose to 104°F during a healing reaction. After that point, I just got better and better," Sandra says. "I took no other medication or nutritional supplementation other than what the Gerson diet prescribes—the niacin, coenzymeQ_{10}, thyroid, potassium, acidol/pepsin, pancreatin, and liver. These simple supplements, the diet itself, the juices, and the detox worked for me. I am alive and thriving today, fourteen years after being diagnosed with the cancer, because of my faithfully following the Gerson Therapy [see the photograph below showing how Sandra Whitwell appears today].

"The detoxification is difficult to take and people should be aware of what to expect. I kept a diary so that I know what I went through and how to cope with the flareups. Perhaps you would want some of my suggestions for achieving a successful Gerson Therapy," wonders Sandra Whitwell. "Would you?"

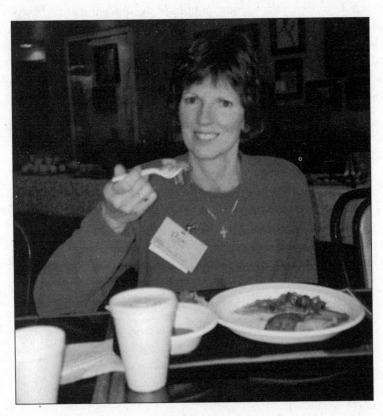

Sandra Whitwell

Sandra's Suggestions for a Successful
Gerson Therapy

Having faithfully pursued the Gerson Therapy full-time for two years, and still making it her total lifestyle, Sandra Whitwell affirms that this procedure has saved her life and restored her health. During that time almost fifteen years ago Sandra accepted the Gerson program as her anti-ovarian-cancer treatment, and nothing else. She still eats, juices, and cleanses according to the Gerson therapy's regulations and occasionally returns to the nearest Gerson facility for further program updates. She looked the picture of robust health when we visited with her at the Gerson hospital for one full week in November 1999.

"Two years is not so long to ensure that you will live, and during the process you are renewing every cell in your liver—the main portion of one's immune system," says Sandra. "The Gerson method is not for wimps; however, it takes fighters! This natural and nontoxic treatment is difficult, because you're not just popping a pill or having some health professional do something to you or for you. Instead, you must help yourself and call for personal assistance from family or friends when needed, at least in the beginning. Most of us are too accustomed to eating fast foods, looking for fast fixes for what ails us, and taking the easy way out. Not so with the Gerson Therapy; it's a life-changing treatment!

"From my experience, I put together some suggestions for achieving success with conquering cancer and other chronic illnesses by use of the Gerson Therapy. In no particular order of importance, my suggestions follow:

- Keep a diary to record your emotional swings, healing reactions, deviations from the Gerson program, responses of outsiders to how you are eating or what you're doing. You'll discover what you've done to bring on a flare-up. And from their comments, you'll learn who are your real friends.
- Try to prepare foods and procedures in advance of the next day after drinking your last daily juice. Not enough time is left to spare during each day for making coffee, taking 'coffee breaks,' engaging in castor oil enema days, fixing the medications, taking in organically grown produce shipments, cleaning the veggies, studying recipes, and planning meals. Being organized is a plus for your self-treatment.
- Watch the Gerson videos, read the Gerson books, listen to the

Gerson audiotapes. After almost fifteen years of participating in the Gerson Therapy, I still do this and learn new information every time.

- On castor oil days, start early with drinking the terrible stuff. Use the little medicine cups as dosage forms. (Use of castor oil is not for anyone who has been pretreated with chemotherapy.) I always put one tablespoonful of cranberry juice or apple juice in my cup first and then add the required two tablespoonfuls of castor oil. The mixture goes down more readily with juice added. Then, after swallowing the mixture, I taste the juice rather than the oil. Always drink one cup of hot coffee directly after swallowing the castor oil mixture to speed up the process of the oil going through your gastrointestinal tract.

- Next after drinking the castor oil, eat a piece of fruit and take your first coffee enema. Undoubtedly this will be a 'yucky-feeling' day, but tomorrow you will definitely feel much better! In my opinion, drinking the castor oil is easier on the body than taking a castor oil enema.

- To prepare the castor oil enema, my suggestion is slightly different from the Gerson regulation. Put warm distilled water in the bucket and run that water through the tube into the tub or shower. Then shut off the tube leaving the warm water in it. Pour out the excess water that remains in the bucket. Put castor oil and ox bile mix (no soap) in the bucket. Now open the tube and allow water to flow out into the tub or shower (or toilet); as the water flows out it pulls the oil mixture into the tube. The tube should hold the full amount of mixture needed. Shut off the tube! Now fill the bucket with the coffee mixture, and you are ready for your castor oil coffee cleansing. This enema is usually hard to hold—don't worry! Hold as long as possible and still benefit from taking a castor oil cleanse. As it happens, this method which had been recommended previously is now discontinued by the Gerson hospital, but I find it still works well for me.

- Chamomile tea enemas are always welcome to take when you have released toxins causing you to feel unable to hold the coffee during a cleansing. Chamomile taken rectally is soothing, and on castor oil days especially, may be easier to hold.

- Never become upset when you can't hold the coffee enema. Sometimes you just need to try again or maybe wait until your next coffee-cleansing time. Just keep trying until you become practiced at doing the enema and look forward to the good feeling with which it leaves you.

- A trick I use for those rare times when I'm having a hard time holding the coffee enema is to slow down the flow. I feel fewer spasms if it takes about five minutes to flow in. Slow the flow by lowering your bucket or closing the valve on the tube and opening periodically.

- If you have tried slowing the enema flow but still feel spasms, put a teaspoonful of potassium into the four cups of coffee solution. At the beginning of using the Gerson approach, your body may well be potassium-depleted which manifests itself by abdominal spasms.

- To reduce or eliminate niacin flush, take this vitamin B$_3$ only on a full stomach. Alternatively, let the niacin tablet melt in your mouth or under the tongue. That's what I do.

- If you hire help for daily assistance, employ two or three people so that if someone doesn't show for the work shift, you'll have a backup person to do a double shift. If the absent person is sick, you won't want him or her around anyway since you're fighting enough against illness.

- Don't play the mind games thrown at you by your subconscious or by other people. Think positively, play good music, count your blessings, think of the troubles others are experiencing, and realize that yours are surmountable. Self-pity will get you nowhere. As I've suggested, your diary is the place to write down your thoughts to get rid of them from your head. Then you can dwell on better things. Tomorrow, when you reread your diary, you will wonder why you were in such a bad state of mind.

- Each phase in this step-by-step process—juices, food, medications, coffee—is important. Work hard! Stay with a stick-to-it attitude! Be disciplined! Succeed!

- Finally, remember that God never gives you more than you can handle. There is a reason for going through this tribulation. After coming out from under your trouble, you may be the one to save someone else's life beside your own!"

—Sandra Whitwell, Stuart, Virginia

Pancreatic Cancer Remains Gone for Almost Fifteen Years

In September 1985, pneumonia developed for forty-six-year-old Mrs. Ronald (Patricia) Ainey of Nanaimo, British Columbia, Canada. Despite her being a cigarette smoker and alcoholic beverage drinker, she had sustained good general health throughout her life until that 1985 date. Then, in January 1986, internist Bennett A. Horner, M.D., F.R.C.P.(C), also of Nanaimo, using CAT scan guidance, had a biopsy performed (tissue drawn out with a fine needle) from a tumor site on Pat Ainey's pancreas. The object of this scan and biopsy was to differentiate pancreatic cancer from several other conditions: benign pancreatitis, pseudocyst, islet cell carcinoma, or lymphoma. Dr. Horner confirmed the woman's diagnosis by letter to her family physician in the same town, A. C. Baird, M.B., CH.B, C.C.F.P. Dr. Horner's letter stated: "Mrs. Pat Ainey returned to see me today, January 28, 1986. I informed her that she does have adenocarcinoma of the pancreas; there is no specific treatment indicated presently. . . if she has a lot of pain or discomfort, we'd be glad to help her any way we can."

Dr. Horner gave the patient and her husband Ron, who were one month away from celebrating their thirtieth wedding anniversary, more personal advice too. "The medical specialist told me, 'Go home, get your life in order, the cancer is so bad it is inoperable,'" remembers Mrs. Ainey. "I went through all the anguish, the crying, and I finally resigned myself to my own death."[8]

She had learned that the malignancy had metastasized to her gallbladder, liver, and spleen. In just a few weeks she lost more than forty-five pounds and regularly vomited blood. She was classified as being in cytology class (stage) III–IV pancreatic cancer (which has a projected five-year survival of 1 percent or less). There were no curative therapies and no proven adjuvant treatment; only palliation could be offered by orthodox oncologists to provide some pain control or ascites reduction. She did have ascites, jaundice, pleural (chest wall) effusion, alcoholic hepatitis, and pain. Any chemotherapy probably would kill Pat Ainey faster than the cancer itself.[9]

"When you're told by the medical profession that your days are done, that's who you believe," admits Mrs. Ainey. But then she read in the *Nanaimo Times* newspaper about a Victoria, B.C., man who had been cured of pancreatic cancer by engaging in the Gerson Therapy. "I decided

I wasn't going to just bugger around crying and dying. I was going to try to live the last few months as well as I could for myself and for my family."

While skeptical at first, wondering if the Gerson hospital in Tijuana, Mexico, was a scam designed to bilk desperate people, "It was the only hope I had. What I needed was a miracle," the woman says. "And my husband stomped his foot down and said, 'Dammit lady, pack your bag, we're catching the eleven o'clock boat to the mainland and going to Mexico to try this damn Gerson thing.'"

Ron and Pat Ainey spent two weeks at the Gerson hospital in Playas, a suburb of Tijuana, where they learned to make her organic juices, what kinds of foods were appropriate, and how to self-administer five coffee enemas a day. She explains, "It wasn't any fun, especially those 'coffee breaks' as we called them. But what choice did I have except to try?"

The Aineys had reserved two weeks to engage in the treatment, and in ten days she began to feel considerably better than she had in months. Knowing that she would be required to live stringently on the Gerson program for a minimum of two years, Mrs. Ainey took up the challenge to conduct the Gerson therapy at home. And it worked well.

"In December 1986 my doctor told me he thought I had the cancer licked."

A letter Dr. Baird wrote in February 1990 on another health matter states: "Mrs. Ainey was diagnosed as having a malignancy of her pancreas. She received treatment of her disease outside of Canada, and I am pleased to say that as of the present time she has no evidence of recurrence of the disease, and what evidence of malignancy was present in 1985 has now gone."

In a follow-up letter he wrote to an insurance company's law firm on that other matter, Dr. Baird added: "In conclusion, I would like to comment that Mrs. Ainey has survived what is generally a fatal illness and now lives life to the full."

We spoke with Patricia Ainey on November 20, 1999, at which time she acknowledged, "I feel good, excellent in fact. I've had these past fifteen years to live happily and well, which I was not supposed to have. I've watched my grandchildren grow up and had a lot of good times in those years." While Mrs. Ainey has been free of pancreatic cancer for all of this fifteen-year period, she still drinks lots of fresh, organic vegetable juices and takes a daily coffee enema. She also has regular blood tests and cancer markers taken, which she sends to the Gerson hospital for evaluation.

Friends and family sometimes ask why she continues these practices if she is cured. Says husband Ron Ainey: "Pat had been looking for a lifeline and once you've found one it's very hard to let go."

A GERSON PATIENT WHO THOUGHT HIMSELF "PERFECT"

(Retitled from the *Gerson Healing Newsletter*,
vol. 14, no. 5, Sep.–Oct., 1999)
by Charlotte Gerson

It has frequently occurred to me that, in order to really be sure Gerson patients understand and follow the Gerson Therapy exactly, I ought to follow them around their house and kitchen for twenty-four hours. A situation that arose recently for a particular Gerson patient amply illustrates this point. Please allow me to tell you of my experience, for it's my desire to have you learn from it for doing the Gerson Therapy right. I was surprised and shocked by certain deviations from the program.

The patient in question (whom I'll call "Phillip") was not only very much interested in the Gerson Therapy for his own recovery; he believes so strongly about spreading the word of healing that he organized a Gerson Convention Day. Phillip also invited me to stay at his lovely home overnight so that I could be spoiled with good, organic Gerson food and juices. Truly, he is a delightful person to be around, and Phillip's wife is too.

Their house is located in a wooded area, with beautiful huge trees, and sitting at the edge of a small lake. In other words, the air is clean and fresh and the atmosphere relaxing—no problem there. This patient's business is organized and runs quite well with minimal attention, allowing him to get a lot of rest and live on a fine income. There is help in the household, so no pressures exist relating to juice and food preparations. Even so, there are at least four major problems in Phillip's application of the Gerson Therapy which I shall describe:

1. The water piped into his home is "hard"; it contains minerals. Like other people in the area, therefore, the patient's home is equipped with "water softener" equipment. Phillip's very warm, concerned and cooperative wife is doing everything in her power to help her husband fully recover from melanoma with metastases to the liver; yet, she told me that she brings in "sacks of salt" for adding to the water softener! As part of the process of removing the unwelcome

hard water minerals, such water-softening equipment replaces these with sodium. What happens as a result is that the patient washes and bathes in "softened water," loaded with salt.

Salt is very easily absorbed through the skin and should never be used by a Gerson patient. The sodium in salt is an enzyme inhibitor and the Gerson Therapy is designed to remove excess sodium. Salt, in fact, is needed for fast growth of tumor tissue. It is also the basis for the "tissue damage syndrome," when normal cells lose their ability to hold potassium while sodium penetrates their protoplasm, causing edema and loss of function. This tissue damage is, according to my father's findings, the beginning of all chronic disease. Naturally, for a cancer patient, bathing in salt water (even in the ocean) must be avoided at all costs.

2. At Phillip's home we were served a very delicious and attractive lunch which included a lovely salad loaded with avocados. I immediately asked if the patient, too, was eating them. He was! This was another serious mistake, since avocados contain a fairly large percentage of fat. The reason avocados and other fat-containing foods are forbidden is that fats tend to stimulate new tumor growth! The lady of the house said that she thought that avocados were served at the Mexican Gerson hospital, but she is wrong. They are not! The problem here is that the patient or caregiver should not rely on memory or rumor alone but should refer to the published information authorized by the Gerson Institute.

All these items are clearly set down in Dr. Gerson's A *Cancer Therapy* and several other sources; and avocados are the second item on the "Forbidden Foods" list.

3. As part of the lunch, we had a very nice vegetable soup. It contained some zucchini, peas, celery, onions, and a few other vegetables. The patient asked me how I enjoyed the "Hippocrates soup." I had to state that the soup we were eating was not Hippocrates soup as Dr. Gerson describes it in his book. The combination of ingredients that are supposed to be in that soup are clearly described in A *Cancer Therapy* as well as the *Gerson Therapy Handbook* (formerly, the *Gerson Therapy Primer*), and the ingredients listed are very specific.

Hippocrates (referred to by the medical profession as "the father of medicine") understood that this special combination of ingredients in the soup has a beneficial, detoxifying effect on the kidneys. For this reason, Dr. Gerson had made use of them. He concluded that the soup ingredients were so important he wanted patients to eat the "special soup" twice daily to benefit the kidneys and help them clear toxins from the body. Occasionally, one can add extra tomatoes to give the soup a different flavor; or one can cut up and roast some onions on a dry cookie sheet (*no* fat, butter, or oil) in the oven. Then these extras can be added to the same basic soup recipe for a tasty treat. However, the basic recipe should remain unchanged.

4. Phillip's wife also thoughtfully offered me some enema coffee, which I gladly accepted. When I picked it up for use, however, I seriously wondered whether it was the proper strength. I have used enemas for many years and know pretty well what the coffee should look like. The solution being provided seemed too weak to be considered "concentrate" for a usual dilution of 4 to 1. The lady "thought" that she used the recipe in the *Handbook* and that it was right, but again she was wrong. My suggestion is that the caregiver must be sure each enema contains the equivalent of three rounded tablespoons of coffee (see A *Cancer Therapy*, p. 247). If a concentrate is prepared, each portion *must* contain the three tablespoonfuls of coffee. The coffee enema, too, is so very important that it is imperative the mixture or solution be correct. Please check and recheck the preparation of the coffee concentrate created for internal cleansing.

5. Somewhat less important than the above four points is another one. Phillip does enjoy eating some bread with his meals—quite acceptable. But it is also important to understand that the main requirements for nutrition are the salads, soup, potato, vegetables, and fruit. If all those foods have been consumed, it is all right for the patient to also have one slice of unsalted rye bread. Even so, be aware that bread should never be the main part of a meal.

I have discussed Phillip's type of problem with the most experienced Gerson Therapy medical doctors whom I know. They affirmed that subtle aspects of patient noncompliance cause them difficulties. Aside from the above, there are other problems we have run across. The Gerson doctors as well as myself (when I talk to patients) meet some serious obstacles to healing. When we ask various patients about their compliance with the Gerson Therapy directives (such as the above patient who made serious errors), for instance, they will assure us that they're doing everything "perfectly." Such patients don't seem to realize what is wrong with their version of the therapy. Phillip, too, thought he was "perfect."

When Gerson therapists try to help, heal, and direct patients on the Gerson Therapy, we are relying on the various tools that we have specially created to give patients and families every possible help and guidance: the food preparation videotape (Tape III); the recipes in the *Handbook;* the other four-hour, two-part workshop tapes (Tape II) discussing in detail as much of the treatment as we can; and, most important, Dr. Gerson's original book. At this point, I need to stress again that the patient must familiarize himself very thoroughly with this material and review it over and over again. As Sandra Whitwell pointed out in her suggestions, you always learn something new when restudying the Gerson Therapy information.

One problem area that keeps coming up is the food preparation. Just boiling the vegetables and putting them on a plate is not good enough. The Gerson Therapy Video: vol. 3: Food Preparation initiates the cook into various ways to make foods tasty. For example, cooked beets when peeled and sliced can be reheated a little with some freshly made applesauce and stirred. The vegetable then resembles Harvard beets. Or the sliced beets can be dressed with onions, some green pepper strips, and vinegar with flaxseed oil dressing for a beet salad. During the summer months, these salads (also potato salad, string bean or butter bean salad, etc.) are very welcome, refreshing, and stimulating to the appetite.

There are many suggested recipes in the back of the *Gerson Therapy Handbook* that have unfortunately been disregarded by some patients. As a result, the Gerson Institute occasionally receives reports from caregivers that the patients are weak, losing weight, and doing poorly. Almost always, it turns out that they have "cravings" for pizza, enchiladas, or some other greasy, salty, forbidden food. They are simply hungry because they are not eating well-prepared healing and nutritious *Gerson* meals.

Gerson meals offer a distinct advantage: if the patient (or family member for that matter) eats fresh, organic food, it is truly satisfying. Frequently we hear further reports that patients' companions who participate in the Gerson program lose their personal cravings for sweets or heavy desserts. But the key to success is eating tasty food that is prepared with imagination and inspiration from the recipes provided.

I must remind patients frequently that when they are on a nutritional therapy such as this one, they are on nothing if they don't eat! If patients eat properly, most will gain weight if they are emaciated. Those who are too heavy will lose weight on the same regimen.

Fruits that are in season in the summer, such as cherries, apricots, peaches, nectarines, plums, pears, and grapes, are especially valuable—they are high in the best nutrients: vitamins, potassium, and enzymes. Not far behind are apples, which are available virtually all year round. Patients (unless they are diabetic or suffer from candidiasis) should always eat much fruit at night, first thing in the morning, and anytime between meals.

Yet one summer food presents a problem: corn. It is perfectly fine to eat fresh corn. The difficulty arising with corn is that nearly everyone loves it and during the season is likely to eat it to the exclusion of other vegetables. That is a very bad idea. The vegetables should provide variety and a large selection of special healing plant chemicals (phytochemicals) and trace minerals. Eating mostly one vegetable is not acceptable and does not fulfill the purpose. Let the guiding spirit of the patient be: "I'll do the best possible to help my sick body heal" rather than "I'll see how little I can do and still get away with it."

References for Chapter Twenty-One

1. Batchelder, T. "Qualitative research on patient experiences and implications for long-term care facilities." *Townsend Letter for Doctors & Patients* 196:56–61, November 1999.

2. Diamond, W.J.; Cowden, W.L.; Goldberg, B. *An Alternative Medicine Definitive Guide to Cancer*. Tiburon, Calif.: Future Medicine Publishing, 1997, p. 212.

3. Kleinman, A.; Eisenberg, L.; Good, B. "Culture, illness and care: clinical lessons from anthropologic and cross-cultural research." *Annals of Internal Medicine* 88:251–258, 1978.

4. Margolis, L.W.; Meyler, T.S. "What happens in radiation therapy." In *Everyone's Guide to Cancer Therapy: How Cancer Is Diagnosed, Treated, and Managed Day to Day*, rev. 3rd ed. by M. Dollinger, E.H. Rosenbaum, and G. Cable. Kansas City, Mo.: Andrews McMeel Publishing, 1997, pp. 49–56.

5. *Ibid.*

6. *Ibid.*

7. Stern, J.L. "Ovary." In *Everyone's Guide to Cancer Therapy: How Cancer Is Diagnosed, Treated, and Managed Day to Day*, rev. 3rd ed. by M. Dollinger,

E.H. Rosenbaum, and G. Cable. Kansas City, Mo.: Andrews McMeel Publishing, 1997, pp. 600–610.

8. Welburn, L. "Alternative medicine." *Nanaimo Times*. April 21, 1992.

9. Rosenbaum, E.H.; Dollinger, M. "Pancreas." In *Everyone's Guide to Cancer Therapy: How Cancer Is Diagnosed, Treated, and Managed Day to Day*, rev. 3rd ed. by M. Dollinger, E.H. Rosenbaum, and G. Cable. Kansas City, Mo.: Andrews McMeel Publishing, 1997, pp. 616–622.

Chapter Twenty-Two

RECIPES

This final chapter contains recipes for dishes prepared only with certified organically grown fresh fruits, dried fruits, vegetables, grains, and sweeteners. Especially important here are the following items:

- Hippocrates soup, recommended by Dr. Max Gerson in the first edition of his book
- Juices as described
- Salads of all types
- Many kinds of salad dressing
- Cooked vegetable dishes of all types
- Potatoes baked or prepared in different ways
- Vegetarian loaves
- Soups based on the Hippocrates soup
- Many kinds of fruit dishes
- Dairy dishes of several types (when allowed)
- Breads of organic rye with little whole wheat, unsalted
- Desserts of many types of fruit, raw or stewed

NOTE 1: The recipes that follow were compiled and edited with the co-operation of Christeene Lindsay-Hildenbrand to be used in conjunction with the Gerson Therapy videotape "Charlotte Gerson Demonstrates Basic Gerson Food Preparation."

NOTE 2: Recipes marked with a [YN] were contributed by Yvonne

Nienstadt, director of health services at Cal-a-Vie, Vista, California. Recipes marked with a ^{SD} sign were contributed by Susan DeSimone of the Gerson Institute. Recipes marked with an ^{MZ} were contributed by Marisol Zuniga of the Hospital Meridien in Tijuana, Mexico. Recipes marked with a ^{GSG} were contributed by the Gerson Support Group in England. The recipes marked with ^{RC} were contributed by Richard Crowell. Recipes marked ^{DAIRY} contain restricted dairy ingredients; instructions for their preparation should be followed carefully. The recipes with an asterick (*) can be found in the Dairy section of the *Gerson Therapy Handbook*.

GERSON THERAPY RECIPES

The Gerson Therapy offers a diet containing a large variety of vegetarian foods ingested in huge quantities. Eating them in the recommended amounts will enable a consumer to reach an ideal weight level and remain there. And one's metabolism will achieve only homeostasis as well. But these two healthy situations are attained only when ingestion is done under certain conditions.

First, use only certified organically grown fresh fruits, dried fruits, vegetables, grains, and sweeteners. We repeat: Use strictly fresh fruits and vegetables and absolutely no canned fruits or vegetables.

Second, the produce should not be peeled or scraped unless indicated. To clean the foods, use only lukewarm water and a brush.

Third, sweeten only with Gerson-approved light honey, maple syrup, or sugar. Dried organic cane sugar (Sucanat®), which has a molasses flavor, may be added in recipes calling for brown sugar. Some cooks may prefer other sweetening options.

Special Soup (Hippocrates Soup)

For one person use a 4-quart pot, assemble the following vegetables, then cover with distilled water:

1 medium celery knob (or 3 to 4 stalks of celery), 1 medium parsley root (if available), garlic as desired, 2 small leeks (if not available, replace with 2 medium onions), 1½ lbs tomatoes or more, 2 medium onions, 1 lb potatoes, and a little parsley.

Do not peel any of these special soup vegetables; just wash and scrub them well and cut them coarsely; simmer them slowly for 2 hours, then put them through a food mill in small portions; only fibers should be left.

Vary the amount of water used for cooking according to taste and desired consistency. Keep well covered in refrigerator no longer than 2 days. Warm up as much as needed each time. Note: For recipes that call for soup stock, use the liquid from this special soup.

PREPARATION OF JUICES

Juices are always freshly prepared. (As a reference, see the classic book *A Cancer Therapy*, p. 240.) Please be aware that it's not acceptable to prepare the full day's juices in the morning.

Carrot-Apple (8 oz juice)

3 carrots (6 oz) and 1 large green apple (6 oz).

Green Juice

Obtain as many as possible of the following kinds of leaves (no others): romaine lettuce, Swiss chard, beet tops (young inner leaves), watercress, some red cabbage, green pepper ($1/4$ of small one), endive, and escarole. Add 1 medium apple for each glass when grinding.

Orange Juice

Squeeze only with a reamer-type juicer made of glass, plastic, or porcelain. Do not use any juice press into which the orange is inserted with the skin (if the skin is also pressed out, it will emit harmful fatty acids and aromatic substances contained in its surface). Do not use an aluminum juicer.

JUICERS

Use a separate grinder and a separate press for juicing or a juicer that incorporates both. Do not use liquefiers, centrifuges, juice mixers or masters, and so on.

Pressing Process

Take 1 or 2 coarsely woven nylon cloths, 12" square, and place a cupful of pulp into center of moistened cloth, fold in thirds in both directions, and press.

Rinse cloths in cool water after each juice preparation.

Do not allow juice to dry on the cloths.

Wash thoroughly each night in warm or hot water; rinse thoroughly.

Keep the pressing cloths overnight in a freezer.

It is essential to clean the machine and cloths very well.

If juice retains the taste of cloth, use a new cloth.

Allow 2 cloths per juicing.

Have 1 set of cloths for each type of juice.

Leftovers of all pressings can be used only for compost or as animal food.

If the patient goes to work again after healing, apple and carrot juice only may be taken and kept in a thermos for no longer than 4 hours to drink on the job.

SALADS AND DRESSINGS

Raw fruit or raw vegetables, when finely grated or shredded, must be used fresh, as quickly as possible.

Raw living tissues may not be stored after any kind of preparation (please see A *Cancer Therapy*, p. 189).

The following vegetables are very important to consume (finely grated if necessary, or chopped; mixed or separate): knob celery, tomatoes, escarole, cauliflower, romaine, chives, green peppers, apples, carrots, lettuce (all types), chicory, watercress, radishes, scallions, and endives.

Buttermilk Dressing^{YN} *

1 cup churned buttermilk (not cultured), 1/3 cup nonfat yogurt cheese (Quark), 1/4 tsp horseradish powder, 2 tsp honey, 1 tsp cider or wine vinegar, pinch of dill, and tarragon or savory.

Hand beat or buzz in blender until smooth. Leftover dressing may be kept in a tightly covered jar in the refrigerator for 48 hours.

Garlic and Onion Dressing

1/2 tsp lemon juice or wine vinegar, 2 tsp water, 1 tsp brown sugar, a little diced onion, 1 clove garlic, and a small amount of permitted herbs.

Mix ingredients together, allow time for flavors to mingle, and serve on salad.

Herb Dressing

2$\frac{1}{3}$ cup apple cider vinegar, 1 tsp brown sugar, $\frac{2}{3}$ cup water.

Mix these three basic ingredients together and add some or all of the following herbs (optional) and leave them to infuse: tarragon (pushed in stalk first), shallots or spring onions chopped finely, 2 cloves garlic peeled and crushed with the back of a knife, and 1 fresh bay leaf.

Orange Dill Vinaigrette[RC]

$\frac{1}{2}$ cup vinegar, 3 cloves peeled garlic, 1 cup orange juice, $\frac{1}{2}$ cup water, 1 green onion, 2 tbsp honey, $\frac{1}{2}$ tsp dried dill, and $\frac{1}{4}$ red bell pepper.

Blend all ingredients in Osterizer. Makes 1 pint of zesty and sweet dressing.

Variation: Substitute juice of 1 lime or lemon for orange juice; increase water. Substitute sage or thyme for dill.

Spinach Dressing[YN] *

1 cup nonfat yogurt, 2 cups spinach chopped raw or 1 cup spinach cooked, 3 green onions chopped, 1–2 tsp vinegar, $\frac{1}{2}$ tsp dill weed, a pinch of mace.

Place in a blender and spin until smooth.

Yoguefort Dressing*

$\frac{3}{4}$ cup dry, fat-free and unsalted cottage cheese, 1 cup yogurt (or churned buttermilk), $\frac{1}{4}$ cup vinegar or lemon juice, 2 tsp honey, 1 clove garlic crushed, $\frac{1}{4}$ tsp tarragon, marjoram, or dill, $\frac{1}{4}$ cup chives or green onions chopped, and 2 tbsp linseed oil (optional).

Blend the first 5 ingredients in blender until smooth.

Add herbs and chives.

To thin mixture, add more yogurt.

Chill before serving.

Summer Cole Slaw*

1 stalk celery finely chopped, $\frac{1}{4}$ cup minced red onion, 1$\frac{1}{2}$ cups shredded cabbage, $\frac{1}{4}$ cup shredded carrot, pinch of fresh dill, and 2 cups nonfat yogurt.

Combine all ingredients in bowl and toss well.

Serve chilled.

Artichoke Salad

1 purple onion, 1 tomato, 2 tbsp apple cider vinegar, 1 artichoke, 1 green bell pepper, 2 carrots, and 3 tbsp flaxseed oil.

Wash the artichokes well and boil in covered pot for 45 minutes to 1 hour.

When ready, peel them until you can see the center.

Remove the "chokes" with a spoon and discard.

Cut the artichoke heart and other vegetables into bite-sized pieces.

Combine and toss with vinegar and oil.

Bessarabian Nightmare[SD]

2 tomatoes sliced, 1 small onion sliced, 1 red or green pepper (or both) sliced, 2–3 cloves of garlic crushed, and permitted herbs to taste.

Layer each ingredient in a glass Pyrex® baking dish.

Bake at 350° until tender.

Cool and add flaxseed oil to taste when cool enough.

Celery Root (Knob) Salad

Remove loose roots from 2 celery knobs and scrub clean.

Boil knobs in jacket about 1 hour; peel and slice.

Add: 1 medium chopped raw onion, scallions (green onion).

Toss with Herb or Garlic and Onion Dressing.

Cold Broccoli Salad[YN] *

2 lbs broccoli cut into bite-sized pieces.

Stew over a low flame in a heavy pan with a tight-fitting cover until barely tender, about 25–30 minutes. Chill.

Add: 1 cup cherry tomatoes, ½ cup shallots or green onions, 1 cup buttermilk dressing, 2–3 tsp chives, and 2–3 tsp parsley.

Combine broccoli, tomatoes, and shallots in bowl.

Mix in dressing.

Serve on bed of endive and garnish with chives and parsley.

Eggplant Salad[SD]

1 eggplant baked for one hour at 350° F (180° Celsius).

Let eggplant cool, then chop into bite-sized pieces.

Combine with: 1 small onion chopped, 1 tbsp cider vinegar, chopped parsley, 2 sliced tomatoes, and flax oil.

Fruity Winter Salad ^{GSG DAIRY}

½ white cabbage, 2 medium carrots, 2 red apples, 1 oz raisins, 1 oz dried figs, 1 oz dried apricots, 10 tbsp nonfat yogurt, 1½ lemon, and chopped parsley.

Soak dried figs and apricots in bowl of water overnight.

The next day, empty water and add finely shredded cabbage, coarsely grated carrots and apples, and raisins.

In a separate bowl, combine yogurt, lemon juice, and parsley.

Combine contents of each bowl and toss together until well mixed. Serve chilled.

Italian Salad

Cauliflower, broccoli, celery, tomatoes.

Wash and cut up all vegetables, then toss with Herb or Garlic and Onion Dressing.

Peach Salad^{SD}

Mix together the following: 1 tomato chopped, 1 red pepper chopped, 1 green pepper chopped, 1 peach chopped, ½ cup green and red seedless grapes, and a few mint leaves.

Dress with lemon and garlic dressing: equal parts lemon juice and water.

Add a little brown sugar (Sucanat) and crushed garlic.

Potato Salad, Basic (#1)

Boil potatoes in jackets until soft (1 hour); peel and slice.

Add: onions, scallions, celery, green peppers, Herb or Garlic and Onion Dressing.

Potato Salad, Fancy (#2)

4 potatoes, 1 white onion, ¼ cup celery, 3 grated carrots, flaxseed oil, 2 bay leaves, 1 purple onion, parsley, 3 tbsp apple cider vinegar, and 1 green bell pepper.

Boil the potatoes, in their jackets, with the bay leaves on slow heat.
Cut the vegetables and sauté with the apple cider vinegar (can use wok).
Use *no* oil!

Once the potatoes are cooked, peel and cut them into small cubes and add the cooked vegetables.

Add the flaxseed oil after the mixture is cooled.

Rice Salad[SD]

Mix cooked, organic, brown rice (with bay leaf and a little rosemary) with plenty of chopped vegetables including tomatoes, celery, zucchini, radishes, fresh garden herbs, and lemon and garlic dressing (see under Peach Salad).

Rose, borage, or marigold petals look beautiful sprinkled over the salad.

Add apricots that have been soaked in water and chopped (if desired).

Raw Grated Carrots and Apples

Grate by putting through food grinder or Norwalk juicer: 2 or 3 carrots,1 apple peeled.

Add ¼ cup raisins, juice of ½ orange or lemon.

Red and Green Salad[YN]

Combine the following ingredients and serve with spinach dressing:
1 head romaine lettuce, 2 cups shredded savoy or green cabbage, 3 green onions, 1 cup sunflower greens, 2 kohlrabi cut in shoestring strips or peeled broccoli stems, 1 thinly sliced yellow crookneck squash, and 1 pint cherry tomatoes or 1 large sweet red pepper cut in strips.

Sunchoke (Jerusalem Artichoke) Salad

Combine: 2 cups sunchokes (cooked or raw), ½ cup celery sliced diagonally, ¼ cup green peppers, and ½ cup salad dressing.

Tomato and Pepper Salad[SD]

1 green pepper cut into thin rings, 2 tomatoes firm but ripe and sliced or chopped.

Dress with lemon juice and crushed garlic, fresh herbs, and chopped celery leaves.

Add flax oil to taste.

Beet Salad

Boil beets in water for 1 hour.
Peel and cut tips off; slice thin.
Add chopped onions and either Herb or Garlic and Onion Dressing.

COOKED VEGETABLE DISHES

Preparation of Vegetables

All vegetables must be cooked slowly, over low flame, with little or no added water. In order to preserve the natural flavor of the vegetables and keep them easily digestible, the slow cooking process is very important. All vegetables should be "done" or tender. Valuable components are lost in fast cooking by excessive heat. Because the components' cells burst, the minerals go out of their colloidal composition and become more difficult to be absorbed. A stainless steel "flame tamer" may be used to prevent burning. And a little of the Special Soup (see above) may also be used, or tomatoes, apple slices, or chopped onion may be placed at the bottom of the pan to produce more fluid. In some cases this addition also improves the flavor. Only spinach water is too bitter, contains too much oxalic acid, and must be discarded.

Tomatoes, leeks, zucchini, and onions should be stewed in their own juices, as they contain an abundance of fluid by themselves. Red beets should be cooked like potatoes, in their peel, in water. All vegetables must be carefully washed and cleaned. Peeling or scraping is forbidden, because important mineral salts and vitamins are deposited directly under the skin.

The pot (not aluminum) must close tightly, to prevent escape of steam. Don't use a pressure cooker. Lids must be heavy and fit well into the pots. Cooked foods (soup and fruit) may be kept in the refrigerator for 48 hours. Baked vegetables should be slow cooked in a "low" oven (180–190° F; use oven thermometer) for 2 to 2½ hours, in a covered casserole with a tightly fitting lid. This method of baking is virtually waterless. Use onions or tomatoes, or sprinkle vegetables with lemon to add moisture when necessary.

Stewed vegetables are cooked in a heavy pot with a tightly fitting lid on top of the stove over a low flame, slowly with little or no added liquid.

Simmered vegetables are cooked on the top of the stove over a low flame in a tightly covered pan with a small amount of liquid. The temperature is kept just at the boiling point.

Boiled vegetables (like corn and artichokes) are cooked on the top of the stove in a heavy pot with a tightly fitting lid. Place 1" of cold water in the bottom of the pot, add the washed vegetables (do not peel or scrape), and cover. Cook over medium heat, slowly bringing the liquid to a boil (bubbles breaking on the surface and steam given off). Lower the flame as much as possible, keeping the liquid boiling.

Note: Bring liquids to a boil only if the recipe specifically calls for it.

Tightly Fitting Lids

Saucepans must be tightly covered to prevent steam from escaping. Covers must be heavy and close-fitting.

You may have to place wax paper under the lid to aid the seal.

Artichokes

Cut artichoke ends and rinse in the center.

Bring 2 inches of water to a boil.

Add artichokes.

Lower temperature, cover, and simmer for approximately 1 hour.

Serve with salad dressing on the side as a dip.

Asparagus

Bake in covered casserole with a small amount of soup stock or lemon juice in low oven 1 hour, or simmer with ½" soup stock for 30 minutes or until tender.

Beautiful Borscht[SD]

1 onion, 3 garlic cloves, 1 cup Special Soup, 6 small beets with tops, 1 large potato, 1 carrot, 4 red cabbage leaves, 2 bay leaves, 3 cups water, and 2 tomatoes.

Run all the vegetables through your grinder and add the water and bay leaves.

Cook for 30 minutes on low heat.

Serve with a dab of nonfat yogurt.

Beets

Bake or boil beets in their jackets.

Glazed Beets[YN] (serves 6–8)

Scrub 9 large beets and boil in 1" water until tender, approx. 1 to 1$\frac{1}{2}$ hours.

Peel in cold water.

Slice or cut into bite-sized pieces.

Glaze for Beets:

Combine: $\frac{2}{3}$ cup fresh orange juice, 1 tsp cornstarch, 1$\frac{1}{2}$ tsp cider vinegar, and 1 tsp honey or crude brown sugar.

Cook over low flame until thick.

Add beets and mix well.

Variation: Use $\frac{1}{2}$ cup apple juice and 3 tsp lemon juice in place of orange juice.

Beets, Cooked and Creamed[DAIRY]

3 cooked beets, 6 tbsp nonfat yogurt, 1 tbsp fresh snipped chives, 2 tbsp finely chopped onion, finely chopped parsley.

Put cooked, chopped beets into a saucepan with the yogurt, chives, and onion and heat gently.

Put into serving dish and sprinkle with chopped parsley.

Broccoli

Bake in a covered casserole in low oven with onions or a small amount of soup stock for 1–2 hours.

Serve with tomato sauce.

Broccoli and Herbs[MZ]

2 bunches of broccoli, 4–6 cloves of garlic, $\frac{1}{2}$ onion sliced, $\frac{1}{4}$ tsp dill, and $\frac{1}{4}$ cup Special Soup broth.

Wash broccoli and peel stems.

Put garlic and onion in one pot and cook until onion becomes translucent.

Add cut broccoli crowns and stems, dill, and broth.

Cook on low heat until broccoli is tender.

Festive Broccoli[YN] (or Festive Green Beans)

1 large bunch broccoli (or 3½ cups sliced green beans), 1 clove garlic minced, 1 small onion diced, 1 medium sweet red or yellow bell pepper cut in strips, 2 tsp lemon juice (optional), and ¼ tsp dried or 1 tsp fresh dill weed.

Select dark green bunch of broccoli with no yellowing.

Wash well and cut into spears, peeling tougher stalks at base.

Place onion and garlic in pot.

Cover and stew on low flame for 45 minutes or until tender.

Add pepper strips for last 20–25 minutes of cooking.

Add lemon just before serving (lemon will discolor broccoli if added during cooking).

Sprinkle vegetables with dill and serve.

Cauliflower

Wash cauliflower and break into sections.

Add 2–3 tomatoes, sliced and cut into chunks.

Stew together for approximately 45 minutes (or until tender) on low heat.

Cauliflower and Carrot Sauce

1 small cauliflower, 3 carrots, and flaxseed oil.

Separate the cauliflowerets and place in a baking dish with a little water and cook until soft at 250° F.

When ready, drain off the water.

At the same time, simmer the carrots on low heat with enough water until they are soft.

Blend carrots in blender with the oil.

Pour sauce over the cooked cauliflower, and place in warm oven (turned off) for 5–10 minutes, before serving.

Carrots and Honey

Wash carrots, cut off ends, and slice.

Do not peel or scrape.

Stew in a small amount of soup stock for 45 minutes or until tender.

Last 5–10 minutes of stewing add: ½ tsp honey for slight flavoring.

Chard Rolls, Stuffed[MZ]

1 bunch of chard, 6 medium potatoes, 4 carrots, ½ onion sliced, and 3 large cloves of garlic minced.
Cook onions and potatoes separately.
In another pot, cook carrots and garlic.
When done, puree each potful separately, then mix together.
Put chard leaves in very hot water, being sure not to overcook.
Spread each leaf and remove tough center stem.
Then place puree in center of leaf and roll tightly.
Display on tray and serve with ketchup (see recipe, p. 85 of the *Gerson Therapy Handbook*).

Corn

Corn may be baked in the husk wrapped in foil.
Bake in low oven for 1 hour or place in boiling water for approximately 7 minutes.

Corn with Mixed Vegetables

3 stalks of celery, 2 carrots, 2 ears of corn, and 2 zucchini squash.
Wash the corn well and husk it.
Cut the kernels off.
Slice the other vegetables into smaller pieces.
Put the corn in a baking dish and add the vegetables.
Bake in the oven at 200° F for 1 hour.

Creamed Corn

3 ears of corn and 1 green bell pepper.
Husk corn and cut off the kernels.
Put kernels from 2 ears in a blender and blend.
Add the kernels from the third ear to the blended corn.
Place in a baking dish and on the top place sliced green pepper.
Bake in the oven 1½ hours at 200–250° F.

Corn with Orange Juice

2 ears of corn and 1 glass of orange juice.
Wash the corn well, husk, and cut off the kernels.

Put this in a baking dish with a lid and bake in the oven at 250° F until done.

Pour the corn juice off, and add the orange juice.

Let set 5–10 minutes before serving.

Dilly Beans^{YN}

3 cups green beans, ⅓ cup onion sliced in half rings, ½ tsp dill weed, 2 tsp lemon juice, and green or white cabbage.

Combine in pan: ½ cabbage, shredded thinly, pinch marjoram, 3–4 tsp apple cider vinegar, 1 large tomato, chopped sage, and 1 onion diced.

Combine and bake in low oven in a covered casserole until tender.

Stew approximately 1 hour, until tender.

Do not add water.

Eggplant, Baked

Put some soup stock in bottom of large covered baking dish.

Add in layers: 1 chopped onion, 1 eggplant sliced, plus 2 tomatoes sliced and skinned.

Cover and bake in low oven for 2 hours.

Eggplant, Stewed

Combine in a stew pot: 1 eggplant cut into cubes, 2 onions chopped, and 3 tomatoes (peeled and chopped).

Stew approximately 30 minutes (until tender).

Do not add water.

Eggplant Roulades^{DAIRY} with Red Pepper Sauce

The Sauce:

1 red pepper quartered and deseeded, 1 onion finely chopped, 2 tomatoes chopped, 1 clove garlic crushed, and 6 tbsp water.

To make the sauce, cook the pepper, onion, tomatoes and garlic in the water, and simmer for 20 minutes.

Put through the food processor or blender.

The Roulade:

2 eggplants, 16 oz of cottage cheese (unsalted, nonfat), 2 tomatoes skinned and chopped, plus herbs (such as parsley or coriander).

For the roulade, cut the eggplants lengthwise into 1/4 inch slices.

Put in an oven-proof dish and cook a little in the oven to soften them.

In the meantime, mix together the cottage cheese and herbs and prepare the tomatoes.

Then spread a little cottage cheese over each partially cooked piece of eggplant, scatter with tomatoes and roll up.

Place back into the oven-proof dish and cook for 15–20 minutes.

Serve hot, garnished with the pepper sauce.

Fennel Treat[SD]

1 bulb of fennel, 1 large tomato cut into ¼" slices, and 2–3 cloves garlic peeled and sliced thin.

Cut off stalks and leaves from fennel.

Slice bulb in half lengthwise so you have two flat halves.

Rinse halves under running water to remove sand and put them in a baking dish with cut side up.

Cover halves with tomato slices and place garlic slices on top of tomatoes.

Cover dish and bake at 250° for 1–2 hours.

Serve with a baked potato and a salad of grated carrots on a bed of pretty greens.

Green Chard Rolls

4 leaves of green chard, 2 carrots, ¼ head broccoli, 2 cloves garlic, ½ cup rice uncooked, ¼ head cauliflower, 2 small zucchini squash, 1 ear of corn (cut kernels off), and 1½ tomatoes.

Wash the vegetables well.

Put the chard leaves in hot water long enough to wilt them so they will bend.

Cut the other vegetables into small pieces, and put them in a pan with a little bit of water to boil on low heat.

When cooked, drain the water off.

Make a sauce in the blender with the tomatoes and garlic, and pour this sauce on top of the vegetables and raw rice.

Place some of the vegetables-rice mixture in the center of each leaf and roll them up.

Put these in a baking dish with a lid and bake in the oven for 1 to 1½ hours at 250° F.

Green Peppers

2–4 sliced green peppers and 2–4 sliced onions.
Stew in tightly covered pot approximately 30 minutes (add no water).

Lima Beans and Zucchini

1 large onion, 1 clove garlic, ½ cup soup stock, 1 cup fresh lima beans, 3 cups zucchini, 4 med. tomatoes, ½ tsp cornstarch, 4 sprigs fresh parsley, a dash of thyme and sage or a pinch of dried parsley.
Mix all ingredients except herbs.
Simmer about 15 minutes (until tender).
Thicken with cornstarch mixed with a little water.
Just before serving add herbs.

Onions and Raisins

1 onion peeled and chopped plus ¼ cup raisins.
Stew in tightly covered pot approximately 30 minutes.

Onions, Cheese Marinated*

2 tbsp lemon juice, 3 oz pot cheese (unsalted, nonfat), ½ tsp brown sugar, and 2 cups onions sliced thick.

Stuffed Pepper[SD] *

1 large green or red pepper, 4 oz pot cheese, ¼ onion, 1 zucchini, 1 small carrot, 3 tomatoes, 1 small turnip, 1 clove garlic, 1 tbsp fresh mixed herbs, and 4 oz Special Soup.
Put the pepper in a saucepan with a little water and cook over low heat (covered) until tender.
Remove from the pan and leave the pepper upside down to drain and cool.
Finely chop the onion, zucchini, carrot, herbs, tomatoes, turnip, and garlic.
Place in a small saucepan with the soup and simmer over low heat for 45 minutes to an hour.
Core the pepper with a sharp knife, removing all seeds.
Mix the pot cheese with the cooked vegetables and fill the pepper using a small spoon.

Stand the pepper in a suitable baking dish and bake for 40 minutes at 350° F.

Serve with French Tomato Sauce, baked potato, and a green vegetable.

Potatoes

Potatoes are most often boiled slowly in a covered pot over medium-low heat approximately 1 hour until tender.

Baked Potatoes

Baked potatoes should be thoroughly washed, not scraped or peeled.

Bake in a low-heat oven for 2 or 2½ hours or, alternatively, bake for 50 minutes to 1 hour at 350° F.

Mashed Potatoes

Peel and cube potatoes.

Place in pan with one small onion and enough water to bring to a boil and simmer until done.

When done, there should be no water left.

Mash with enough nonfat yogurt to make smooth.

Mashed Potatoes and Chard

Take one bunch of chard, green or red, wash and shred, and put in pan.

Add small amount (4–5 tbsp) of water or soup stock, and start to boil.

When boiling, turn down to simmer.

Meantime, peel 3 large or 4 medium potatoes; cube and place on top of the chard.

Let simmer until potatoes are soft and done.

Remove water if any remains, and add approximately 6–8 oz of nonfat yogurt.

Mash all together.

Add a little more yogurt if the mixture is too dry.

The same recipe can be used with kale. When using kale, remove central stems by stripping them before shredding into pan.

Parsley Potatoes

Boil several potatoes in their skins until done.

Remove the peel and roll in some chopped parsley after slightly brushing with flaxseed oil.

Potato Puffs (Note: this is marginal food; eat rarely)

Take a baking potato and cut it into thin (½") slices.

Place the slices on the oven rack and, without any addition, bake at high heat (425° F) to puff, turn over, and lower heat to 325° F (with oven door cracked open).

Bake for another 20 minutes.

The slices puff up and become crisp and tasty, almost like fried potatoes.

Done when shiny brown on both sides.

Scalloped Potatoes

Take a glass baking dish and place one whole chopped onion in bottom.

Slice potatoes and place one layer on top of the onion.

Then place a layer of sliced tomato on top, another layer of sliced or chopped onion.

Sprinkle with a dash of marjoram and/or thyme and bake in a low oven 1–2 hours or until done.

Potatoes and Carrots, Westphalian Style

6–8 small carrots sliced or 4–5 large carrots sliced, 3 medium potatoes or 2 large potatoes, 1 large onion, and 3–4 tbsp of soup stock.

Wash and slice carrots into pan.

Peel and slice potatoes and chop onion.

Add all together in pan with soup stock.

Let simmer until done, adding a bit more soup stock if necessary.

When done, no water should remain in pan.

Red Cabbage

Combine in pan: ½ cabbage shredded, 3 tsp vinegar, 3 large chopped onions, 2 bay leaves, and a little soup stock.

Stew over low heat approximately ½ hour.

Last half hour add: 3 apples peeled and grated plus 1 tsp raw sugar.

Spinach

After cutting off roots wash 3–4 times.

Put in large, tightly covered pot that has a layer of onions on the bottom of the pan.

Do not add water.

Stew over a low flame until spinach wilts.

Pour off excess juice.

Serve chopped with slice of lemon.

Stuffed Holiday Squash[YN]

1 large kabocha squash (about 4½ lbs), ¾ cup raw brown rice, ¼ cup raw wild rice, rye or wheat berries, or more brown rice, 2½ cups vegetable stock or purified water, 1 cup onion diced, 3 cloves garlic minced, 1½ cup fresh peas shelled, or sprouted lentils, ¾ cup celery diced, ¾ cup yellow or red bell pepper diced, ½ cup unsulphured raisins or prunes (pit prunes and chop), 1 tsp each of sage and savory, 2 tsp thyme, ⅓ cup fresh parsley finely chopped, and ¼ cup fresh orange juice.

Yvonne Nienstadt says: "I love the texture and taste of this Japanese squash. It's very meaty and sweet, but you could use pumpkin, turban, or acorn squash too (cut the latter in half and seed). You may also use 2 or 3 smaller-sized squashes rather than a large one. This makes a very attractive presentation, especially if the squash are of different sizes."

Cook rice and wild rice together in vegetable stock for 45 minutes or until rice is done.

Using stock to cook the grain adds both nutrition and flavor.

Just save your vegetable trimmings, for carrots, parsnips, chard stems or greens, celery, celery root, onion all work well.

Avoid cabbage family veggies as they impart a strong flavor.

Cover with pure water and simmer until done.

Use in soups, to make sauces or what have you.

Carefully cut the top off of the squash as you would when carving a pumpkin.

Remove seeds.

Place squash face down on baking pan together with the squash lid and prebake for 25 to 30 minutes in a 350° F oven.

Take care not to overcook; a mushy squash cannot be stuffed.

Place onion, garlic, peas, and celery in a pot and cook on low for 20 minutes to barely tenderize.

Add diced pepper, raisins, herbs, citrus juice, and cooked rice, mixing well.

Fill squash with stuffing, packing it down.

Return to oven and bake 25 to 30 minutes, or until squash is tender, but still firm.

If there is extra filling, bake in a covered casserole with a tablespoon of stock or juice, or fill a bell pepper or two and do the same.

To serve, arrange a platter with fresh kale or other leafy greens.

Place squash in center of platter and artistically prop squash lid up against squash.

Spoon out each helping, making sure to get some of the delicious squash meat.

Alternatively, if squash is cooled a bit before serving, it may be sliced in wedges.

Ladle Parsley Yogurt Sauce (see recipe below under Sauces and Dips) over each portion, if dairy is allowed; otherwise, a squeeze of orange juice adds a bit of zing. Enjoy!

Stuffed Squash[YN]

3–4 acorn squash, ½ cup onion diced, ½ cup celery diced, ½ cup carrot diced, 1¼ cup cooked brown rice, ½ cup lentils sprouted, ¼ cup raisins or chopped prunes soaked and drained, 3 tsp fresh parsley minced, ½ tsp rubbed sage, ½ tsp thyme, and 1 large clove of garlic crushed.

Slice squash lengthwise and remove seeds.

Combine remaining ingredients; fill squash halves.

Cover and bake at 300–325° F for 1½ hours, or until squash is tender.

Delicious with Apricot Sauce or Golden Gravy (see under Sauces and Dips).

Try using 6–8 whole cloves garlic for a delicious mild flavor. Crushing the fresh garlic releases its strong aromatic oils, whereas using garlic uncut imparts a very mild flavor.

Stir-Steamed Snow Peas Medley*

1 lb snow peas, 1 bunch bok choy, 1 medium zucchini, 1 medium crookneck yellow squash, 1 small red onion, 1 carrot, 1 leek, 1 cup orange juice, 1 tbsp honey, 1 tbsp vinegar, and 1 tsp of allspice.

Clean all vegetables, removing stem from snow peas, slicing white stalk and green leaf of bok choy into strips, slicing yellow squash lengthwise and then into half circles.

You can make attractive planks out of the zucchini by trimming off each end, and then cutting in half, then half again.

Stand each barrel of squash on end and slice down into ⅛" planks.

Dice red onion, then slice carrots oriental style as thin as possible at a 45-degree angle into ovals.

Slice leek in similar fashion across stalk into ovals.

Put orange juice, honey, allspice, and vinegar into a blender, then pour into a suitable-sized steam pot.

Cover with all the vegetables and simmer 15–20 minutes until tender. Very succulent!

String Beans

1 lb green beans (cut tips, wash, and cut into any size piece desired).

Add: 1 onion chopped, some soup stock (just enough to keep beans moist).

Stew approximately 50 minutes (until tender).

Sweet Potato

Cut off tips and wash.

Perforate potato with knife to let steam escape and place in casserole (covered for soft skin, uncovered for crisp skin).

Bake in low oven for 2 to 2½ hours.

Tomatoes, Grilled

Slice tomatoes in half.

Put in pan, sliced side up, and cover each half with chopped onions.

Bake in a low oven 1 hour.

Save juice to put into soup.

Green Tomato Mincemeat

1 qt green tomatoes, 2 oz golden raisins, ½ cup brown sugar, ¼ cup water, 2 oz seeded raisins, ¼ tsp cloves, ¼ cup wine vinegar, along with 1 pt of tart apples.

Put tomatoes through coarse chopper.

Combine all ingredients except apples.

Heat to tender about 30 minutes, stirring.

Add chopped apples and cook until thick.

Tomatoes Stuffed with Mixed Vegetables

4 tomatoes (hollowed out as the vessel), vegetables: a variety, as much as desired, 2 tomatoes and 6 garlic cloves (the sauce).

Wash tomatoes well.

Hollow out the 4 tomatoes.

Cut the vegetables into small pieces and boil in a little water for half an hour.

Put cooked vegetables in the tomatoes and place them in a baking dish without the lid.

In the blender, blend the 2 tomatoes and garlic.

Spread sauce on top of each tomato.

Preheat oven to 350 degrees for 10 minutes.

Turn it off and put tomatoes in for another 10 minutes.

Zucchini

Combine: sliced zucchini, raw chopped onion, chopped tomatoes, and a touch of soup stock.

Stew for 20 minutes or cut squash into small pieces and place in a baking dish. In the blender, blend the tomatoes, onion, and 4 garlic cloves.

Pour sauce over squash and bake 1½ hours at 200–250° F.

Zucchini and Rice

½ lb organic brown rice, 1 carrot, 1 zucchini, and 2 garlic cloves.

Wash the rice and vegetables well.

Put rice in a baking dish and add chopped up parsley, carrot, celery, and zucchini squash.

At the same time blend tomato and garlic in the blender and spread on top of the rice and vegetables.

Bake in the oven for 1½ hours at 250°F.

Zucchini and Tomatoes[SD]

6 small zucchini sliced, 1 medium or large onion chopped, 2–3 tomatoes chopped, plus garlic and herbs to taste (thyme, mace, marjoram).

Saute onion, tomatoes, and seasonings in a little water.

Add zucchini when half done, and simmer.

Serve as a vegetable or potato topping.

Spaghetti with Beetballs[YN]

Wash 1 medium spaghetti squash and cut in half.

Scoop out seeds and place cut side down on baking sheet.

Bake in low oven for 2 hours or until tender.

Or, place cut side up in a large covered pot with 1" water and steam over low flame for 1 hour or until done.

Note: Spaghetti squash is a yellow hard winter squash developed by a Japanese farmer some 30 years ago. When cooked, it comes out in strands like spaghetti. It is now widely available especially in organic growers' circles.

Spaghetti Beetball Sauce

2 lb ripe tomatoes (6–8 large), 3–5 cloves garlic minced, 1 medium onion diced fine, 1 green pepper diced, 2 stalks celery diced, or 1 small fennel bulb diced, 2 small zucchini sliced, or 1 cup eggplant cubed, 4 tsp fresh parsley minced, pinch each of rosemary, thyme, sage, and marjoram,* and ½ tsp fennel seeds.

Cook whole tomatoes over a low flame for 30–35 minutes or until tender. To ensure a thick, rich sauce, pour off the extra juice drawn from the tomatoes during cooking.**

Put drained tomatoes through food mill or sieve to remove skins and seeds.

Pour sauce back into pot and add remaining veggies and seasonings.

Cover and stew over low flame for 1 hour or until veggies are done to your liking.

For a little extra bite add a dash or two of wine vinegar with a tsp of honey.

*Basil and oregano, both favorite Italian seasonings, are not allowed on the Gerson Therapy owing to the aromatic oils they contain.

**Please be sure to keep extra tomato liquid for soup or gravy, or better still, drink as a hot broth immediately. It's delicious.

Beetballs

2 tsp parsley minced, 1 small onion minced, 1 medium beet grated, and 3–4 medium carrots grated. Or, 1 cup eggplant ground, ½ cup Essene

rye bread or saltless and fatless rye, 1½ cup of 2-day-old lentils germi-nated,* 1 small bunch endive, spinach or young chard finely chopped, and 2–3 cloves garlic minced.

Put lentils and eggplant (if used) through food grinder or Norwalk® juicer using grid #2.

Mix with bread crumbs and remaining veggies.

Mix well.

Form into 2" balls and place on baking sheet well sprinkled with oat or rye meal to prevent sticking.

Cover and bake in low oven for 1 hour.

Uncover and bake 1 hour more.

Arrange cooked spaghetti squash on a plate with one or two beetballs, cover with sauce and enjoy!

Variations of this recipe: Use 3 large white or 3 medium sweet potatoes in place of ground lentils.

Boil sweet potatoes until tender, then put through food mill or grinder with skins. Proceed as with above.

Replace bread crumbs with ½ cup cooked brown rice or ⅓ cup oat flakes ground in the Norwalk juicer.

*Cover lentils with distilled water and allow to soak (germinate) overnight. Drain.

Veggie Loaf^{YN}

Grind in the Norwalk® juicer or in a food grinder: 2 cups lentils germi-nated, ¼ cup fresh parsley, 1½ cups eggplant diced or parsnips or yams.

Add: 1 cup onions diced fine, ¾ cup beets grated, ¾ cup carrots grated, 1 cup celery diced fine, 3 cloves garlic minced, 1½ cups cooked brown rice, pinch thyme, pinch of rubbed sage, pinch of tarragon, and 1 tsp lemon juice.

Bake in covered pan in low oven for approximately 2 hours.

Uncover and baste with Golden Sauce or Tomato Sauce.

Bake another 30 minutes to 1 hour.

Serve with extra sauce.

Veggie Stroganoff^{YN}

1 cup onion diced, 1 cup eggplant diced, 1½ cups cauliflowerets or cab-bage, 1½ cups sliced carrots or tomatoes, 1 cup broccoli or green pepper, and 1 cup celery or zucchini sliced.

Stew vegetables for 1½ hours until tender (you may want to add soft veggies like tomatoes and zucchini last).

Set aside and let cool to 140° F while making sauce as follows: combine 3 tbsp wine or cider vinegar, 1 tsp dillweed, 2 cups yogurt, 1 cup cottage cheese (nonfat, saltless), and green onions or parsley for garnish.

Blend sauce until smooth.

Mix with warm veggies.

Serve over a bed of baked spaghetti squash or cooked brown rice. Garnish with chopped green onions or parsley.

Soups

Potato Soup

1 large onion, ½ small celery knob, parsley, 2 large potatoes, 1 leek, plus 2 stalks celery and 2 quarts water.

Clean and dice all vegetables.

Place in covered saucepan with water.

Bring to boil.

Lower heat.

Cover. Simmer 2–3 hours.

Mash through food mill.

Special Soup (also called "Hippocrates soup"—see its recipe cited at the start of this chapter or see the *Gerson Therapy Handbook*, page 80)

Tomato Soup with Lemon and Garlic

2 to 3 large tomatoes, 1 clove garlic, 1 bay leaf, juice of ½ lemon, 2 onions, 1 tsp oat flakes, 1 tsp brown sugar, and ½ cup soup stock (see Special Soup recipe above).

Dice all vegetables.

Place vegetables, soup stock, sugar, and lemon in covered saucepan and cook for 1 hour.

Mash through food mill.

Replace in saucepan.

Add oat flakes and cook 5 more minutes.

Tomato and Mint Soup[GSG]

2 lbs tomatoes (Roma preferably), 5 green onions (scallions), 2 small cooking apples, 5 tbsp cider vinegar, 1 tsp brown sugar, 2 large lemons, 6 or 8 sprigs fresh mint, and 200 g (6–8 oz) of nonfat yogurt (optional).

Chop tomatoes, slice spring onions, core and slice apple.

Put these into a saucepan with the cider vinegar and sugar.

Bring to a boil and simmer gently for 30 minutes.

Put through food mill.

Either leave to cool, adding last ingredients later, or add the lemon juice and beat in the yogurt (if used) immediately.

Just before serving, add the chopped mint, leaving some scattered over the top of the soup for decoration.

Makes 4 generous or 6 small servings.

Tomato Soup with Potato and Onion

2 large tomatoes, 1 medium onion, 1 tsp brown sugar, 2 medium potatoes, 1 tsp wine vinegar, and a small piece of bay leaf.

Wash and dice all vegetables.

Place all ingredients except sugar in covered saucepan with water to cover.

Cook over low flame for 1 hour.

Mash through food mill and add sugar to taste.

SAUCES AND DIPS

Apricot Sauce

¼ cup dried apricots unsulfured, 1 cup pure water heated, and ½ cup fresh apple or orange juice.

Wash and drain apricots.

Combine with water and soak for several hours.

Add juice and stew over low flame until apricots are very tender, about 1½ hours.

Puree sauce in blender or by putting through Foley food mill or the Norwalk® juicer.

Baba Ghanoush

1 large eggplant, 2 cloves garlic, 1 tsp lemon juice, 1 tbsp chopped parsley, and lemon wedges.

Bake eggplant for 1 hour and when cool enough, peel, and drain off excess liquid, squeezing gently.

Blend with garlic until fairly smooth, add lemon juice and parsley.

Mix well.

Serve with raw dipping vegetables such as celery, carrots, cauliflower, and peppers.

Golden Gravy

1 small potato quartered, 4 carrots sliced, 2 tsp cider vinegar or lemon juice, 1 cup soup stock or water, 1 small onion diced, 1/4 tsp dill, marjoram or thyme, and 1 tsp parsley minced.

Combine ingredients and stew over low flame for 1 1/2 to 2 hours or until tender.

Remove potato skins and puree.

Golden Sauce

Combine in a covered casserole: 1 small sweet potato or yam quartered, 2–3 carrots coarsely chopped, 1 small onion diced, 1/2 cup soup stock, 1/2 cup tangerine or orange juice, and a pinch of thyme and rosemary.

Bake in low oven until tender (approx. 2 hours).

Put through Foley food mill or spin in blender adding more juice to achieve desired consistency.

Add 2 tsp parsley and serve.

Ketchup/Catsup

3 tomatoes, 1/2 head of garlic, 1/2 onion, 1/16 cup (1/2 oz) vinegar, 1/4 tsp dill, and 1/2 cup Sucanat (organic brown sugar).

Place all ingredients in pan and bring to a boil.

Cook until tender and put through food mill or liquefier until smooth.

Parsley Yogurt Sauce^{DAIRY}

½ cup minced onion, 1 tsp fresh grated horseradish or ½ tsp dried horseradish (optional), 1 cup nonfat yogurt, 1 tbsp lemon or lime juice, 1 tsp maple syrup or honey, and ¼ cup minced parsley.
Cook onions over low heat until tender and translucent.
Remove from heat and let cool slightly.
Blend onions with horseradish, yogurt, citrus juice, and sweetener in blender until smooth.
Stir in parsley.

Plum Sauce

½ lb plums, ½ tsp lemon juice, 1 slice toast diced, 1 tsp brown sugar, and 2 tsp bread crumbs.
Wash plums.
Remove pits and place in saucepan with water to half cover.
Cook 15 minutes and strain through food mill.
Add sugar, bread crumbs, and lemon juice.
Replace in saucepan.
Cook 3 minutes longer.
Serve over toast if desired.

Tomato Salsa

1 medium tomato finely chopped, green onions or 1 medium red onion, 2 tbsp fresh coriander leaves (cilantro) chopped, and 3 tbsp lemon juice.
Combine ingredients (don't overdo the lemon juice), cover, and chill.
Best eaten fresh but can be kept for up to 2 days in the refrigerator.

Tomato Sauce, No-Wait (this sauce is raw)

1 lb Roma Tomatoes cut into pieces, 3–4 cloves of garlic, 3 sprigs of parsley herbs, and 1 tsp linseed oil.
Place linseed oil in blender and start.
Begin adding pieces of tomato and other ingredients a little at a time.
Allow to whip for a minute or so until all ingredients are mixed.
Yields about 2–3 cup of sauce.

Tomato Sauce

Combine in large pan: 4–6 large tomatoes, 4–5 large onions peeled and sliced, 1 large or 2 medium potatoes with skin diced, 2–3 cloves garlic, a pinch of marjoram, and a pinch of thyme.

Stew and let simmer for 1 hour and pass through Foley food mill.

One can also add a little celery or green pepper for taste.

Tomato Sauce, French

1 onion, ½ stick celery, ½ small carrot, 1½ pounds tomatoes, a few sprigs of flat leaf parsley, 1 clove garlic, and 1 bay leaf.

Cook chopped onion, carrot, celery tomatoes, parsley, garlic, and bay leaf.

Puree and serve hot or cold.

Makes 1¼ pints.

FRUITS AND DESSERT

Fruits

Most fresh fruits can be eaten unpeeled when ripe.

Of course, fruits like oranges and bananas should be peeled.

Always wash fresh fruit.

Dried fruits should be washed in clean, lukewarm distilled water and soaked overnight in water (little more than to cover).

Use the same water and cook in covered saucepan until tender.

Dried fruits must be unsulfured.

The following fruit recipes are taken from Dr. Max Gerson's personal files.

Desserts

Desserts should never replace the meals or juices of the therapy.

At the risk of sounding like your mother, we advise to "clean your plate before dessert, dear!"

Do not eat or use as ingredients in desserts: ice cream, fat, white flour, baking soda, candy, chocolate, cream, or salt. Have fun!

Sugar

Use only brown (Sucanat) or raw sugar, light honey, maple syrup, or un-sulfured molasses.

Syrup

Boil 1 lb brown sugar in 1 quart of water and 1 cup apple juice until dis-solved.

Keep in covered jar.

Apples, Baked

2 medium apples, 1 tsp raisins, and 2 tbsp water.

Wash, core, and cut apples in half.

Place with raisins in pan or baking dish in oven for about 15 minutes until done then broil under flame until golden brown about 5 minutes.

Apple halves should stay whole.

Honey may be added to raisins to taste.

Apple and Banana

½ cup applesauce, ½ raw sliced banana, and juice of ½ lemon.

Serve raw or place applesauce and banana in covered saucepan and heat slowly.

Serve with lemon juice.

Apple Cake with Maple Yogurt^{DAIRY}

1½ lbs cooking apples, 1 lemon, 1 oz rolled oats, 1 oz oatmeal, 2 oz sul-tanas or raisins, 4 oz brown sugar, 4 oz whole wheat flour, 1 tsp potassium baking powder, ½ cup fresh apple juice, yogurt, and maple syrup.

Put peeled and chopped apples into a large bowl and sprinkle with lemon juice.

Combine rolled oats, oatmeal, raisins, sugar, flour, and baking powder and mix well.

Stir this mixture into the apples.

Pour mixture into cake pan and bake at 350° F for 20–35 minutes or until lightly browned on top.

Serve with yogurt mixed with 1–2 tbsp maple syrup.

Applesauce, Cooked

3 medium apples pared, cored, and sliced.
Add honey or brown sugar to taste.
Put apple slices in saucepan half covered with cold water.
Boil until soft, about 15 minutes.
Put through food mill and mix with honey.

Applesauce, Fresh

3 medium apples pared, cored, and sliced.
Add honey or brown sugar to taste.
Run apples through the grinder portion of the juicer.
Season to taste and enjoy.

Apple Spice Cake[YN]

Combine: ¼ cup honey or maple syrup, 1 cup fresh applesauce, 1½ cups oat flour, and ¾ cup whole wheat flour or triticale flour.

Sift together: ¾ cup crude brown sugar, a pinch of allspice, a pinch of mace, ¼ tsp coriander, and 1 tsp Featherweight sodium-free baking powder* (optional).

Add: 2 cups raisins or chopped dates.
Combine wet and dry ingredients.
Pour into nonstick oblong bake pan.
Mix crumb topping and sprinkle on top.
Bake at 325° F for 40 minutes or until cake tests done.
Serve with a spoonful of fresh applesauce or nonfat yogurt. Enjoy.

*This is a potassium-based baking powder. If you are a cancer patient, check with your health professional first before using it.

Crumb Topping for Apple Spice Cake

⅔ cup rolled oats, ⅓ cup maple syrup or honey, a pinch of allspice, and a pinch of mace.

Buzz oats briefly in blender to make a finer flake.
Mix spices with oats.
Mix in enough sweetener to make a crumbly mixture.

Apple Streusel Pie

One 8" or 9" pie crust (see below), 12 medium green apples sliced thin, 1/3 cup crude brown sugar or 1/4 cup honey, 2 tsp. cornstarch or oat flour, 2–3 tsp lemon or orange juice, 1/2 cup dried currants or chopped dates, plus a pinch of coriander, mace, and allspice.

Combine dry ingredients.

Coat apples.

Drizzle on honey (if used) and juice.

Fill pie crust.

Sprinkle on topping.

Bake at 300–325° F for 1 hour and 15 minutes or until apples are tender.

Crumb Topping for Apple Streusel Pie

2/3 cup oat flour, 3 tsp crude brown sugar, pinch allspice, and 1/3 cup honey or maple syrup.

Apple–Sweet Potato Pudding

1 tsp raisins, 1/2 cup bread crumbs*, 1/2 cup orange juice, 1 sweet potato (boiled, peeled, sliced), 1 apple (raw, peeled, sliced), and 1 tsp of brown sugar.

Place sweet potato slices in baking dish with apple slices and raisins spread with bread crumbs, sugar, and orange juice and bake in 350 degree oven for 30 minutes.

Serve hot with 3 tsp buttermilk or yogurt if permitted.

*Never use commercial bread crumbs (see recipe for bread crumbs in the bread section that follows in this chapter or on p. 100 of the *Gerson Therapy Handbook*).

Apple Tart DAIRY

1/2 cup warm water (105–110° F), 1 tbsp crude brown sugar (Sucanat), 1 package dry yeast, 2/3 cup churned buttermilk, nonfat yogurt or apple juice*, 1/2 cup crude brown sugar (Sucanat), 2 1/2 cups oat flour, 1 cup whole wheat or triticale flour, 9–10 medium apples (Gala, Pippin, and Golden Delicious are good), 4 tbsp maple syrup, or liquid Fruit Source**, 4 tbsp brown rice syrup†, 1/2 cup date sugar (dried ground dates), 1 1/2 tsp of allspice, and 1/4 tsp mace or coriander.

*Use only apple juice if patient is not yet allowed dairy.
**Fruit Source is a sweetener derived from natural fruit sugars.
†Rice syrup, derived from malted rice, is a thick and creamy syrup that needs to be thinned by either the maple syrup or Fruit Source.

Sprinkle yeast onto warm water into which 1 tbsp crude brown sugar has been dissolved.

Let stand for 5 to 10 minutes or until frothy.

Warm buttermilk, yogurt, or juice to 100°F.

Add crude brown sugar and stir until dissolved.

Stir buttermilk into yeast mix, then add oat flour and beat vigorously.

Stir in enough of the remaining flour to make a stiff dough.

Knead on a floured bread board, adding only enough flour to keep dough from sticking.

Knead until smooth and elastic, approximately 5 to 10 minutes.

Place in a bowl, cover with tea towel, and let rise in a warm place until double in bulk, about 1½ hours.

Punch down and let rise again.

Divide dough in half.

On floured board, press each part into a 15" x 9" rectangle.

Place on separate nonstick bake sheets, or regular sheets that have been thoroughly coated with oat flakes to prevent sticking.

Prick surface with fork, leaving ¼" border around the edges.

Cover and let rise until doubled, approximately 40 minutes.

Quarter, core, and slice apples, arranging each sliced quarter over dough, as you cut it.

Place the flat side down and the skin side up, fanning the slices out slightly.

Leave about a ½" border.

Mix maple and brown rice syrups.

Using a pastry brush, coat the apples with the syrup.

Combine date sugar and spices and sprinkle over apples.

Bake at 325°F for 30 minutes or until bread is lightly browned.

Serve as is or with a spoonful of nonfat yogurt or yogurt cheese (see below) lightly sweetened with honey or maple syrup.

Note: Non-Gerson family members could enjoy this dessert with a scoop of nonfat fruit sweetened frozen yogurt—Cascadian Farm Vanilla (the milk is organic) or Stars Vanilla Bean are two brands enjoyed in moderation.

Yogurt cheese is made by draining non-fat yogurt through a stainless steel or nylon sieve lined with a cotton tea towel or cheese cloth with a bowl beneath to catch the whey.

Refrigerate and drain until desired consistency is achieved, anywhere from 2 to 8 hours. A short drainage period will yield a thickened yogurt;

longer periods will produce a cream-cheese-like texture. For our purposes, a thickened yogurt texture is what we want.

Apricots

½ lb fresh apricots, 1 tsp cornstarch dissolved in 2 tsp cold water, and 2 tsp brown sugar.
   Cut apricots in halves and remove pits.
   Place in pot with boiling water and cook for 10 minutes.
   Add cornstarch during last 2 minutes.
   Add sugar when cool.

Banana (Broiled)

1 banana and 1 tsp brown sugar.
   Cut banana in half lengthwise, then add 1 tsp brown sugar and a few drops lemon.
   Place in pan and broil under low flame for 10 minutes.
   Serve hot.

Banana and Apple

1 banana (peeled and finely mashed), 1 apple (peeled, cored, grated), and 10 tsp of raisins.
   Mix banana and apple beating thoroughly with fork or eggbeater.
   Add raisins and serve.

Banana and Figs

1 banana, 3 figs (fresh), and juice of 1 orange.
   Chop banana and figs fine and mix well with orange juice.
   Fill orange peel with this mixture and serve.

Cherries (Stewed)

½ lb cherries (washed, stemmed), 1 tsp potato starch, and 2 tsp brown sugar.
   Place cherries in saucepan with water to cover.
   Cook 10 minutes over low flame.
   Add potato starch dissolved in 2 tsp cold water.
   Add to boiling cherries.

Cook 2 minutes longer.

Chill and serve.

Currants

¼ lb red currants and 3 tsp brown sugar.

Clean and wash currants thoroughly before removing stems.

Place in dish, add sugar, and serve.

Buttermilk or yogurt (if permitted) sweetened with brown sugar may be used for sauce.

Fruit Combination

3 cups fresh cherries and apricots (halved, sliced, pitted), 2 cups water, ½ cup brown sugar, and 2 tsp cornstarch dissolved in ⅓ cup cold water.

Place fruit with water and sugar in saucepan.

Boil gently, slowly for 10 minutes.

Add cornstarch.

Cook 3 minutes longer.

Cool and serve.

Glazed Pear Halves

4–5 ripe pears and 4 tbsp honey or Sucanat (organic dried cane sugar).

Cut ripe pears into halves, and core.

Add about 4 oz of water to honey or Sucanat and mix well.

Place pear halves in baking dish and pour sugar mixture over fruit.

Bake in slow oven (275°F) until done.

Baste with juice if necessary.

Frozen Yogurt[SD DAIRY]

¼ cup stewed fruit (cherries, apricots) and 1 lb fat-free yogurt.

Spoon yogurt into a thin mesh strainer that has been lined with two layers of cheesecloth, and place it over a deep bowl.

Let it drain into the bowl in the refrigerator for about 30 minutes.

Spoon the drained yogurt into ice cube trays and freeze.

Mix fruit and yogurt cubes in a food processor or the grinder of your K & K juicer or Norwalk® juicer until the consistency is thick and smooth.

Serve immediately.

Oatmeal Cake

4 cup oatmeal (dry oats), 2 grated or blended carrots, honey and raisins as desired.

Combine all the above ingredients in a baking dish.

Put in the oven without a lid and bake for 45 minutes at 250°F.

Oatmeal Cookies^{DAIRY}

1 cup applesauce, 1 cup rye flour, 1 cup raisins, ½ cup churned butter-milk, ½ cup brown sugar, ½ cup molasses, 2 cups oatmeal, and 1 pkg yeast.

Mix and let stand 10 minutes.

Drop from teaspoon and bake in moderate oven about 20 minutes.

Pasha^{YN} (Uncooked Cheesecake)^{DAIRY}

¼ cup fresh orange juice strained, ½ cup chopped dried fruit, 4 cups soft or medium curd cottage cheese, ½ cup honey or ¾ cup brown sugar, plus raisins, dates, papaya, peaches, prunes, etc.

Mix all ingredients.

Pour batter into a strainer or colander lined with a clean cotton cloth (muslin).

Cover with a plate to weight it down.

Place in a bowl or pan and refrigerate for 5–10 hours or until dry and firm.

Turn out onto a plate and slice.

Good as is, or on a slice of Essene bread.

Peaches

½ lb peaches (skinned) and 2 tsp brown sugar.

Wash peaches.

Place in boiling water ½ minute, drain and peel.

Cut in halves.

Remove pits and place in saucepan with boiling water.

Cover. Simmer for 10 minutes.

Cool.

Add sugar and serve chilled.

Pears

1 large pear (peeled, cored, halved) and 1 tsp brown sugar.
Place pears in saucepan with water to half cover.
Add sugar and cook 30 minutes

Plums

½ lb plums and 2 tsp brown sugar.
Wash plums, cut in half, and remove pits. (Plums can also be cooked whole.)
Place in saucepan with water to cover.
Cook 15 minutes.
Remove, cool, and add sugar.
Serve chilled.

Prune and Apricots (Dried)

½ lb of each of the prunes and apricots plus 1/3 cup barley.
Soak prunes and apricots overnight in water to cover.
Use same water and boil with barley.
Cool and serve.

Prune and Banana Whip

1 cup dried prunes (soaked, cooked), 2 small bananas, ¼ lemon juice, and 1 tsp brown sugar.
Whip together thoroughly and put in refrigerator for 1 hour.
May be served in slices decorated with sweetened yogurt (if permitted).

Pumpkin Pudding Pie[YN] (Unbaked)

Pinch of allspice, pinch of coriander, pinch of mace, 2 tsp unsulfured molasses (optional), one 8" or 9" pie crust, ½ cup tapioca, 1½ cup dates, pitted and chopped, 1⅓ cup apple juice or water, and 1½ to 2 cups mashed pumpkin.
Soak tapioca and dates in juice overnight.
In morning, stew over low flame using a burner pad to diffuse heat.
Cook for 30 minutes until thick, stirring frequently to prevent sticking.
Purée tapioca and pumpkin in Foley food mill or processor.

Add spices and molasses.

Pour into prepared pie crust and chill thoroughly (may put in freezer for several hours until very firm); otherwise cutting will be a problem.

Serve with a dollop of honey-sweetened yogurt cheese (see under Apple Tart) if desired (and permitted by physician).

Variation: Use cooked squash, yams, or sweet potatoes in place of pumpkin.

Thin Buttermilk Crust^{DAIRY}

1¼ cup oat flour, ⅓ cup churned buttermilk, apple juice or water (cold), 2 tsp honey, pinch allspice or mace, and 1 tsp Featherweight (sodium-free) baking powder (optional).

Mix dry ingredients.

Add honey and just enough liquid to make a stiff dough.

Knead lightly to mix.

Roll out on floured board or between layers of waxed paper.

Carefully place in 8" or 9" pie plate which has been thoroughly coated with oat flakes to prevent sticking.

Trim excess dough and flute edges or make indentations with fork.

Chill crust, then bake at 325°F for 10–15 minutes or until lightly browned.

Note: This will not be your traditional flaky crust, so roll out thin.

Raised Pie Crust^{YN}

1 cup oat flour, ½ cup potato flour (or use more oat flour), 1 cup triticale or whole wheat flour, 1 tsp honey or brown sugar, ½ cup warm water, and 1 tsp baker's yeast.

Sprinkle yeast into warm water mixed with honey.

When frothy add flour and mix well.

Let rise in a warm place for 1 hour.

Knead on floured board for 5 minutes.

Let rest for 10 minutes and roll out on floured board.

Place in 8" or 9" pie plate that has been thoroughly coated on the bottom with rolled oat flakes.

Flute edge.

Let rise for 15 minutes.

Bake at 375°F for 20–25 minutes.

Variation: Omit yeast; use just enough cold water to make a stiff dough.

Roll out between sheets of floured wax paper.

Carefully place in pie plate.

Chill crust.

Then bake at 350°F for 10–12 minutes.

Essene Bread Crust[YN]

2 cups Essene bread crumbs, ¼ cup honey, and 3 tsp oat flour.

Toast slices of bread in slow oven until lightly brown.

Let cool.

Grind coarsely by running through grinder or Norwalk®.

Add flour, then honey.

Press into pie plate that has been well coated with rolled oat flakes.

Chill for 1 hour.

Bake at 350°F for 10–12 minutes.

Roll, then fill.

Rhubarb

½ lb rhubarb (washed and cut into 1" pieces), 2 to 3 tsp brown sugar (to taste), and 1 tsp cornstarch (if desired).

Place washed rhubarb in saucepan.

Simmer 15 to 20 minutes.

Dissolve cornstarch in a little cold water.

Add to rhubarb and allow to stew a few more minutes.

Cool and add sugar.

Note: Combine rhubarb with other sweet fruits such as apples, peaches, or apricots (fresh or dried).

Stewed Fruit Combinations

Together, use pears and plums, plums and applesauce, peaches and plums, apricots and plums, apricots and sliced apples, or peaches and pears.

Note: Stewed fruits may be served on toasted rye bread by placing a thick layer of fruit on top and allowing it to soak through for ½ hour before serving.

Sunshine Smoothie[SD]

In a blender or food processor container, combine 1 cup nonfat organic yogurt, ½ cup orange juice, 2 tbsp honey, 1 cup cut-up fresh fruit, and ½ cup crushed ice (made from distilled water); process until smooth.

Sweet Potato and Apple Bake[GSG]

12 oz sweet potatoes, 3 eating apples, allspice, a little brown sugar, and a little water.

Cook the sweet potatoes gently in their skins until tender.

Allow to cool.

Slice and put into baking dish, alternating with layers of apple.

Over each layer, sprinkle some water, a little sugar, and some allspice.

Bake covered for 20 minutes at 350°F, then remove cover and bake for an additional 10 minutes.

Sweet Potato Stuffed Oranges

3 lbs sweet potatoes (or yams), freshly made applesauce, 8 orange peel halves, and 4 oz orange juice.

Boil sweet potatoes (or yams) until done.

Peel and mash with orange juice and applesauce to make it a smooth, stuffing paste.

Put stuffing into orange peel halves and put a dab of applesauce on top.

Can be reheated in a cake tray.

Makes 4 servings.

Recipe may actually stuff 10 or more orange peels and may make more than 4 servings.

Sweet Rice[MZ]

1½ cups organic brown rice, 4 cups water, 1 cup organic brown sugar (Sucanat), and 1 cup organic raisins.

Wash the rice and put into pot with the water.

Once the water begins to boil, add the sugar and raisins and reduce the heat.

Maintain on low heat until the rice is tender.

DAIRY

Dairy is temporarily forbidden in the beginning of the Gerson Therapy.

Consult with your Gerson-trained health professional or physician before adding any dairy to your diet.

After 6 to 12 weeks on the therapy, upon doctor's orders, animal proteins are cautiously added to the diet in the form of pot cheese, yogurt and cottage cheese, and churned (not cultured) buttermilk, all made from *nonfat* milk (preferably raw) and *without salt*.

When starting the proteins, it must be done slowly and carefully. Just one tablespoon at lunch and supper of the solid proteins and ½ cup of the buttermilk per meal.

After 3 to 4 days, these levels can be increased until, at 3 weeks, one cup of of yogurt or churned (not cultured) buttermilk per meal have been added.

While adding the dairy proteins, a Gerson patient needs to watch for signs that the body is tolerating these new foods. Indigestion, flatulence (intestinal production of gas), and nasal mucus production are signs the enzyme activity cannot yet handle the dairy products. The patient should reduce or, after consulting the Gerson-trained physician, eliminate the proteins for several more weeks.

Yogurt DAIRY

Combine: 2 quarts raw nonfat (not low-fat) milk heated to 118°F, 1 pkg "Bulgarian Yogurt Culture" or 3 tsp yogurt (purchased or saved from a previous batch).

Pour mixture into sterilized glass jar(s).

Incubate at 110°–115° F for 4–8 hours by one of the following methods:

- Electric yogurt maker
- In gas oven, above pilot light
- In electric oven, low heat (gauge heat with thermometer)
- In a thermos
- In a covered pan set in a container of warm water (change water to keep warm)

Incubation time may vary, depending upon temperature.

The yogurt is ready when a toothpick inserted point first into the yogurt doesn't fall over.

The yogurt becomes set a little more firmly after refrigeration.

This is a thin yogurt because it has no fat or processed dried milk added.

Be sure to save 3 tbsp for the starter for the next batch.

Yogurt Cheese^{DAIRY}

Yogurt cheese is made by hanging nonfat yogurt in a muslin sack over a sink or bowl or in a muslin-lined strainer until it thickens to the consistency of cream cheese, without the fat, in about 6 to 8 hours.

Cottage Cheese Loaf^{YN DAIRY}

1 cup dry Essene or rye bread crumbs, 1 tbsp lemon juice or vinegar, 1–2 tsp dried parsley, ½ tsp dill weed or tarragon, ½ tsp dry horseradish (1 tsp if fresh), 2 cups mashed potatoes, 2⅓ cups dry curd cottage cheese, ½ cup sweet red or green pepper, ½ cup celery diced, and 1 small onion diced.

Combine all ingredients except the last two.

Form into a loaf.

Place on garnished platter.

Top with decorative veggie slices.

Use watercress or endive for garnish plus slices of carrot, tomato, onion, and green or red pepper for top.

Cottage Cheese^{YN DAIRY}

½ gallon unpasteurized, nonfat milk (which may not be available). Makes approx. 9 oz (1 cup) cheese.

Warm milk to body temperature (98° to 100°F) by placing unopened bottle of milk in sink of warm water.

Incubate in warm place (near pilot light or in oven with light on).

It is best to leave milk in original container to prevent airborne bacteria or molds from contaminating culture.

The incubation period ranges from about 24 to 30 hours. (Culture longer for a sharper-tasting cheese.)

Shake several times during this period.

When curd has formed, it will rise to the top.

A harder curd can be formed by putting cheese (still in bottle) in sink of warm water and gradually increasing temperature to 110° for soft curd, and to 120° for farmer-style cheese.

Be careful not to overheat or you will destroy precious enzymes and beneficial bacteria.

Use a thermometer to be safe.

Pour cheese into a strainer or colander lined with muslin or several layers of cheesecloth.

Gather the corners of the cloth and press out whey.

You may place a weight on top to speed the process.

For cream-style cottage cheese add approx. ¼ cup thick yogurt per cup of finished cheese.

For herbed cottage cheese, season with any of the following: fresh chives, crushed garlic, tarragon, parsley, dill weed, dill seed.

Let set for ½ hour before serving.

Variations: Add the juice of 1 or 2 lemons or ⅛ cup yogurt to the fresh milk instead of letting it clabber naturally. These additions result in different flavors and textures. Experiment to find the one you like the best. Enjoy!

Cottage Cheese Sour Cream^{YN DAIRY}

½ cup yogurt, 1 tbsp lemon juice, and 1 cup dry curd cottage cheese. Blend ingredients in blender.

Add any or all of the following: pressed garlic, grated horseradish, chives or green onion, fresh mint, or dried dill weed.

Use to top baked potatoes or as dip for veggies.

BREADS

Bread can be used as a snack, after breakfast, or with a meal if the patient has a good appetite.

Do not replace potatoes and vegetables with any of the breads.

Sourdough

Sourdough is sour fermented dough used as leaven. Don't be put off by the name, because sourdough breads don't taste sour. They have a tangy flavor.

Sourdough is a white substance over which a colorless or gray liquor called hooch collects. Hooch enables sourdough to complete its fermentation.

You have to feed sourdough and keep it in the refrigerator because it is a living thing that's full of microorganisms. Colonies of these microorganisms can live for many decades with proper care and feeding. You can use a starter batch obtained from someone else to get your own colonies going or buy a dehydrated starter or make it from scratch.

There are many different kinds of sourdough starters: white, yogurt, whole wheat, sour rye, and so on. For patients on the Gerson Therapy, rye sourdough is the recommended variety.

Sourdough Starter

1 tsp active dry yeast, 3 cups warm water (105°–115°F), and 3½ cups rye flour.

Dissolve yeast in warm water in a large mixing bowl. Set aside for about 5 minutes.

Gradually add flour, stirring until smooth with a wooden spoon.

Cover with cheesecloth; leave on counter in warm, draft-free place.

In about 24 hours the mixture will start to ferment.

Cover tightly with plastic wrap and leave for another 2 to 3 days.

Stir starter 2 or 3 times a day.

Starter should be foamy at the end of this time. Put into a plastic container, glass jar or crock with at least a 1-quart capacity.

Stir and cover but not with a tight-fitting top.

Feeding Sourdough

Put 1 cup sourdough in mixing bowl.

Add 2½ cups flour and 2 cups warm water. (This combination is known as feeding.)

Mix thoroughly.

Leave on counter for 8 hours or overnight.

Be sure to replace 1 cup sourdough in the jar in the refrigerator.

Try to feed sourdough once a week or every 10 days.

Feeding is necessary to keep the culture alive and may add tang to its flavor. (Note: Sourdough can be frozen).

General Rules Pertaining to Sourdough

- Use glass, stoneware, or plastic bowls. Don't use metal. Wild yeast produces acids that can corrode metal and thus kill the starter.
- Use a wooden spoon.
- Clean container about every week so that unwanted bacteria will not grow and ruin your sourdough.
- Wipe up spilled sourdough immediately. It can stick like glue or cement.
- Keep covered with a loose-fitting cover in refrigerator.

Wholegrain Rye Bread

6 cups lukewarm water, sourdough starter, and 3 lbs rye flour or a 70/30 ratio of rye flour to whole wheat flour.

Mix sourdough in water, add flour.

Leave covered and warm (180°F) for 12–24 hours.

Replace 1 cup sourdough to refrigerator as starter for next time.

Add: 2 cups lukewarm water, 2 lbs rinsed whole rye grain, and 2 lbs rolled rye (use enough rye flour, maybe 2 lbs, to hold dough together).

Roll and cut dough to fit loaf pans.

Smooth the surface with a wet hand and leave dough in a warm place to rise for 2–5 hours.

The taste gets stronger the longer it is left to rise, and it will rise only a little.

Cut a furrow down the middle, about ¼" to ½" deep.

Bake for 1½ hours at 385°F.

Take out of pans immediately and wrap in towels and turn upside down.

Do not cut for about 12 hours.

Bread can be frozen when lukewarm.

Bread Snack

1 slice of bread, spread with cottage cheese, topped with tomatoes, and radishes or sprouts or 1 slice of bread topped with honey.

Bread Dressing

1 part chopped onions, 1 part chopped celery, 2–3 parts cubed grain bread, ½ part chopped parsley, ½ to 1 cup water, plus sage, garlic, and thyme.

Place in an uncovered casserole and bake in low oven for 2 hours.

Bread Crumbs

Toast leftover bread in the oven.
Run it through the food grinder.
Store in covered container in the refrigerator.

Sour Rye Bread (Black Bread Russian Style)

Note: Sour rye is a different sourdough culture.

You will need to make the sour rye sourdough starter from scratch and keep it separate from your other starter.

8 cups freshly ground whole rye flour, 3 cups warm water, and ½ cup sourdough culture.

Mix 7 cups of the rye flour with water and sourdough culture.

Cover and let stand in a warm place 12 to 18 hours.

Remove and save ½ cup of dough as a culture for next baking, and keep the saved culture in a tightly closed jar in refrigerator.

Add remaining cup of rye flour and mix well.

Divide dough in half.

Form oblong loaf smaller than size of pan in lightly floured hands (using rye flour).

Place gently into stainless steel baking pans.

Do not press; allow space around sides of loaf.

Try dusting stainless steel pan with flour or rye meal, no oil.

Let rise for approximately ½ hour.

Bake at 350°F for 1 hour or more.

Makes two 2-lb loaves.

Store tightly wrapped in refrigerator.

Sourdough Culture

In a wide-mouthed glass jar at least 1 quart in size, mix well the following ingredients: 1 cup lukewarm distilled water, 2 tsp baking yeast, 1 tsp raw sugar, and 1 cup rye flour.

Stir well once daily with a wooden spoon (never leave a metal spoon in starter).

Allow to sit for 3 to 5 days until sour odor is detected.

May cover loosely after 2nd day.

Remove ½ cup for bread recipe above.

Store covered in refrigerator adding half cup from dough after first rising.

Bring to room temperature 1 hour before starting each new recipe.

Sourdough Potato Rye Bread[YN]

1 cup sourdough starter, 2 cups warm mashed potatoes, 1⅓ cups potato cooking water, 2 cups whole wheat or rye flour,* ¼ cup molasses (unsulfured), and ⅓ tsp caraway or fennel seed.

Mix ingredients in large nonmetal bowl.

Cover and let stand in warm place for several hours (or overnight for a very sour loaf).

Add the following: 1½ to 3 cups rye flour as needed to make a workable dough.

Turn onto floured board and knead for 5–10 minutes.

Let dough rest for 5 minutes, then form into round or baton-shaped loaves.

Place on nonstick bake sheet, or regular bake sheet (ungreased) that has been well coated with raw oat flakes to prevent sticking.

Let bread rise until almost double (when bread does not spring back when lightly touched).

Bake at 350°F for 50 minutes to 1 hour.

For a very chewy crust, place a pan of water in bottom of oven to create steam, or baste bread several times during baking with water.

For soft crust, do not steam or baste.

Immediately wrap loaves in cotton towels after removing from oven.

Let bread cool before cutting.

*Dr. Gerson allowed patients to use ⅓ wheat to ⅔ rye flour. The bread is delicious with or without wheat.

Sourdough Squash Rye Bread

1 cup sourdough starter, 2 cups puréed cooked squash (such as butternut or kabocha),1⅓ cups water, 2cups rye flour, ¼ cup honey, and ¼ cup potato flour.

Mix dry ingredients in ceramic or plastic bowl.

Cover and let stand in warm place to rise (85 to 95 percent is ideal.)

Add 2 cups rye flour, then 1½ to 3 cups more rye flour until achieving workable dough.

Turn onto floured board and knead for 5–10 minutes.

Let dough rest for 5 minutes, then shape into loaves or rolls.

Sprinkle bottom of baking pans with raw oats, then let rise for 2 hours or until doubled in size.

Bake at 350°F for an hour.

Let loaves cool before slicing.

Carrot Raisin Quick Bread[YN]

1½ cups triticale or rye flour, 1½ cups brown rice or oat flour, 1 cup whole wheat or rye flour, 5 cups carrots grated, 2½ cups orange pulp, ⅓–½ cup honey, 2 cups raisins, ½ tsp each of allspice and coriander, plus approx. 2 large navel oranges, peeled and ground.

Sift dry ingredients together.

Stir in raisins.

Mix the remaining ingredients, then gradually stir into dry mix.

Dough should be rather firm.

Divide in half and fill two nonstick bake pans.

Bake at 325°F for 50 minutes or until toothpick comes out clean.

Let cool before removing from pan.

Essene Bread[YN]

This naturally sweet cakey bread is made with only sprouted grain.

The original Essene Bread recipe comes from *The Essene Gospel of Peace*, a 2,000-year-old Aramaic text, which reveals the process of sprouting wheat as follows: "Moisten your wheat, that the angel of water may enter it. Then set it in the air, that the angel of air may also embrace it. And leave it from morning to evening beneath the sun, that the angel of sunshine may descend upon it." This modern version differs from the original only in the use of oven heat instead of the sun's.

For 1 loaf use: 1 quart of 2-day-old wheat, rye, or triticale sprouts.

Refrigerate sprouts for 1 day, uncovered, to dry slightly.

Do not rinse before grinding or you will wind up with more of a pudding than bread.

Grind in hand or electric grinder or in the Norwalk® using the #2 grid (second to the largest).

Feed sprouts gradually or they will become like cement in your grinding mechanism.

Shape into 1½"-to-2" high loaf.

Place on nonstick or regular baking sheet well coated with oat flakes to prevent sticking.

Bake at 250–300°F for 1½ to 2½ hours (loaf should be nicely browned). Cool thoroughly before slicing (chilled is best). Use serrated knife with a gently sawing motion. It also helps to dip knife in cold water before slicing bread.

VARIATIONS IN BREAD

Fruit Bread

Add: ⅓ or ⅔ cup raisins or other chopped dried fruit, ½ tsp coriander, and mace or allspice.

Onion or Garlic Herb Bread

Add: 2 or 3 tbsp finely minced onion, or 2–4 cloves pressed garlic, ½ to 1 tsp dill, thyme, and caraway or fennel.

Wafers or Crackers

Form into ¼" patties or roll out on floured board and cut into squares.

Bake wafers or crackers on a nonstick or oat-coated baking sheet at a temperature of 250–300° F for 45 minutes to 1 hour.

Appendixes

GERSON THERAPY
FINANCIAL
AND CONTACT
INFORMATION

You may have wondered: How much does the Gerson Therapy cost, and how long does the treatment last?

At the present time, the cost at a Gerson cancer facility is U.S.$5,500 per patient per week. This price includes room and board for a companion to assist in learning the treatment to help the patient on his return home to self-administer the nutritional/detoxifying program. Bringing a caregiver is necessary. A companion shares the patient's room (twin beds are provided in each room) and meals are included. The patient's cost includes all physicians' fees, nursing care, all medications, coffee for enemas, teas, weekly blood and urinalysis tests, hyperthermia treatments, laetrile, all meals, and thirteen glasses daily of the approved juices, prepared from fresh, organically grown produce. Also included are lectures, several Gerson books and teaching videotapes, and a counseling session each week with a nutritionist. Extraordinary items are charged separately, such as surgery, permanent need for oxygen, blood transfusions, and any diagnostic and treatment procedures performed at a different location.

Some of the additional cost incurred happens after the patient returns home. For instance, it costs approximately $1,400 for going-home medicine for a three month supply. Also, the Gerson Therapy requires thirteen glasses of juice a day and much other produce for soups, vegetables, fruit plates, and so on. Remember that in this particular natural and nontoxic treatment, food is medicine. These nutritional items cost more than ordinary foods, depending also on the patient's location. Costs are lower on the West Coast, but higher in the Northeast, Midwest, and other places where organic foods must be shipped in quickly to maintain freshness.

Seriously ill patients usually spend a minimum of three weeks at the Gerson hospital before returning home. If a patient is not in an advanced pathological condition, two weeks at the hospital may be satisfactory and sufficient. Still, in order to fully restore the body, the patient must continue the strict therapy for a suggested minimum of two years. The treatment may need to be extended if the patient has received chemotherapy treatments, has extensive bone metastases (which heal more slowly), or is suffering from a disease that responds slowly, such as multiple sclerosis. The time required for total healing, therefore, varies according to the degree of disease, the patient's age, how faithfully the healing program is followed, and other variables.

Patients not suffering from cancer may heal more easily. On the other hand, patients with kidney damage may need to stay "very close to the therapy" for the rest of their lives.

Many private health insurance companies do cover costs for the Gerson Therapy, but health maintenance organizations (HMOs); in-house insurance plans such as the one at Kaiser; and Medicare, CHAM-PUS, and other government insurance programs mostly do not provide reimbursements.

To inquire about enrollment as a patient at a medical facility licensed by the Gerson Institute, or to acquire information about any of the other programs offered below, contact the nonprofit Gerson Institute (a.k.a. the Cancer Curing Society) at:

THE GERSON INSTITUTE
1572 Third Avenue, San Diego, CA 92101
Tel. (619) 685-5353
Tel. toll free (888) 4-GERSON
Fax (619) 685-5363
Email: *info@Gerson.org*

Here are some additional programs offered by the Gerson Institute:

- Referral to a trained Gerson practitioner
- Practitioner training courses
- Caregivers' training weekends

- Gerson support groups
- Recovered Gerson patient referral list
- Recovered Gerson patient support network
- Outreach program for schools and businesses
- Membership
- Calendar of events
- National and international seminars
- Library donation program
- Subscription to the bimonthly *Gerson Healing Newsletter*
- Free literature about additional aspects of the Gerson program
- Purchases from a selection of Gerson Institute videotapes, audio-tapes, and book titles in addition to the current one
- Gerson Therapy Products Resource List
- Mind/Body/Spirit Resource Guide
- At home Gerson Therapy followup program packet

The Gerson Institute does not own, operate, or control any treatment facility. Instead, it maintains a licensing program with hospitals or clinics to ensure that patients are receiving true, 100 percent Gerson-recommended care. Be sure that the clinic or hospital chosen for therapy is Gerson Institute Approved. Readers are invited to call the Institute for discussions about how the Gerson Therapy may help you or your loved one.

GERSON THERAPY DIETARY PREPARATION SUMMARIZED

The Gerson Therapy is a totally integrated system of nutrition and detoxification to help the body restore all the essential organs and defenses. Therefore, it has many facets and complex directions to cover all areas including food preparation.

Always keep in mind that the basic problem of all chronic disease is twofold: toxicity and deficiency. It is essential to address and reverse both of these. Our modern agriculture and food-processing systems contribute toxins to the food supply in many ways: pesticides and fungicides, preservatives, dyes, coloring, and emulsifying materials. But there are other ways the body is poisoned too: alcohol; nicotine; prescription, over-the-counter, and street drugs; toxins in the air, water, and soil; and in day-to-day work and home environments. There are also industrial chemicals in paints, textile chemicals, glues, polishes, benzene fractions, and so on. In order to heal and detoxify the body, all these have to be eliminated.

It also stands to reason that in the Gerson diet all foods should be organically (or biochemically) grown on soil fertilized by natural composted materials—free of pesticides, herbicides, and so on and rich in the best nutrients. All foods must be freshly prepared, unsalted, and fat-free. Aluminum and Teflon-coated cooking utensils must be avoided. Stainless steel, enamel, ironware, and glass containers may be used in cooking. Microwave ovens change the foods so that they are poorly assimilated, besides emitting radiation into the kitchen and "cooking the cook." Avoid cooking in microwaves and never heat water in them. Some crockpots may be safe; some have been found to contain toxins in their glaze.

Dr. Gerson found that juicers that work on a centrifugal system do not extract minerals efficiently. Besides, they tend to kill enzymes. He insisted that the best juices with the highest mineral content can be made using a two-process juice-extracting system: first grind the materials to be pressed in an electric food triturator; mix them well in a bowl; then place the ground, mixed material in a strong cloth and put it under pressure in a press. This juice is rich and homogeneous (does not easily separate), and the process helps to extract the largest amount of juice and minerals—up to 50 percent more than a centrifugal juicer!

FOOD PREPARATION

Necessary Foods

Fruit
Juices of fruit, vegetables, and leaves
Vegetables, salads
Special soup
Potatoes
Oatmeal, salt-free rye bread

Dr. Gerson added that the above foods are easily and quickly digested; the body needs larger portions and more frequent servings. The patient is to eat as much as possible, even during the night when awake. As the body rebuilds, some patients are ravenously hungry and food should be available at the bedside: a fresh fruit plate, some fruit salad, applesauce, and so on. Since patients are not supposed to drink water, peppermint tea should be placed at the bedside. If the patient awakens during the night and is thirsty, some warm tea should be available as well as food.

Forbidden Foods

All manufactured (processed) foods—bottled, canned, frozen, preserved, refined, salted, smoked, and sulfured items—must be avoided. They are harmful.

Alcohol	Cream	Pineapples
Avocados	Cucumbers	Spices (pepper, paprika)
Berries	Epsom salts	Soybeans and products
Bicarbonate of soda in	Flour (wheat)	Meat
toothpaste and gargle	Fish	Milk
Butter	Eggs	Tea (black)
Cheese	Ice cream	Drinking water
Candy	Mushrooms	Fats
Cake	Coffee (including	Nuts
Sugar (white)	decaffeinated)	
Commercial beverages	Oils	

Other Absolutely Forbidden Items

Fluorides in water, toothpaste, gargle
Hair dyes, permanents
Cosmetics: underarm deodorants, lipstick, lotions

JUICE PREPARATION

Citrus Juices

Use only a reamer-type juicer—do not use a juicer into which a half or-ange or lemon is inserted with the skin. Pressing the skin of citrus extracts harmful fatty and aromatic acids into the juice.

Apple and Carrot Juice

Use apples and carrots in approximately equal proportions. Wash ap-ples; do not peel. Cut and remove core. Wash carrots; use a brush but do not peel or scrape.

Grind apples and carrots into a bowl; mix thoroughly, place in juicer cloth, and press.

Apple/carrot juice may be kept for 2–3 hours in a thermos if patient goes back to work.

Green Leaf Juice

Obtain as many of the items mentioned below as possible. During certain seasons, only two or three may be available. *Do not substitute* items not on the green leaf juice materials list.

Escarole	Lettuce	Watercress
Endive	Red lettuce	Swiss chard
Romaine	Beet tops (young	Red cabbage (2–3 leaves)
Green pepper	inner leaves)	

Add 1 medium apple per glass when grinding. Grind, press, drink immediately. Wash all juice cloths regularly. If pores are clogged and pressing is difficult, discard and use a new cloth.

PREPARATION OF VEGETABLES

Use *all* vegetables except mushrooms, mustard greens, and carrot greens. Vegetables should be cooked with a minimum of water or soup stock (perhaps 2 to 3 tablespoonfuls) slowly on low heat until *well done*. To prevent burning, place on metal mat, and place cut tomatoes and/or onions at the bottom of the pot. These generate juice and make the food tasty. You can also use celery. Certain vegetables (squashes) contain a lot of water and need no additional water. Spinach releases much water in cooking—discard this water. It is bitter and should not be used. Certain other vegetables (beets, corn) cannot be cooked without water. Beets should be cooked in their jackets and peeled when done.

SPICES

Since spices, like other aromatic items (such as pineapples and berries) can interfere with the healing reaction, Dr. Gerson allowed only certain relatively mild spices and warned patients to use *very small quantities*. Use only those spices on the list below; *no others*.

Allspice, anise, bay leaves, coriander, dill, fennel, mace, marjoram, rosemary, sage, saffron, tarragon, thyme, sorrel, and summer savory.

Chives, onions, garlic, and parsley can be used in larger amounts.

SALADS

It's imperative for the patient to eat as much as possible of raw vegetables in the form of salads. These items can be finely grated, chopped, or minced, mixed or eaten separately. Here are the vegetables:

Apples and carrots	Watercress	Green onions	Knob celery
All lettuce greens	Cauliflower	Endives	Chives
Chicory	Radishes	Green peppers	Tomatoes

Salad Dressing: Dilute organic red wine or apple cider vinegar with water to taste. Add a little spray-dried organic cane juice (Sucanat), some herbs, onion, or garlic.

Special Soup

This special (Hippocrates) soup is extremely important, and Dr. Gerson ordered his patients to have it at both lunch and dinner. Since much of the Gerson Therapy is directed toward cleansing the liver, this soup is specially designed (and Hippocrates did acknowledge its effectiveness) to help cleanse the kidneys. After patients become used to eating without salt (usually in one to two weeks after starting the Gerson Therapy), the special soup is tasty and a delicious start for every meal.

The following vegetables should be used, thoroughly washed, *not* peeled, cut into cubes, covered with water, and cooked for 1½ to 2 hours. Put through a food mill and allow only fibers and peels to remain. (This should form a thick, creamy soup, not a clear broth!) Allow soup to cool before storing in refrigerator. Make only enough for about two days. The ingredients include:

1 medium celery knob (root), 2 medium onions (if not in season, substitute a *little* parsley only and 3–4 stalks of branch celery), 1½ lbs tomatoes, 1 lb potatoes, 1 medium parsley root (rarely ever available; if not, omit but more if desired during the summer season), 2 small leeks (if not available, substitute 2 medium onions), several cloves of garlic.

Until patients are used to salt-free eating, raw garlic should always be offered with a garlic press to add a "kick" to soup, vegetables, salad, and so on.

Potatoes

Baked potatoes are the most valuable. Potatoes should be used at lunch and dinner and should only rarely be replaced by organic brown or wild rice. Pasta should be avoided because it is made from processed flour that has no nutritional value. Potatoes can be baked, boiled in their jackets, mashed with a little soup, peeled after being boiled in their jackets, or cut up and mixed with salad dressing into a potato salad. Potatoes can also be baked in a casserole with onion, tomatoes, celery, and so on. After 6–10 weeks, if nonfat yogurt is permitted, add onions, chives, or garlic to the yogurt for a great dressing for your baked potato. Sweet potatoes may be used once a week.

Oatmeal

A large portion of oatmeal should be eaten for breakfast, made from organic rolled oats, 1/2 cup of oats to 1 cup (or a little more) of water. Cook slowly until done. Other cereals should *not* be used; the oats have a special purpose: they provide good B vitamins; they are rich in proteins but have a special property: they provide the patient's intestinal tract with a soft cushion (rather than harsh and grainy cereals) for all the juices to come. You can vary the flavor by adding different fruit: raw grated apples, papaya or other fruit; honey or 100 percent pure maple syrup; unsulfured blackstrap molasses; stewed prunes or other dried fruit, fresh raw or stewed apricots, apples with raisins, peaches, bananas, and so on.

Bread

You may use some salt-free and fat-free rye bread *only after consuming the full meal* (rye is more nourishing and easier to digest than wheat, which is low in nutrients and often causes allergic reactions). Remember that bread should not be the main part of any meal. When bread is dry, it can be grated and used in recipes requiring bread crumbs. Occasionally you may also use potato flour, tapioca, and cornstarch.

SUGAR AND SWEETENERS

Use organic brown sugar, maple syrup, organic light honey, or unsulfured molasses up to 2 teaspoons a day (provided there is no hypoglycemia or diabetes).

PEPPERMINT AND OTHER HERB TEAS

Peppermint tea relieves nausea, flatulence, and upset stomachs (during
healing flare-ups) and helps digestion. Other herb teas (linden blossom,
tahebo, licorice root, essiac, etc.) are all permitted and can often be useful
in overcoming problems. Herb teas such as chamomile and valerian are
soothing and can help induce restful sleep. Since the patient should not
drink water, a thermos bottle of peppermint or other herb tea should be
provided at bedside in case the patient awakens at night and is thirsty.

SAMPLE MENU

Breakfast

1 glass (8 oz) of orange juice
Large portion oatmeal with choice of fruit sauce
Organic 100 percent rye bread, unsalted and fat-free, toasted and
spread with honey if desired

Lunch

Plate of salad
1 glass (8 oz) of warm special soup
1 glass apple/carrot juice
Baked potato or other (boiled in jacket, potato salad, casserole, etc.)
with yogurt dressing, when permitted
Freshly cooked vegetables
Dessert: raw or stewed fruit

Dinner

Same as lunch. Vary meals by using different vegetables, different methods of preparing potatoes, other kinds of salads.

Organic brown rice may be used once a week.

Organic sweet potatoes may be used once a week in the place of potatoes.

GERSON THERAPY SUPPLY RESOURCES

The Gerson Institute endeavors to provide Gerson Therapy resources and referrals that are useful and well researched. All information provided at the time of printing is accurate. The Gerson Institute does not own or operate any of the clinics or related businesses listed and cannot claim responsibility for the services they provide, their products or their business practices. Please let the Gerson Institute know if you encounter any difficulties.

When making your Gerson Therapy choices please ensure that any individual, clinic, support group or business offering the Gerson Therapy or claiming to be associated with the Gerson Institute is in possession of a current "Gerson Institute Seal of Approval." Please contact the Gerson Institute for more information.

For a possible discount from any of these resources, mention that you are a Gerson Therapy patient who learned of the resource from this book.

RECOMMENDED JUICERS

Specific requirements for the proper juicer were devised by Dr. Max Gerson. He discovered that centrifugal juicers were unacceptable and that a separate grinder and press provide the best juice extraction. Consequently the following are superior:

The most popular juicing device among Gerson patients is the Norwalk® Model 270 Ultimate Juicer manufactured by Norwalk Sales & Service, P.O. Box 829, or 808 South Bloomington, Lowell, Arkansas 72745.

Please be aware that to order, you will be referred by Norwalk Sales & Service to the Norwalk® juicer's worldwide distributor, Richard Boger; therefore, it's best to contact this accommodating person directly at:

NORWALK® JUICER, Distributor Richard Boger
493 Quail Gardens Lane, Encinitas, CA 92024
Tel. (800) 405-8423

GERSON THERAPY MEDICAL SUPPLIES

STAT S.A., Owner Ann Ocello
Apartado Postal No. 2392
Tijuana, B.C.N. 22000, Mexico
U.S. 1st-class postage to Mexico: 46 cents
International tel. (52) 66-801103; Local tel. 6-80-14-40; FAX (52) 66-802529

KEY COMPANY
1313 W. Essex Ave.
St Louis, MO 63122
Tel. (800) 325-9592 or (314) 965-6699

LIFE SUPPORT
P.O. Box 4651
Modesto, CA 95352
Tel. (209) 529-4697

ORGANIC COFFEE

ROYAL BLUE ORGANICS/CAFÉ MAM
P.O. Box 21123, Eugene, OR 97403
(888) CAFE-MAM or (541) 338-9585

Organic Dried Fruits

INTERNATIONAL HARVEST, INC. Owner Bob Sterling
71-40 242nd Street,
Douglaston, New York 11362
Tel. (800) 277-4268
Warehouse (914) 631-3165

Gerson Therapy Organic Sourdough All-Rye Saltfree Bread

RUDOLPH'S SPECIALTY BAKERIES
390 Alliance Avenue, Toronto, Canada M6N 2H8
Tel. (800) 268-1589

Nature's Path Foods, Inc. makes an organic rye-carrot-raisin bread found in health food stores.

Information About Fresh Organic Produce

CO-OP DIRECTORY SERVICES, attention Kris Olsen
(For a self-addressed stamped envelope, Co-op Directory Services
refers you to food co-op stores and food buying clubs)
919 21st Avenue South, Minneapolis, Minnesota 55404

NATIONAL CO-OP DIRECTORY, an $8.50 Guide to U.S. Co-operative
Natural Food Retailers, send payment to The CO-OP NEWS NET-
WORK, P.O. Box 57, Randolph, Vermont, 05060; Tel. (802) 234-9293.

RAWMA's ORGANIC & LIVING FOODS RESOURCES (O&LFR), $12
in U.S.A., $14 to Canada, send payment to O&LFR, P.O. Box 15632, San
Diego, California 92195; FAX (619) 698-5969

CENTER FOR SCIENCE IN THE PUBLIC INTEREST
(Provides a list of U.S. mail-order businesses that sell organic food)
1875 Connecticut Avenue, NW, Suite 300, Washington, D.C. 20009-
5728; Tel. (202) 332-9110

CO-OP AMERICA
(publishes National Green Pages listing businesses offering organic food products)
2100 M Street, N.W., Suite 403, Washington, D.C. 20037
Tel. (800) 424-2667

DIAMOND ORGANICS (ships organic produce via FedEx)
Tel. (888) ORGANIC (674-2642)

FLAXSEED OIL SUPPLIES

OMEGA NUTRITION
5373 Guide Meridian, Building B, Bellingham, Washington 98226
Tel. (800) 661-3529 (from the U.S. and overseas)

WATER DISTILLING DEVICES

THE CUTTING EDGE, Owner Jules Klapper
P.O. Box 5034, Southampton, New York 11969
Tel. (800) 487-9516 or (516) 287-3813; FAX (516) 287-3112

AQUA CLEAN MD-4
(Contact this main office for your local Aqua Clean distributor.)
3725 Touzalin Avenue, Lincoln, Nebraska 68507
Tel. (402) 467-9300

PURE WATER, INC., Owner Steve Norvell (distributes Aqua Clean MD-4)
11760 Sorrento Valley Road, San Diego, California 92121
Tel. (619) 792-8275

Shower Filters

THE CUTTING EDGE, Owner Jules Klapper
P.O. Box 5034, Southampton, New York 11969
Tel. (800) 487-9516 or (516) 287-3813; FAX (516) 287-3112

SPRITE INDUSTRIES, INC.
1827 Capital Street, Corona, California 91720
Tel. (909) 735-1015

Ozone Machines and Air Purifiers

THE CUTTING EDGE, Owner Jules Klapper
P.O. Box 5034, Southampton, New York 11969
Tel. (800) 487-9516 or (516) 287-3813; FAX (516) 287-3112

AIR PURIFIERS, INC.
220 Reservoir Street, Suite 22, Needham Heights, Massachusetts 02194
Tel. (800) 442-1237; FAX (781) 449-8099

Nontoxic Paints, Sealers, Adhesives, and Household Cleaners

AMERICAN FORMULATING & MANUFACTURING
300 West Ash Street, Suite 700, San Diego, California 92101
Tel. (619) 239-0321

Nontoxic Carpeting

SUTHERLIN CARPET MILL
3653 Vine Street, Norco, California 91760-1866

GERSON THERAPY SUPPORT GROUPS

THE GERSON THERAPY PATIENT SUPPORT NETWORK

The Gerson Institute offers a means of contacting others who are currently on the Gerson Therapy as a means of exchanging ideas, tips, and hints during the difficult recovery period. If a Gerson patient wishes to be listed for communication with others and receive their names and locations, please contact the Gerson Institute to receive the appropriate release and authorization for disclosure and distribution.

CONTACTS FOR A GERSON THERAPY SUPPORT GROUP

A number of Gerson Therapy Support Groups exist in the United States and throughout the world. These groups are organized by long-term recovered patients. They offer local seminars, orientation programs and advice to callers considering or doing the Gerson Therapy. The Gerson Institute maintains a current list of Support Groups. Please contact them to be referred to a group near you or if you wish to establish a group of your own.

PATIENT HOURLY SCHEDULE

	Enema	Meal	Flaxseed Oil	Acidoll	Juice	Potassium Cpd.	Lugol	Thyroid	Niacin	Pancreatin	Liver Caps.
6:00 AM	Coffee										
8:00 AM		Breakfast		2 caps.	Orange	4 tsp.	3 drops	1 gr.	50 mg.	3 tabl.	
9:00 AM					Green	4 tsp.	—				
9:30 AM					Car/apple	4 tsp.	3 drops				
10:00 AM	Coffee				Car/apple	4 tsp.	3 drops	1 gr.	50 mg.		
11:00 AM					Carrot						2
12 Noon					Green	4 tsp.					
1:00 PM		Lunch	1 tblsp.	2 caps.	Car/apple	4 tsp.	3 drops	1 gr.	50 mg.	3 tabl.	
2:00 PM	Coffee				Green	4 tsp.					
3:00 PM					Carrot						2
4:00 PM					Carrot	NO					2
5:00 PM					Car/apple	4 tsp.	3 drops	1 gr.	50 mg.	3 tabl.	
6:00 PM	Coffee				Green	4 tsp.					
7:00 PM		Dinner	1 tblsp.	2 caps.	Car/apple	4 tsp.	3 drops	1 gr.	50 mg.	3 tabl.	
10:00 PM	Coffee										

Make yourself a blank schedule to be filled in later as the medications change and the frequency of enemas will be reduced.

Castor oil enemas: to be taken every other day as per Gerson doctor's order.

NUTRITION REPORT: THE CHINA STUDY

An exciting book came out in January 2005, titled *The China Study: Startling Implications for Diet, Weight Loss and Long-term Health,* by T. Colin Campbell, Ph.D., with Thomas M. Cambell II (BenBella Books, Dallas, TX 75206). Dr. Campbell's many years of in-depth research prove many of Dr. Gerson's ideas.

Dr. Campbell, a Professor of Nutrition at Cornell University, states that his thinking was originally very much "establishment." However, over thirty years of in-depth nutrition studies have changed his ideas. When we first heard him speak some six years ago, we were so impressed that we wrote up the content of the tapes we had made of his lectures. We subsequently published an extract in our Newsletters Vol. 17, #3 May/June 2000 and Vol. 17, #4 July/August 2000. Reproduced below is a paragraph from one of those articles on the subject of animal proteins in relation to cancer. Our article is taken from Dr. Campbell's new book on the subject of sugar.

"Dr. Campbell and his team were sent to study nutrition in the Philippines: the idea was to develop a way of self-help for the starving children, and it was assumed they needed protein. They were supposed to find a good source. Then some surprising facts came up: the advisors were told that kids who consumed the most proteins got the most liver cancer. Other studies, some done by physicians in India, also showed in rats that 30 experimental animals fed a 20 percent protein diet all developed liver cancer. Those that were fed a 5 percent protein diet got none. It seemed unbelievable. Further, liver tumors grew faster in those animals that received a 20 percent protein diet. When switched to a 5 percent protein diet, the tumors in the sick animals shrank. It became very clear: appropriate nutrients control growth. Less protein leads to less cancer."

With Dr. Campbell's permission, we quote freely here from his new book:

"The recommendation on added sugar is as outrageous as the one for protein. [When] this FNB (Food and Nutrition Board) report was being released, an expert panel put together by the WHO (World Health Organization) and the FAO (Food and Agriculture Organization) was completing a new report on diet, nutrition and the prevention of chronic diseases. Professor Phillip James was a member of this panel and a panel spokesperson on the added sugar recommendation. Early rumors of the report's findings indicated that the WHO/FAO was on the verge of recommending an upper safe limit of 10 percent for added sugar, far lower than the 25 percent established by the American FNB group.

"Politics, however, had entered the discussion early, as it had done in earlier reports on added sugars. According to a news release from the Director-General's office at the WHO, the U.S.-based Sugar Association and the World Sugar Research Organization, who 'represent the interests of sugar growers and refiners, had mounted a strong lobbying campaign in an attempt to discredit the WHO report and suppress its release . . .' According to the *Guardian* newspaper in London, the U.S. sugar industry was threatening to 'bring the World Health organization to its knees' unless it abandoned these guidelines on added sugar. WHO people were describing the threat as 'tantamount to blackmail.' The U.S.-based group even publicly threatened to lobby the U.S. Congress to reduce the $406 milllion U.S. funding of the WHO if it persisted in keeping the upper limit so low at 10 percent. There were reports . . . that the Bush Administration was inclined to side with the sugar industry."

Dr. Campbell concluded: "So, for added sugars, we now have two different upper 'safe' limits: a 10 percent limit for the international community and a 25 percent limit for the U.S." (!!)

This recalls the horrific scandal involving the drug VIOXX, which was withdrawn from the marketplace after it was found to have caused some 50,000 deaths, then was subsequently *reestablished as a permitted drug* by the FDA (Food and Drug Administration). As we can now see, that is obviously not the only instance of huge industry interests threatening the public's health.

THE ANTI-CANCER INGREDIENTS IN THE GERSON THERAPY

In 1994, Dr. Michael Gearin-Tosh, a professor of English literature and an Oxford University don, was diagnosed with multiple myeloma (bone marrow cancer) and was offered chemotherapy to extend his life expectancy to possibly one to two years. Without it, he was told, he might not survive six months.

Professor Gearin-Tosh decided to investigate alternatives. In time, his research led him to the Gerson Therapy. In 2002, his delightful book, *Living Proof: A Medical Mutiny*, was published by Scribner in Great Britain. It not only details his search and his adventures while recovering, but at the end there is a most interesting research report by Dr. Carmen Wheatley, of "Orthomolecular Oncology," also reviewed by Dr. Peter Gravett, Professor Ray Powles, and Dr. Robert Kyle, all connected with prestigious oncology clinics (*Living Proof*). Dr. Wheatley, a good friend of Prof. Gearin-Tosh, was most interested in his illness, research and subsequent recovery.

We are interested here in Dr. Wheatley's report. She studied the Gerson Therapy intensively in connection with her work, specifically its "anti-cancer" ingredients. She expressed amazement about Dr. Gerson's selection of specific foods that are now proven to be cancer fighters. At the time of Dr. Gerson's work, the cancer-fighting benefits of these ingredients were not known, so Dr. Wheatley came to the conclusion that Dr. Gerson worked with a great deal of intuition. He was also a thorough observer and insisted that "the results at the sickbed are conclusive."

We quote from Dr. Wheatley's notes:

"The Gerson diet highlights a number of foods in which modern research has identified some key cancer-fighting components, i.e., flaxseed oil containing Omega-3, which oppose the bad eicosanoids (fats) and appear to interfere with metastasis and promote apoptosis (the breakdown of tumor cells) and Omega-6, promoting Tumor Necrosis Factor."

Dr. Wheatley further details some specific foods, for instance apples, which are rich in quercetin. This substance, according to Dr. Patrick Quillin of Cancer Treatment Centers of America, has the potential to revert a cancerous cell back to a normal healthy cell and is also capable of producing apoptosis. Quercetin also interferes with metastasis. Apples, Dr. Wheatley continues, "are just one component of Gerson's fruit list. The vegetables, particularly of the cruciferous family, can modify carcinogen activation. Garlic is a natural detoxifier, while onions, leeks, scallions and chives are all good sources of the allium family, which has been demonstrated to enhance DNA repair mechanisms" (pp. 278-279). Dr. Wheatley wonders how Gerson, "without this scientific knowledge, empirically devised a method which ensured that a large range of these compounds would be delivered to the cancer patient *intact and in pharmacologically active doses*" (p. 280). There are many more examples given but it would lead too far to quote them all.

HOUSEHOLD CHEMICALS: ANOTHER SOURCE OF TOXICITY

We are always very anxious to keep a clean house. Probably, this feeling gets even more intense when there is a seriously ill person in the home. As a result, the householder does a lot of cleaning, using all kinds of advertised chemicals. Actually, that is a very bad idea! It would be a far better idea to consider a "clean" house one that contains *no toxic chemicals*. Use simple soaps, for instance.

The problem is that most cleaning chemicals are quite toxic, some more than others. An immediate offender is the spray can, especially the aerosols. Spray bottles aren't safe, either: for example, once you spray a window cleanser, there are droplets in the air that one inhales. If the patient is in the area, those droplets can go into his bloodstream! Cleansers containing chlorine are also a bad idea. Furniture polishes containing solvents, coloring, waxes, etc., are toxic. Paints, including art materials, are very toxic—the list is virtually unending!

The worst things to use, of course, are pesticides, including sprays to kill cockroaches, mosquitoes and flies. These not only kill insects, they are clearly toxic to humans as well. So, what to do?

Avoid all aerosols, since they contain fluorocarbons, which are highly toxic to humans as well as damaging to the ozone layer in the atmosphere.

There are many soaps and even cleansers that do not contain chlorine or other harmful additives. Instead of using pesticides to kill roaches, sprinkle boric acid powder where they are seen. They may not die immediately—it may take several days—but they can be controlled without harm to the patient. If you have flies in the house, even old-fashioned sticky flypaper is quite safe and effective. To control mosquitoes, you'll need screening. *Don't* put any advertised chemicals on your skin! And if you clean windows, simply pour some liquid on a cloth—*don't spray.*

There can also be trouble from the outside: your next-door neighbors may use pesticides in their gardens and the wind can blow theses toxic chemicals your way. Stay indoors for a day or so while they are doing this and use a room ozone generator or air purifier. Also, while a patient is using the Gerson Therapy, *do not paint the inside of the house!* The outgassing solvents are very toxic. Also avoid acrylic materials. Examine any and all chemicals and cleansers regarding their content and be careful.

COSMETICS: ANOTHER SOURCE OF TOXICITY

As we have seen, it is imperative to eliminate all new sources of toxicity. Since the body becomes toxic from being exposed to so many toxins in the environment—in the soil, air, water, food, not to mention from smokers and other sources—and since the Gerson Therapy is greatly concerned with removing these toxins, it is obvious that all *new* sources of toxicity have to be eliminated.

One such source is cosmetics. All substances sprayed or rubbed on the skin travel promptly into the bloodstream. Orthodox medicine utilizes this fact with the application of "patches" in order to deliver substances (mostly painkillers) into the bloodstream. It doesn't occur to most people that powders, creams, ointments, sprays, etc., are also delivered into the bloodstream! For that reason, we simply tell our female patients that "if you wouldn't eat or drink it, *don't* put it on your skin (or lips)." We are willing to make one tiny concession: it is permissible to use an eyebrow pencil.

One of the most offensive cosmetics is the underarm deodorant. Many of the brands offered contain mercury, which, is severely toxic. But what of those creams or sticks that are sold as "organic"? They are still not acceptable because they interfere with the body's attempt to eliminate poisons by the simple act of perspiration. Many patients experience "night sweats," an attempt by the body to "detoxify" when at rest. Others experience severe sweats during the healing reactions. These eliminations are also embarrassingly "smelly," and the patients first try to clear this "problem" with baths or showers. But that often isn't sufficient—the offensive odor returns! So, of course, they reach for the deodorant cream or spray or stick. That is a serious mistake! When the body attempts to detoxify, one must absolutely not interfere by stopping or blocking this perspiration! Blocking the underarm passages will return the toxic materials into the lymphatic system around the chest and shoulders, and increase the chance for breast cancer—even in men! Male breast cancer is increasing and we have to assume that much of the problem can be related to the use of underarm deodorants.

"So what can I do to overcome the problem?" If baths and showers are inadequate, here is the answer: "Don't eat or drink materials that are toxic (not organic), *and* detoxify the much more efficient way with coffee enemas!"

We are not only addressing women on the subject of cosmetics, but men! Another toxic item that is used by both women and men is hair dye, which is very easily assimilated through the scalp into the bloodstream. This is because the scalp is thoroughly "vasculated;" that is, many blood vessels close to the surface can absorb poisons. Gerson patients must avoid dyes, permanents, and any substances used on the hair other than the mildest of shampoos. Gerson patients should also avoid perfumes (which contain aromatics), and men should avoid aftershave lotions and aerosol shaving creams (see the previous section on household chemicals).

WHY ARE CHILDREN ON ANTIDEPRESSANTS?

While I was recently on a lecture tour in England, on September 20, 2003, a large headline appeared in the *Guardian*: "50,000 Children Taking Antidepressants." A sub-headline read: "Drug withdrawn over fears it made youngsters want to kill themselves."

This was a double shocker! Come to think of it, why are such a huge number of children "depressed"? A number of decades ago, this problem was virtually nonexistent! Why should children now be depressed? They should be living the happiest, most carefree time of their lives. In the UK, as well as in the United States, few children are hungry or homeless. Besides, poor children are not the ones who are medicated with antidepressants. Their parents cannot afford them.

This brings to mind a study that was done in 1994 at the University of North Carolina at Chapel Hill, and was described in *Gerson Healing Newsletter*, Volume 9, #3, Sept./Oct. 1994. The researchers reported at the time that children who ate more than 12 hot dogs a month developed childhood leukemia more than nine times as often as normally expected. Also, children born to mothers who ate at least one hot dog a week during pregnancy had double the normal risk of developing brain tumors.

Clinical depression is presently described in *Current Medical Diagnosis and Treatment* (Krupp & Chatton) as having the following symptoms:

- lowered mood, sadness to intense feelings of guilt and hopelessness,

- difficulty in thinking, inability to concentrate, inability to make decisions,
- loss of interest, less involvement with work and recreation,
- headache, disrupted sleep, change in appetite,
- anxiety,
- suicidal tendencies.

It would follow that present-day food—loaded with pesticides and fungicides, as well as food additives, sugars, dyes, emulsifiers, and preservatives, foods that are depleted in and lacking nutrients—would have to be the culprit. Children are simply suffering from severe deficiencies and toxicity. The brain, this incredibly delicate organ, responds to the burden by decreased function.

Sarah Bosely, health editor, the author of the article in the *Guardian*, reports further that one major antidepressant is being given to some 3,000 children *even though doctors are told that it should not be given to anyone under 18 years of age.*

Another drug, Seroxat, distributed by GlaxoSmithKline (drugs have different names in different countries) was also banned for anybody under 18 years of age. This drug was shown to be able to cause children to have suicidal thoughts or to become "hostile"—this word is used in clinical trials instead of "homicidal".

There is worse news. The article continues: "Data which suggests these drugs could be causing children to feel murderous and suicidal has been in drug company hands for several years."

The drug described, Seroxat, belongs to a group known as "selective serotonin reuptake inhibitors" or SSRIs, of which the one best known in the U.S. is Prozac. It is not licensed for children.

These drugs also admittedly cause "emotional liability"—this term is used to describe potentially suicidal behavior as well as self-harm.

At the end of a lengthy report is the story of a young lady, Holly Workman, who was first medicated at age 14. She had previously felt "low," but had never felt like killing herself. After a few weeks on the drug, she began cutting her arms with knives and other sharp instruments, and her family had to hide all such items from her. She tried several times to commit suicide, even though "she hardly knew the person who was doing these things." When she stopped taking the drug, she felt better, but her G.P. (General Practitioner) felt she needed to continue it and persuaded her to go back on it! She eventually found out for herself that her nightmares stopped when she was off the drug for good.

IMMUNIZATION—
VACCINATION

Due to the current "flu epidemic," there is a great deal of interest in immunization and vaccination. Checking into my files, I find innumerable books and articles written on the subject. The list is much too long to include here.

But let's look at the story. It started with Edward Jenner, M.D. (1749-1823), a British physician. He observed that milkmaids who frequently contracted cases of cow pox had a mild outbreak of the pox and were subsequently immune to smallpox. This led him to assume that a mild form of a disease produces immunity to a more deadly form. It was a correct assumption; however, in future attempts to repeat the results, it was never taken into consideration that the immune milkmaids were young and presumably healthy! Thus, their immune systems were able to respond!

Since then, generations of youngsters have been vaccinated against smallpox and by the 1980s, the medical authorities declared that smallpox was no more!

Louis Pasteur (1822-1895) used the idea of weakening bacteria and germs to clear them and produce "clean" products. Hence, the pasteurization of milk that is now almost universal in the "developed" world. Still, on his deathbed, he is quoted to have stated, "The germ is nothing, the terrain is everything," meaning that the person's immune system makes the difference in whether he or she develops the disease or not. This statement is not widely known. For one, pasteurization is a huge business and the milk industry would oppose any change. Also, vaccination has developed into an important industry and is certain to continue to find support in government and medical circles. It has also not been publicized that "pasteurized" milk is heat damaged, causing the protein content to be poorly assimilated. This has been demonstrated by Dr. Francis M. Pottinger, M.D., in his *Cat* book. (See the article on "Milk—the White Poison" in the *Gerson Healing Newsletter*, Vol. 19, #1, Jan./Feb. 2004.)

But there is more—much more! Babies are no longer just vaccinated against smallpox: for years, they have been receiving the DPT (Diptheria-Pertussis-Tetanus) injections at a younger and younger age. Dr. Robert Mendelsohn, head of the Pediatric Society of the U.S., and head of the Chicago Pediatric Hospital, wrote extensively about his research into that problem. He never stopped warning against immunization of babies in his lectures and articles in medical journals. He pointed to the many children who were permanently injured by disease, including extensive brain damage. Eventually, he was able to demonstrate that some 85% of SIDS (Sudden Infant Death Syndrome) occurred within 48 hours after injection of DPT, while the rest of the deaths occurred within two weeks after the immunization! Nobody listened; however, eventually, the U.S. government had to guarantee the safety of DPT injections since the pharmaceutical companies that were producing them had so many lawsuits on their hands for damage and death caused by the shots. This means that our tax money supports the problem.

The DPT shots are still being administered in the U.S. Their use is actually unscientific, since a new baby does not yet have his or her own immune system and is therefore unable to respond by producing immunity to diseases! A baby is born with about six months' worth of the mother's immunity. Yet, pediatricians continue to start immunization with DPT in babies at two to three months of age!

In Japan, it turns out, the doctors have become aware of the reason for the problem with immunizing babies too early and, we are told, they are now forbidden to give vaccination shots to babies before the age of two years. As a result, there is no more SIDS in Japan.

New and even worse vaccinations have been introduced and schools force kids to be vaccinated or not admitted! These are the vaccines supposedly guarding against hepatitis C. They reportedly contain a mercury compound that is extremely toxic to brain tissue and they have produced a large number of brain-damaged children.

In the United States., former President Ford, shortly after he was nominated by outgoing President Nixon, wanted to "do something for the

American public." It was the time when the flu season was about to start and the virus that was identified at that time was the "swine flu" virus. President Ford ordered a large number of immunizing shots against the swine flu to be made available, particularly to "individuals at risk"—the elderly, young people, and people suffering from chronic diseases. The result of this well-meaning activity was a disaster: a number of people died and many became paralyzed due to the swine flue shots!

We come to the true problem of immunization: people whose immune systems are weakened due to age or disease, particularly due to chemotherapy, or people who have to be medicated with immune suppressants due to organ transplants—those people are unable to respond to immunization and are severely damaged if not killed by their use.

Another problem is the use of vaccines against tumors in cancer patients. One first has to understand that a cancer patient has a weakened immune system—or else he would have no malignancy! A functioning immune response kills developing malignant cells without the host being aware of any activity. So we have to assume that this type of patient is hardly able to respond to immunization. The John Wayne Cancer Center in California has experimented with immunization against cancer for some time, rather ineffectively. However, Dr. Gerson is regularly being misquoted as having supported immunization against cancer. In his book *A Cancer Therapy—Results of 50 Cases*, Dr. Gerson discusses the introduction of cancer cells into patients suffering from malignancies. He admits that a very few dramatic results (not long lasting) were obtained; however, most experiments, including those of the famous Dr. William B. Coley, remained "quite uncertain and sparing"(page 128).

In a reported experiment, one man with advanced colon cancer was given immunization injections of the vaccine every six weeks. Within 12 weeks, the tumor had disappeared. However, "He was part of a national trial being conducted at USC/Norris in L.A. Federal rules require that patients participating in research studies receive "proven" treatments before they receive experimental therapies. Because this means the body has already had its immune system devastated by chemotherapy, it is amazing that they got this kind of result." (In even one case!) The above was taken from an article in the *L.A. Times* of March 17, 2003.

It also needs to be remembered that in a cancer patient, a large number of malignant cells are present and there is no need to introduce more. Further, in order to get a true response, it should be the physician's duty to first of all activate the patient's immune system by detoxifying and replenishing all the organ systems. Once this has been achieved, there is no further need to inject cancer cells because of the presence of tumors in the patient! There is one other problem that Dr. Gerson discusses: it is not sufficient to try to activate the body's defenses temporarily with immunizations. The body needs to recover sufficiently so that its immune activity remains strong and permanent. Then, long recovery without recurrence can be achieved.

The current flu "epidemic" started much earlier than usual and was already well underway in early to mid-December. The flu season is generally expected to become quite virulent by February/March. What is particularly disturbing are the reports of children dying of the flu! And here, I suspect that a great deal of blame goes back to the reports of children's worsening eating habits. We reported in our *Gerson Healing Newsletter*, Vol. 18, #3, on the increasing "addiction" of kids to Chicken Nuggets, and on the frightening lack of nutrition in "fast foods." *The Wall Street Journal* of March 18, 2003, reported on the problem under the heading "Heart Disease Hits the Preschool Set." That article states, "Children's diet is becoming more and more restricted. They develop a taste for the deep-fried salted nuggets and refuse other foods." Is this the ultimate destruction of their immune systems that adds to the problem of early heart disease? It might well be.

In the meantime, a large portion of the population is suffering from the flu. Schools are closing early because kids are sick, and teachers are affected as well. I suspect that nutrition in general is worsening and people will be getting sicker every year.

Again, as I have done so often, I urge our readers, family and friends, to eat fresh, organic, body-building foods in order to remain active and healthy.

THE ROOT CANAL AND DENTAL AMALGAM COVER-UP OF CANCER AND OTHER DEGENERATIVE DISEASES

The Root Canal Coverup (ISBN 0-945196-19-9, U.S.$23) is a 1993 book written by George E. Meinig, D.D.S., F.A.C.D. It is available from him directly by sending payment to his company, Bion Publishing, 323 East Matilijia Street, #110-151, Ojai, California 93023. The book can also be obtained from the Gerson Institute.

Dr. Meinig admits to having installed many root canal fillings while he practiced dentistry and founded the Association of Root Canal Specialists, which he chaired for many years. What the dentist learned when he eventually studied the work of oral scientist Weston Price, D.D.S., changed his thinking and professional life forever. Dr. Meinig discovered that patients treated with root canal fillings suffer from a variety of serious chronic illnesses.

In order to treat the root of a tooth, or an abscess that forms at the base of this root, a dentist must drill any loose or infected material from the canal that houses the tooth's nerve. Then the dentist can treat the abscess. But once a nerve is dead and removed, this tooth also dies. Dr. Meinig's book gives the background of extensive and detailed research done on root canals by Weston A. Price, D.D.S., F.A.C.D.

When Dr. Meinig became aware of the dangers inherent in the accepted root canal treatment, he renounced his position at the Association of Root Canal Specialists. Now he spends his time and energies making the public as well as dentists aware of the research conducted by Dr. Price.

The first indication of problems due to root canals came from one of Dr. Price's patients who was bedfast and virtually paralyzed due to rheumatoid arthritis. For necessary reasons, her root-canal-filled tooth was removed although it looked healthy and normal on X rays. Within a few weeks the patient was up; and after some months, she could walk and her health was totally restored—no more rheumatoid arthritis.

Curious at the patient's positive response, Dr. Price recovered that extracted tooth from storage, sterilized it thoroughly, and implanted it under the skin of a rabbit in an in vivo experiment. Within five days, the rabbit was victimized by the same disease, severe rheumatoid arthritis. And in ten days it died of this disease. Dr. Price implanted the same tooth under the skin of thirty-three rabbits. In each case, the tooth caused arthritis to occur in the rabbit and killed the animal.

Going even further, Dr. Price performed more experiments with trying to clear the apparently infectious material from extracted teeth. He autoclaved them (sterilized by steam pressure, at 250°F, or 121°(C). This made no difference. Each rabbit with the "sterilized" (autoclaved) tooth implanted still developed the disease and died, usually within ten days. Then, as a control, Dr. Price implanted a healthy tooth under the skin of a rabbit. The rabbit lived without showing any signs of problems for fifteen years, its normal life span.

He published the results of this laboratory finding. Subsequently, many other patients had root-canal-filled teeth extracted—some suffering from kidney disease, others from cancer, heart disease, or arthritis. In virtually all cases, the patients showed considerable improvement or even total recovery after their offending teeth were removed. However, in each case, the rabbit receiving the tooth died of the same disease that the patient exhibited.

To explain: When the nerve is removed from a tooth, it's no longer living or supplied with nutrients. It is dead. However, the normal structure of the tooth includes tiny "canules" (similar to the capillaries in every human tissue) that carry nutrients to the living tooth. Once the tooth is dead, nutrients stop circulating through these canules; instead the canules become infested with bacteria or viruses. Not only that, but the filling of the nerve canal shrinks a tiny bit, enough for more microorganisms to lodge there too.

None of this infection shows on dental X rays. A dead tooth is thus a potent source of bacterial and viral toxins that spread throughout the body. Many people with a good immune system and powerful defenses can live with this constant source of trouble without showing any symptoms. For others—about 25 percent of all persons having root canals—chronic illness sets in. They come down with various severe diseases or other health difficulties.

Carefully taken and scrutinized, X rays eventually show "cavitation" (hollowing out of the surrounding jawbone) around the root-canal-treated tooth. As the resistant patient ages or is weakened by accidents, colds, flu, or severe stress, the ability to overcome this "focal infection" is reduced and can cause or contribute to a chronic degenerative disease such as cancer. Unquestionably, cancer can come from root canals in your mouth.

CANCER FROM MERCURY
AMALGAM DENTAL FILLINGS

Many Gerson patients are informed about health dangers associated with dental "silver" amalgam fillings. They appear silver because the toxic metal mercury used in them is silver in color. In fact, dental amalgams consist of more than 51 percent mercury mixed with a small amount of silver and other toxic metals (tin, copper, zinc, and sometimes nickel). The problem, of course, is the mercury, a highly poisonous heavy metal with powerful adverse effects on the nervous system. Once installed in teeth, the mercury steadily leaches out into the body and is carried throughout the system by blood circulation.

Some people are a great deal more sensitive to this circulating mercury than others, and it's been proven to cause multiple sclerosis along with vast numbers of other degenerative diseases in many people. Especially, dental amalgam fillings cause cancer. This has been documented in a March 2000 book issued by Hampton Roads Publishing Company, Inc., *Elements of Danger: Protect Yourself against the Hazards of Modern Dentistry* (ISBN 1-57174-146-1), written by Morton Walker, D.P.M. To acquire a copy, send U.S.$18 to the book distributor, Freelance Communications, 484 High Ridge Road, Stamford, Connecticut 06905-3020.

When dental amalgam fillings are removed, it's been observed (as detailed by over one thousand references in Dr. Walker's book) that some chronically ill dental patients tend to recover from their illnesses. While admittedly, other people possessing amalgams in their teeth for many years do not show apparent health problems, it's likely that they actually are experiencing unrecognized subclinical illnesses.

It will not come as a surprise that we who represent the Gerson Therapy urge debilitated patients to remove teeth with root canal fillings and eliminate all dental amalgam fillings.

Important: Seriously ill patients should not have their mercury fillings removed immediately. No matter how well the removal is done, some mercury vapor is released, and temporary mercury poisoning is inevitable. This must be avoided until the patient is strengthened, that is, after nine to twelve months on the Gerson Therapy.

For prevention and as a means of self-treatment, it is highly advisable to eliminate these sources of cancer and other illnesses. To do so, consult a holistic (biological), biocompatible (mercury-free) dentist who belongs to one of the four dental professional organizations offering names, addresses, and telephone numbers of their members. For referrals to such a dentist in your area, see Appendix C in Morton Walker's book *Elements of Danger.*

SELECTED
BIBLIOGRAPHY

Ahringsmann, H. "Historische Bemerkung zu der neuen Diätbehandlung der Tuberkulose nach Gerson-Sauerbruch-Herrmannsdorfer." *Münch. med. Wochnschr.* 76:1565, Sep. 1929.

Alexander, H. "Treatment of pulmonary tuberculosis with salt-free diet." *Münch. med. Wochnschr.* 77:971, Jun. 6, 1930.

Apitz, G. "Treatment of tuberculosis of lungs and of other organs with salt-free diet." *Deutsche med. Wchnschr.* 55:1918, Nov. 15, 1929.

Axmann. "Dietary treatment in tuberculosis of the skin." *Münch. med. Wochnschr.* 77:707, Apr. 25, 1930.

Bacmeister, A. "Interne Behandlung der Lungentuberkulose." *Med. Welt.* 4(14):474–476, Apr. 5, 1930.

Bacmeister, A.; Rehfeldt, P. "Phosphorlebertran und die Gerson-Herrmannsdorfersche Diät zur Heilung der Tuberkulose." *Deutsche med. Wchnschr.* 56(12):480–481, Mar. 21, 1930.

Baer, G.; Herrmannsdorfer, A.; Kausch, H. "Salt free diet in tuberculosis." *Münch. med. Wochnschr.* Jan. 4, 1929.

Banyai, A.L. "The dietary treatment of tuberculosis." *Am. Rev. Tuberc.* 23:546–575, May 1931.

Barát, I. "Gerson's diet in treatment of pulmonary tuberculosis." *Orvosi hetil.* 74:877–879, Aug. 3, 1930.

Barát, I. "Über den Wert der Gersondiät in der Behandlung der Lungentuberkulose." *Beitr. z. Klin. d. Tuberk.* 76:588–591, 1931.

Beck, O. "Herrmannsdorfer dietary treatment of tuberculosis: theoretical basis." *Monatsschr. f. Kndrheilk.* 48:276, Oct. 1930.

Bentivoglio, G.C. "Le variazone del riflesso oculocardiaco nei bambini in seguito al trattamento dietetico di Gerson." *Pediatria.* 41:1457–1483, Dec. 1933.

Bertaccini, G. "A proposito della dieta aclorurata Gerson-Herrmanns-dorfer-Sauerbruch nella tuberculosi: richerche sulla influenza del cloruro di sodio nella infezione tubercolare sperimentale del coniglio." *Gior. ital. di dermat. e sif.* 73:1775–1778, Dec. 1932.

Bertaccini, G. "A proposito della dieta Gerson-Herrmannsdorfer-Sauerbruch nella tuberculosis recherche sulla influenza del cloruro di sodio nella infezione tubercolare sperimentale del coniglio; infezione cutanea." *Gior. ital. di dermat. e sif.* 74:1469–1486, Dec. 1933.

Blumenthal, F. "Treatment of tuberculosis of skin with special considera-tion of dietary therapy." *Med. Klin., Berlin.* 26:1432, Sep. 26, 1930.

Bommer, S. "Dietetic treatment of tuberculosis of skin." *Münch. med. Wochnschr.* 76:707, Apr. 26, 1929.

Bommer, S.; Bernhardt, L. "Dietary treatment of lupus vulgaris." *Deutsche med. Wchnschr.* 55:1298, Aug. 2, 1929.

Bommer, S. "Neue Erfahrungen auf dem Gebiete der Hauttuberkulose mit besonderer Berücksichtigung der Gersondiät." *Strahlentherapie* 35:139–148, 1930.

Bommer, S. "Dietary treatment of skin tuberculosis." *Am. Rev. Tuberc.* 27:209–215, Feb. 1933.

Bommer, S. "Beitrag zur Diätbehandlung von Lupus vulgaris." *Med. Klin.* 28:209–215, Feb. 1933.

Bommer, S. "Capillaroscopic study of skin following administration of Gerson-Herrmannsdorfer-Sauerbruch diet in treatment of injuries to skin." *Dermat. Wchnschr.* 97:1367–1372, Sep. 23, 1933.

Bommer, S. "Zur Frage der Wirkung von Sauerbruch-Herrmannsdorfer-Gerson-Diät." *Deutsche med. Wchnschr.* 60:735–739, May 18, 1934.

Bommer, S. "Salzarme Kost im Gefässystem (G.H.S.-Diät)." *Klin. Wchnschr.* 13:148-158, Oct. 27, 1934.

Brezovsky. "Sauerbruch-Gerson diet in treatment of tuberculosis of skin." *Budapesti orvosi ujsag.* 28:769–773, Jul. 17, 1930.

Bruusgaard, E.; Hval, E. "Gerson-Sauerbruch-Herrmannsdorfer diet treat-ment in skin tuberculosis and its results." *Norsk mag. f. laegevidensk.* 92:1157–1175, Nov. 1931.

Bruusgaard, E. "Über die Herrmannsdorfersche Diätbehandlung von Hauttuberkulose." *Acta dermat.-venereol.* 13:628–642, Nov. 1932.

Bussalai. "La dieta di Gerson-Herrmannsdorfer nel Lupus. (Nota preventi.) Con presentazioni di ammalati, di'preparti microscope e di fotografie." *Gior. ital. di dermat. e sif.* (supp. fasc. 1). 1:10–13, 1931.

Canal Feijoó, E.J. "Régimen ácido Como tratamiento de la tuberculosis pulmonar." *Rev. med. latino-am.* 16:981–992, Apr. 1931.

Canal Feijoó, E.J. "Régimen ácido Como tratamiento de la tuberculosis pulmonar." *Rev. españ. de med. y gir.* 16:124–128, Mar. 1933.

Cattell, H.W. " "Diet in treatment of tuberculosis." *Internat. Clin.* Vol. 1, 41st Series. 1931.

Clairmont, P.; Dimtza, A. "Dietary treatment in tuberculosis." *Klin. Wchnschr.* 9:5, Jan. 4, 1930.

Conrad, A.H. "Lupus Vulgaris." *Archiv. Dermat. Syph.* 24:688, 1931.

Cope, F.W. "A medical application of the Ling association-induction hypothesis: the high potassium, low sodium diet of the Gerson cancer therapy." *Physiol. Chem. Phys.* 10(5):465–468, 1978.

Crosti, A.; Scolari, E. "La dieta di Gerson-Herrmannsdorfer-Sauerbruch nella tuberculosi cutanea. Osservazioni cliniche e recherche biologiche." *Gior. ital. di dermat. e sif.* 72:897–945, Aug. 1931.

Crosti, A. "La dieta Sauerbruch-Herrmannsdorfer-Gerson nella tuberculosi cutanea; reperti clinice, biochimici, istopatologici (con dimostrazioni di fotografie)." *Gior. ital. di dermat. e sif.* (supp. fasc. 1). 1:13–16, 1931.

Csapó, J.; Péterfy, M.; Palfy, E. "Urinalysis in tubercular children kept on Sauerbruch-Herrmannsdorfer-Gerson diet." *Orvosi hetill.* 75:1090, Nov. 7, 1931.

Csapó, J.; Péterfy, M.; Palfy, E. "Harnuntersuchungen bei der Diät nach Sauerbruch-Herrmannsdorfer-Gerson." *Arch. f. Kinderh.* 96:231–235, 1932.

Curschmann, W. "Ein klärendes Wort zur Ablehnenden Kritik der Ernährungsbehandlung der Tuberkulose. Erwiderungen auf die Aufsätze von Sauerbruch und Herrmannsdorfer." *Münch. med. Wochnschr.* 77:2196, Dec. 19, 1930.

Curschmann, W. "Ergebnisse salzloser Diätbehandlung nach Sauerbruch und Herrmannsdorfer bei Lungentuberkulose und Knochentuberkulose." *Beitr. z. Klin. Tuberk.* 77:540–590, 1931.

Curschmann, W. "Beobachtungen bei Gersonscher Diät." *Beitr. z. Klin. Tuberk.* 80:120–131, 1932.

Danholt, N. "Culture of tubercle bacilli from lupus lesions of patients under the Gerson-Herrmannsdorfer-Sauerbruch diet." *Acta dermat.-venereol.* 13:617, Nov. 1932.

(Directives). "Richtlinien für die Heilkostbehandlung der Tuberkulose nach Gerson-Sauerbruch-Hermannsdorfer." *Med. Welt.* 3:1229, Aug. 24, 1929.

de Raadt, O.L.E. "Factor responsible for curative value." *Wien. Klin. Wchnschr.* 43:752–753, Jun. 12, 1930.

de Raadt, O.L.E. "Reply to Korvin's article." *Wien. Klin. Wchnschr.* 45:146–147, Jan. 29, 1932.

Doerffel, J. "Clinical, experimental and chemical studies on the influence of diet on inflammatory changes in healthy and diseased skin." *Arch. Dermat. Syph.* 162:621, Jan. 24, 1931.

Doerffel, J., Goeckerman, W.H. "Effect of a diet low in salt in cases of tuberculosis of the skin." *Proc. Mayo Clinic.* 7(6):73–78, Feb. 10, 1932.

Doerffel, J. "Effect of a diet low in salt in cases of tuberculosis of the skin." *Arch. Dermat. Syph.* 26:762–764, 1932.

Doerffel, J.; Passarge, W. "Lokale Ektebinbehandlung der Hauttuberkulose bei gleichzeitiger Kochsalzarmer Diät (Gerson-Herrmannsdorfer-Sauerbruch)." *Dermat. Wchnschr.* 99:1173–1179, Sep. 8, 1934.

Drosdek-Praktische. "Erfahrungen mit der Gerson-Sauerbruch-Diät." *Beitr. z. Klin. d. Tuberk.* 78:697–723. 1931.

Eckhardt, H. "Die Stellung der Krüppelfürsorge zur Gerson-Herrmannsdorfer-Sauerbruch-Diät bei der Knochengelenktuberkulose." *Ztschr. f. Krüppelfürsorge.* 28:79, May–Jun. 1935.

Egues, J. "Regimen dietetico en los tuberculoses pulmonares." *Rev. Asoc. red. Argent.* 46:1574–1581, Dec. 1932.

Elder, H.C. "The Influence of the Gerson regime on pulmonary tuberculosis." *Trans. Med.-Chir. Soc. Edinburgh.* Nov. 1932.

Eller, J.J.; Rein, C.R. "The value of an equilibrated salt diet in the treatment of various dermatoses: a modification of the Herrmannsdorfer-Sauerbruch-Gerson diets." *N.Y. State J. M.* 32(22):1296–1300, Nov. 15, 1932.

Emerson, C. "Treatment of tuberculosis by altering metabolism through dietary management. (Gerson-Sauerbruch method.)" *Nebr. St. Med. J.* 14(3):104–107, Mar. 1929.

Falta, W. "Ist die Gerson-Diät bei Tuberkulose zu empfehlen?" *Wien. Klin. Wchnschr.* 43:148–149, Jan. 30, 1930.

Falta, W. "Ist die Gerson-Diät bei Tuberkulose zu empfählen?" *Aerztl. Prax.* 99–101, Apr. 1, 1930.

Fishbein, M., ed. "The Gerson-Herrmannsdorfer dietetic treatment of tuberculosis." *J. Amer. Med. Assoc.* 93(11):861–862, Sep. 14, 1929.

Fishbein, M., ed. "Dietetic treatment of tuberculosis." *J. Amer. Med. Assoc.* 93(16):1237, Oct. 19, 1929.

Fishbein, M., ed. "Gerson's cancer treatment." *J. Amer. Med. Assoc.* 122(11):645, Nov. 16, 1946.

Fishbein, M., ed. "Frauds and fables." *J. Amer. Med. Assoc.* 139:93–98, Jan. 8, 1949.

Formenti, A.M. "Studi sulla lipasi ematica nella dieta di Gerson-Herrmannsdorfer-Sauerbruch." *Riv. di. clin. pediat.* 36:319–350, Apr. 1938.

Foster, H.D. "Lifestyle changes and the 'spontaneous' regression of cancer: an initial computer analysis." *Intl. J. of Biosocial Rsch.* 10(1):17–33, 1988.

Francois, P. "Le regime de Gerson-Sauerbruch-Herrmannsdorfer dans le traitement de la tuberculose lupeuse." *Bruxelles-med.* 11:1034–1038, Jun. 28, 1931.

Frontali, G. "La dieta di Gerson nel trattamento della tuberculosis infantile." *Lotta contro. la tuberc.* 5:818–830, Aug. 1934.

Funk, C.F. "Zur Therapie der Hauttuberkulose unter besonderer Berücksichtigung des Lupus vulgaris." *Dermat. Ztschr.* 68:87–96, Nov. 1933.

Funk, C.F. "Einflüsse der Sauerbruch-Herrmannsdorfer-Gerson-Diät auf den Effektoren-Bereich der vegetativen Neuroregulation." *Med. Klin.* 27:1139–1141, Jul. 31, 1931.

Gade, H.G. "Preliminary communication on treatment with Gerson's diet." *Med. rev., Bergen.* 46:385–399, Aug. 1929.

Gerson, M. "Eine Bromoformvergiftung." *Aerztliche Sachverständigen-Zeitung.* (Aus der innern Abteilung des Stadt. Krankenhauses im Friedrichshain zu Berlin). S. 7. 1910.

Gerson, M. "Zur Aetiologie der myasthenischen Bulbarparalyse." *Berl. Klin. Wchnschr.* 53:1364, 1916.

Gerson, M. "Über Lähmungen bei Diphtheriebazillenträgern." *Berl. Klin. Wchnschr.* 56(12):274–277, Mar. 24, 1919.

Gerson, M. "Zur Aetiologie der multiplen Sklerose." *Deutsche Ztschr. f. Nervenh., Leipz.* LXXIV. 251–259, 1922.

Gerson, M. "Über die konstitutionelle Grundlage von nervösen Krankheitserscheinungen und deren therapeutische Beeinflussung." *Fortschr. d. Med., Berl.* 42:9–11, 1922.

Gerson, M. "Die Entstehung und Begründung der Diätbehandlung der Tuberkulose." *Med. Welt.* 3:1313–1317, 1929.

Gerson, M. "Korrespondenzen. Rachitis und Tuberkulosebehandlung." *Deutsche med. Wchnschr.* 55(38):1603, Sep. 20, 1929.

Gerson, M. "Phosphorlebertran und die Gerson-Herrmannsdorfersche Diät zur Heilung der Tuberkulose." *Deutsche med. Wchnschr.* 56:478–480, Mar. 21, 1930.

Gerson, M. "Comment on Wichmann's article of December 17." *Klin. Wchnschr.* 9:693–694, Apr. 12, 1930.

Gerson, M. "Einige Ergebnisse der Gerson-Diät bei Tuberkulose." *Med. Welt.* 4:815–820, Jun. 7, 1930.

Gerson, M. "Grundsätzliche Anleitungen zur "Gerson-Diät." *Münch. med. Wochnschr.* 77:967–971, Jun. 6, 1930.

Gerson, M. *Meine Diät.* Berlin: Verlag Ullstein, 1930.

Gerson, M. "Erwiderung auf die Arbeit; Die Gründe der Ablehnung der salzlosen Diät durch die Tuberkuloseheilanstalten von Prof. O. Ziegler." *Deutsche med. Wchnschr.* 57:334–335, Feb. 20, 1931.

Gerson, M. "Einiges über die Kochsalzarme Diät." *Hippokrates.* 3:627–634, Mar. 1931.

Gerson, M. "Erwiderung auf die Arbeit C. v. Noordens 'Kritische Betrachtungen über Gerson-Diät in Besondere bei Tuberkulose.'" *Med. Klin. Wchnschr.* 45:1116–1117, Sep. 9, 1932.

Gerson, M. "Blutsenkung bei Diätbehandlung der Lungentuberkulose." *Zeitschr. f. Tuberk.* 63:327–337, 1932.

Gerson, M. "Einige Resultate der Diättherapie bei Kavernen nach vorausgegangener chirurgischen Behandlung." *Verhandl. d. deutsche Gesellsch. f. inn. Med. Kong.* 44:222–224, 1932.

Gerson, M. "Diätbehandlung bei Migräne und Lungentuberkulose." *Wiener Klin. Wchnschr.* 45:744–748, Jun. 10, 1932.

Gerson, M. "Psychische Reaktionen während der Gerson-Diät bei Lungentuberkulose." *Psychotherapeut. Praxis.* 1:206–213, Dec. 1934.

Gerson, M. *Diättherapie der Lungentuberkulose.* Leipzig and Vienna: Franz Deuticke, 1934.

Gerson, M. "Unspezifische Desensibilsierung durch Diät bei allergischen Hautkrankheiten." *Dermat. Wchnschr.* 100:441, Apr. 20, 1935.

Gerson, M. "Unspezifische Desensibilsierung durch Diät bei allergischen Hautkrankheiten." *Dermat. Wchnschr.* 100:478, Apr. 27, 1935.

Gerson, M. "Bemerkungen zum Aufsatz von Neumann Ernährung der Tuberkulösen." *Wien. Klin. Wchnschr.* 48:272–273, Mar. 1, 1935.

Gerson, M. "Rückbildung von Entzündungen bei Gerson-Diät unter besonderer Berücksichtigung der Tuberkulösen Entzündung." *Wien. Klin. Wchnschr.* 48:847–853, Jun. 21, 1935.

Gerson, M. "Anmerkung zur obigen Ausführung von W. Neumann." *Wien. Klin. Wchnschr.* 48:1069, Aug. 23, 1935.

Gerson, M.; von Weisl, W. "Lebermedikamentur bei der Diättherapie chronischer Krankheiten." *Wien. med. Wchnschr.* 85:1095–1098, Sep. 28. 1935.

Gerson, M.; von Weisl, W. "Flüssigkeitsreiche Kalidiät als Therapie bei cardiorenaler Insuffizienz." *Münch. med. Wochnschr.* 82:571–574, Apr. 11, 1935.

Gerson, M. "Feeding the German army." *New York State J. Med.* 41:1471–1476, Jul. 15, 1941.

Gerson, M. "Some aspects of the problem of fatigue." *Med. Record.* 156(6):341, 1943.

Gerson, M. "Dietary considerations in malignant neoplastic disease; preliminary report." *Rev. Gastroenterol.* 12:419–425, Nov.-Dec. 1945.

Gerson, M. "Effects of combined dietary regime on patients with malignant tumors." *Exper. Med. & Surg.* 7:299–317, Nov. 1949.

Gerson, M. "Kein Krebs bei normalem Stoffwechsel; Ergebnisse einer speziellen Therapie." *Med. Klin.* 49(5):175–179, Jan. 29, 1954.

Gerson, M. "Diet therapy in malignant diseases (cancer)." Scala, *Handbuch der Diätetik.* Vienna: Franz Deuticke, 1954.

Gerson, M. "Krebskrankheit, ein Problem das Stoffwechsels." *Med. Klin.* 49(26):1028–1032, Jun. 25, 1954.

Gerson, M. "Zur medikamentösen Behandlung Krebskranker nach Gerson." *Med. Klin.* 49(49):1977–1978, 1954.

Gerson, M. "A new therapeutical approach to cancer." *Herald of Health.* Apr. 1957.

Gerson, M. "The cure of advanced cancer by diet therapy: a summary of 30 years of clinical experimentation." *Physiol. Chem. Phys.* 10(5):449–464, 1978.

Gerson, M. A *Cancer Therapy: Results of 50 Cases.* 6th edition. Bonita, Calif.: The Gerson Institute, 1999.

Gettkant, B. "Lungentuberkulose und Gerson-Diät." *Deutsche med. Wchnschr.* 55:1789–1790, Oct. 25, 1929.

Gettkant, B. "Die Heilkostbehandlung der Tuberkulose nach Gerson." *Med. Welt.* 3:1349–1351, Sep. 21, 1929.

Gettkant, B. "Die Gerson-Diät im Lichte der Fachkritik." *Med. Welt.* 4:804–807, Jun. 7, 1930.

Gezelle Meerburg, G.F. "Gerson Herrmannsdorfer diet." *Geneesk. gids.* 8:381–392, Apr. 25, 1930.

Gibbens, J. "Gerson-Herrmannsdorfer diet; summary of recent experiences." *Brit. J. Tuberc.* 25:132–135, Jul. 1931.

Gloor, W. "Dietetic treatment of tuberculosis." *Schweiz. med. Wchnschr.* May 17, 1930.

Golin, A.; Domenighini, R. "La dieta di Gerson-Herrmannsdorfer-Sauerbruch nel trattamento della tuberculosi infantile." *Riv. di clin. pediat.* 33(3):257–300, Mar. 1935.

Grunewald, W. "Untersuchungen über den Wasser und Chlorbestand der Organe des tuberkulosekranken Menschen." *Beitr. z. Klin. d. Tuberk.* 82:189–206, 1933.

Guy, J.; Elder, H.C.; Watson, C.; Fulton, J.S. "Influence of Gerson regime on pulmonary tuberculosis." *Tr. Med. Chir. Soc. Edinburgh.* 1–20, 1932–33.

Hagedorn, K. "Vitamine und Tuberkulose. Eine kritische Besprechung der experimentellen und klinischen Ergebnisse, einschliesslich der Diäten nach Gerson und Herrmannsdorfer." *Zentralbl. f. d. ges. Tuberk.-Forsch.* 34:665, May 2, 1931.

Hagedorn, K. "Vitamine und Tuberkulose." *Zentralbl. f. d. ges. Tuberk.-Forsch.* 34:809, Jun. 27, 1931.

Haldin-Davis, H. "The dietetic treatment of lupus vulgaris." *Brit. J. Med.* 2:539, Sep. 27, 1930.

Hashimoto, M. "Über die Diätetische Behandlung der Knochentuberkulose nach Gerson, Sauerbruch und Herrmannsdorfer." *J. Orient. Med.* 13:54, Nov. 1930.

Harms; Grunewald. "Treatment of pulmonary tuberculosis with salt-free diet." *Deutsche med. Wchnschr.* 56:2–61, Feb. 14, 1930.

Henius, K. "Die wirksamen Faktoren der Gerson-Herrmannsdorfer-Diät und ein Rat zur versuchsweisen Anwendung." *Ztschr. f. Tuberk.* 55:319, 1930.

Herrmannsdorfer, A. "La influencia de una alimantación especial sobre la cicatrización de las heridas y sobre las afecciones tuberculoses graves." *Rev. méd. german.-iber.-am.* 2:677–684, Nov. 1929.

Herrmannsdorfer, A. "Über Wund- und Tuberkulose Diät." *Jahresk. f. ärztl. Fortbild.* (Hft. 8). 20:35–43, Aug. 1929.

Herrmannsdorfer, A. "Über Wund Diätetik." *Ztschr. f. ärtzl. Fortbild.* 26:580–587, Sep. 15, 1929.

Herrmannsdorfer, A. "Dietary treatment in tuberculous diseases." *Med. Klin.* 25:1235, Aug. 9, 1929.

Herrmannsdorfer, A. "Dietetic treatment before and after operation in pulmonary tuberculosis." *Ztschr. f. Tuberk.* 55: 1, Oct. 1929.

Herrmannsdorfer A. "Differences between Gerson and Herrmannsdorfer diets." *Ztschr. f. Tuberk.* 56:257, Apr. 1930.

Herrmannsdorfer, A. "Effect of sodium chloride–free diet on tuberculous process." *Ztschr. f. Tuberk.* 59:97, Dec. 1930.

Herrmannsdorfer, A. "Zehnjährige Erfahrungen mit der Ernährungs-behandlung Lungentuberkulöser. Zugleich ein Kritischer Beitrag zum gegenwärtigen Stande der Gerson-Diät." *Ztschr. f. ärtzl. Fortbild.* 32:673–678, Dec. 1, 1935.

Herrmannsdorfer, A. "Rückschau auf die mit der Sauerbruch-Herrmanns-dorfer-Gerson-Diät erzielten Ergebnisse der Tuberkulosebehand-lung." *Ztschr. f. Tuberk.* 100:316–322, 1952.

Hildenbrand, G.L.; Hildenbrand, L.C.; Bradford, K.; Cavin, S. "Five-year survival rates of melanoma patients treated by diet therapy after the manner of Gerson: a retrospective review." *Alt. Ther. in Health and Med.* 1:4:29–37, Sep. 1995.

Hindhede, M. "Gerson's tuberculosis diet." *Ugesk. f. laeger.* 91:1018–1022, Nov. 14, 1929.

Hoffschulte, F. "Ergebnisse der Gerson-Diät bei Tuberculose." *Med. Welt.* 4:928, Jun. 28, 1930.

Holm, E. "Versuche mit Gerson-Diät." *Acta Ophth.* 10:232–236, 1932.

Hval, E. "Microscopic study of capillaries of patients on Gerson-Herr-mannsdorfer-Sauerbruch diet." *Acta dermat.-venereol.* 13:593–600, Nov. 1932.

Jaffé, K. "Hämatologische Untersuchungen bei Hauttuberkulose während der Behandlung mit Gerson-Herrmannsdorfer-Sauerbruch-Diät." *Münch. med. Wochnschr.* 78:703–705, Apr. 24, 1931.

Keinung, E.; Hopf, G. "Die Bedeutung des Mineralsalzeinflusses für die pathogenische Beurteilung der Hauttuberkulose." *Dermat. Wchnschr.* 99:1397–1406, Oct. 27, 1934.

· Keinung, E.; Hopf, G. "Wirkt kochsalzzusatzfreie Diät Tuberkulose-spezifisch?" *Ztschr. f. Tuberk.* 62:352–356.

Klare, K. "Warum muss die Sauerbruch, Hermannsdorfer Gerson-Diät bei Lungentuberkulose im allegemeinen versagen?" *Deutsche med. Wchnschr.* 57:928–930, May 29, 1931.

Koehler, B. "Dietary treatment of tuberculosis." *Münch. med. Wochnschr.* 77:1832, Oct. 24, 1930.

Korvin, E. "Zur Wirkungsweise der S.H.G.-Diät, Kritik der Ausführungen de Raadts." *Wien. Klin. Wchnschr.* 45:144–146, Jan. 29,1932.

Kremer, W. "Erfahrungen mit der Gerson-Herrmannsdorfer-Diät." *Med. Welt.* 4:354–356, Mar. 15, 1930.

Kremer, W.; Cobet, G.; Frischbier, G. "Erfahrungen mit der Sauerbruch-Herrmannsdorfer-Gerson-Diät bei Lungentuberkulose." *Ztschr. f. Tuberk.* 66:185–203. 1930.

Kretz, J. "Über die Diätetische Behandlung der Lungentuberkulose nach Sauerbruch, Herrmannsdorfer und Gerson." *Wien. Klin. Wchnschr.* 42:993–995, Jul. 25, 1929.

Kulcke, E. "Die Gerson-Herrmannsdorfer-Sauerbruchsche Diät und ihre Beziehungen zur Lahmannschen Diät." *Med. Klin.* 26:196–200, Feb. 7, 1930.

Lambotte. "Le régime de Gerson dans le traitement de la tuberculose." *Liége méd.* 23:1–12, Jan. 5, 1930.

Lana Martinez, F. "La dieta de Gerson Sauerbruch en el tratamiento do las tuberculosis cutáneas." *Clín. y Lab.* 20:550–552, Jul. 1932.

Lassen, O. "Gerson, Herrmannsdorfer diet in pulmonary tuberculosis." *Ugesk. f. laeger.* 92:445–451, May 8, 1931.

Lechner, P. 1984. "Dietary regime to be used in oncological postoperative care." *Proc. Oesterreicher Gesellsch. f. Chir.* Jun. 21–23, 1984.

van Leersum, E.C. "Phosphorlebertran und die Gerson-Herrmannsdorfer-Sauerbruchsche Diät zur Behandlung der Tuberkulose." *Nederl. tijdschr. v. geneesk.* 74:2854–2864, Jun. 7, 1930.

van Leersum, E.C. "Phosphorlebertran und die Gerson, Herrmannsdorfer, Sauerbruch Diät zur Behandlung der Tuberkulose." *Münch. med. Wochnschr.* 77:975–976, Jun. 6, 1933.

Leitner, J. "Blutdruck, Blutstatus und Blutsenkung bei der Diätbehandlung der Tuberkulose nach Gerson-Sauerbruch-Herrmannsdorfer." *Beitr. z. Klin. d. Tuberk.* 78:331–336, 1931.

Levin, O.L. "The treatment of psoriasis by means of a salt-free diet." *Med. Journ. and Record.* 134(4):179, Aug. 19, 1931.

Liesenfeld, F. "Klinische Versuche und Beobachtungen mit der Diätbehandlung der Lungentuberkulose nach Sauerbruch-Herrmannsdorfer-Gerson während 11/2 Jahren." *Beitr. z. Klin. d. Tuberk.* 72:252–259, 1929.

Lorenz, G.F. "Der Kochsalzgehalt der Gersondiät. Entgegnung aus dem Diätsanatorium von Dr. Gerson, Kassel-Wilhelmshöhe." *Med. Welt.* 4(38):1362–1363, Sep. 2, 1930.

Lubich, V. "La dietoterapia della tuberculosis (Rivista sintetico-critica sulle diete Gerson-Herrmannsdorfer-Sauerbruch)." *Lotto. contro. la tuberc.* 3:245–261, Mar. 1932.

Ludy, J.B. "Cutaneous tuberculosis." *Med. Clin. North Amer.* 18(l):311–327, Jul. 1934.

Maag. "Über die Diätbehandlung chirurgischer Tuberkulose nach Sauerbruch-Herrmannsdorfer-Gerson." *Deutsche Ztschr. f. Chir.* 236:603–610, 1932.

Maendl, H.; Tscheme, K. "Beobachtungen bei der Diät nach Gerson-Sauerbruch-Herrmannsdorfer an 40 Fällen von Tuberkulose." *Tuberkulose.* 10: 132–134, Jun. 10, 1930.

Mariette, E. "The dietetic treatment of tuberculosis." *Annals of Int. Med.* 5:793–802, 1932.

Mårtensson, A. "Gerson-Sauerbruch-Herrmannsdorfer diet in treatment of tuberculosis." *Ugesk. f. laeger.* 91:1063–1066, Nov. 28, 1929.

Mathiesen, H. "Gerson's tuberculosis diet." *Ugesk. f. laeger.* 91:1066, Nov. 28, 1929.

Matz, P.B. "Gerson-Sauerbruch dietetic regimen." *U.S. Vet. Bur. M. Bull.* 6:27–32, Jan. 1930.

Mayer, E.; Kugelmass, I.N. "Basic (vitamin) feeding in tuberculosis." *J. Amer. Med. Assoc.* 93(24):1856–1862, Dec. 14, 1929.

Mayer, E. "Salt-restricted dietary with particular application to tuberculosis therapy." *J. Amer. Med. Assoc.* 97(26):1935–1939, Dec. 26, 1931.

McCarty, M. 1981. "Aldosterone and the Gerson diet—a speculation." *Med. Hypotheses.* 7:591–597, 1981.

Mecklenburg, M. "Sauerbruch-Herrmannsdorfer diet in chronic pulmonary tuberculosis." *Ztschr. f. Tuberk., Leipzig.* 57147, Jun. 1930.

Mienicki, M. "An attempt to increase the curative effect of a salt-free diet on lupus vulgaris." *Przegl. dermat.* 29:346, Sep. 1934.

Metz, G.A. "Über die therapeutische Wirkung von Lebertran, Sauerbruch-Herrmannsdorfer-Gerson-Diät und Heliotherapie bei Tuberkulose." *Deutsche med. Wchnschr.* 61:916–917, Jun. 1935.

Meyer, F. "Zur Gerson-Therapie (Medizinische Aussprache)." *Med. Welt.* 4(2)168, Jan. 11, 1930.

Meyer, M.; Irrmann, E. "Considérations sur le traitement diététique de la tuberculose d'après Sauerbruch-Herrmannsdorfer-Gerson." *Strasbourg méd.* 92:169-171, Mar. 15, 1932.

Meyer, M.; Irrmann, E. "Le Régime de Sauerbruch-Herrmannsdorfer-Gerson. Ses Bases Théoriques. Ses Résultats Dans la Tuberculose Externe." *Gaz. d. hôp.* 105(51):957–961, Jun. 25, 1932.

Meyer, M.; Irrmann, E. "Le Régime de Sauerbruch-Herrmannsdorfer-Gerson. Ses Bases Théoriques. Ses Résultats Dans la Tuberculose Externe." *Gaz. d. hôp.* 105(52):997, Jul. 2, 1932.

Michelson, H.E. "Lupus vulgaris." *Arch. Dermat. Syph.* 24:1122, 1931.

Moeller, A. "The dangers of salt withdrawal in pulmonary tuberculosis." *Deutsche med. Wchnschr.* Aug. 15, 1930.

Monzon, J. "Le régime de Gerson; un essai allemand de traitement diététique de la tuberculose pulmonaire." *Presse Méd.* 37:1251–1254, Sep. 25, 1929.

Müller, P. "Über die Behandlung der Lungentuberkulose mit salzfreier Kost und Mineralogen." *Deutsches Arch. f. klin. Med.* 158:34–41, 1927.

Münchbach, W. "Gerson-Herrmannsdorfer-Sauerbruch-Diät." *Beitr. z. Klin. d. Tuberk.* 77:395–411, 1931.

Neumann, W. "Bemerkungen zu der Arbeit von Max Gerson." *Wien. Klin. Wchnschr.* 48:1069, Aug. 23, 1935.

Noorden, C. von. "Kritische Betrachtungen über Gerson-Diät, ins Besondere bei Tuberkulose." *Med. Klin.* 28:743–748, May 27, 1932.

Noorden, C. von. "Reply to Gerson." *Med. Klin.* 28:1062–1063, Jul. 29, 1932.

Noorden, C. von. "Bemerkungen zur Gerson-Diät." *Wien. Klin. Wchnschr.* 45:708–709, Jun. 3, 1932.

Oulmann, L. "Lupus vulgaris." *Arch. Dermat. Syph.* 34:317, 1931.

Ota, M. "Erfahrungen mit der Diätbehandlung nach Gerson-Sauerbruch-Herrmannsdorfer bei Hauttuberkulose." *Jap. J. Dermat. & Urol.* 39:82–85, May 20, 1936.

Pachioli, R.; Gianni, G. "Contributo ala cura della tuberculosi polmonare del bambino medianto il trattamento dietetico di Gerson, Herrmannsdorfer, Sauerbruch." *Riv. d. pat. e clin. d. tuberc.* 5:446–469, Jun. 30, 1931.

Pachioli, R.: Gianni, G. "Richerche sull meccanismo d'azione del regime di Gerson-Herrmannsdorfer-Sauerbruch nel trattamento della affezioni tubercolari." *Riv. di clin. pediat.* 30:664–680, May 1932.

Parreidt, R. "Behandlung der Paradentose durch Diät (nach Gerson)." *Oesterreichische Zeitschr. f. Stomatol.* 27:969–972, Oct. 1929.

Pawlowski, E. "Erfahrung mit der Gerson-Herrmannsdorfer-Diät in der Behandlung der Knochen- und Gelenktuberkulose." *Deutsche med. Wchnschr.* 56:1870–1871, Oct. 31, 1930.

Pennetti, G. "La dieta de Gerson-Herrmannsdorfer-Sauerbruch nella affezioni tubercolari." *Riforma med.* 46:372–376, Mar. 10, 1930.

Pfeffer, G.; Stern, E. "Über die Wirkung der Sauerbruch-Gersonschen Diät bei Lungentuberkulose." *Beitr. z. Klin. d. Tuberk.* 67:742–747, 1927.

Pöhlmann, C. "Influence of Gerson's dietary treatment continued for four months in severe pulmonary and laryngeal tuberculosis." *Münch. med. Wochnschr.* 77:707–708, Apr. 25, 1930.

Popper, M. "Dermatoskopische Befunde bei Lichtreaktionen der Haut unter dem Einfluss Sauerbruch-Herrmannsdorfer-Gersonschen (S.H.G.) Diät." *Strahlenther.* 45:235–246, 1932.

de Raadt, O.L.E. "Gerson diet; factor responsible for curative value." *Wien. Klin. Wchnschr.* 43:752–753, Jun. 12, 1930.

Rieckenberg, H. "Gerson-Diät bei Lungentuberkulose." *Deutsche med. Wchnschr.* 56:746–747, May 2, 1930.

Ritschel, H.U. "Die Diät nach Gerson in der Behandlung der chronischen Lungentuberkulose." *Beitr. z. Klin. d. Tuberk.* 68:394–398, 1928.

Rosen, K. "Herrmannsdorfer-Gerson diet in pulmonary tuberculosis." *Svenska lak. tidning.* 28:305–316, Feb. 27, 1931.

Sachs, W. "Die salzarme Kost nach Gerson-Sauerbruch-Herrmannsdorfer in der Behandlung der Lungentuberkulose." *Beitr. z. Klin. d. Tuberk.* 73:816–824, 1930.

Santori, G. "L'alimentazione di Gerson, Sauerbruch e Herrmannsdorfer nelia cura del lupus vulgare." *Bull. e atti D.R. Accad. med. di Roma.* 56:25–29, Jan. 1930.

Sauerbruch, F.; Herrmannsdorfer, A. "Ergebnisse und Wert einer Diätetischen Behandlung der Tuberkulose." *Münch. med. Wochnschr.* 75:35–38, Jan. 6, 1928.

Sauerbruch, F. "Stellungnahme zu Gerson und Gettkant." *Med. Welt.* 3:1351, Sep. 21, 1929.

Sauerbruch, F. "Erklärung zur Ernährungsbehandlung der Tuberkulose." *Zentralbl. f. Chir.* 56:2306–2307, Sep. 14, 1929.

Sauerbruch, F. "Erklärung zur Ernährungsbehandlung der Tuberkulose." *Beitr. z. Klin. Chir.* 147:501–502, 1929.

Sauerbruch, F. "Erklärung zur Ernährungsbehandlung der Tuberkulose." *Deutsche Ztschr. f. Chir.* 219:381–382, 1929.

Sauerbruch, F. "Erklärung zur Ernährungsbehandlung der Tuberkulose." *Med. Klin.* 25:1272, Aug. 9, 1929.

Sauerbruch, F. "Erklärung zur Ernährungsbehandlung der Tuberkulose." *Deutsche. med. Wchnschr.* 55:1391–1392, Aug. 16, 1929.

Sauerbruch, F. "Erklärung zur Ernährungsbehandlung der Tuberkulose." *Münch. med. Wochnschr.* 76:1363, Aug. 16, 1929.

Sauerbruch, F. "Erklärung zur Ernährungsbehandlung der Tuberkulose." *Zentralbl. f. inn. Med.* 50:802, Aug. 31, 1929.

Sauerbruch, F. "Erklärung zur Ernährungsbehandlung der Tuberkulose." *Chirurg.* 1:933, Sep. 1, 1929.

Sauerbruch, F. "Erklärung zur Ernährungsbehandlung der Tuberkulose." *Med. Welt.* 3:1351, Sep. 21, 1929.

Sauerbruch, F. "Ein Klärendes Wort zur ablehnenden Kritik der Ernährungsbehandlung der Tuberkulose." *Münch. med. Wochnschr.* 77:1829-1832, 1930.

Schade, H., Beck, A.; Reimers, C. "Physiochemical study of action of acid food in wound healing: effect of Gerson diet on wound healing." *Zentralbl. f. Chir.* Leipzig 57:1077, 1930.

Schedtler, O. "Wirkt kochsalzusatzfreie Diät Tuberkulose-spezifisch? Bemerkungen zu der Arbeit von Keining und Hopf." *Ztschr. f. Tuberk.* 63:337–338, 1932.

Scheurlen, F.; Orlowitsch-Wolk, A. "Vitamin therapy of pulmonary tuberculosis." *Münch. med. Wochnschr.* 77:976, Jun. 6, 1930.

Schiller, W. "Zur Frage der Kochsalzarmen Kost nach Sauerbruch-Herrmannsdorfer-Gerson bei Tuberkulose." *Tuberkulose.* 9:70–74, Apr. 1929.

Schlammadinger, J. "Gerson-Herrmannsdorfer-Sauerbruch diet in treatment of tuberculosis and chronic diseases of the skin." *Orvosi hetil.* 74:954–957, Sep. 20, 1930.

Schlammadinger, J.; Szép, E. "Erfahrungen mit der Gerson-Sauerbruch-Herrmannsdorferschen Diät bei einigen tuberkulösen und anderen entzündlichen Dermatosen." *Med. Klin.* 27:508–510, Apr. 2, 1931.

Schlesinger, W. "Die Gerson-Herrmannsdorfer-Sauerbruchsche Tuberkulose Diät." *Wien. med. Wchnschr.* 80:587–589, Apr. 26, 1930.

Schmiedeberg, H. "Herrmannsdorfer diet in tuberculosis in children." *Monatsschr. f. Kndrheilk.* 48:230, Oct. 1930.

Schmitz, H. "Über die Gersonsche Diät bei Lungentuberkulose." *Ztschr. f. Tuberk.* 47:461, 1927.

Schrick, F.G. van. "Haut und Knochentuberkulose unter dem Einfluss der Sauerbruch-Herrmannsdorfer-Gerson-Diät." *Ztschr. f. Orthop. Chir.* 61:388–394, 1934.

Schroeder, M.G. "Modern dietetic problems in treatment of the tuberculous." *Journal of State Med., London.* 39:435, Aug. 1931.

Schwalm, E. "Erfahrungen mit der Gerson-Diät bei Lungentuberkulose." *Klin. Wchnschr.* 8:1941–1943, Oct. 15, 1929.

Scolari, E. "Osservazioni cliniche e richerche sperimentali sulla dieta di Sauerbruch-Herrmannsdorfer-Gerson nella affezion cutanea." *Gior. ital. di dermat. e sif.* 76:665–701, Jun. 1935.

Sellei, J. "Gerson diet in treatment of skin diseases." *Gyogyaszat.* 70:453–454, Jun. 8, 1930.

Sliosberg, A. "Le traitement de la tuberculose par la méthode de Gerson." *Rev. do. phtisiol. méd. soc.* 10:564–574, Nov.-Dec. 1929.

Sossi, O. "Sulla cura dietetica di Sauerbruch-Herrmannsdorfer nella tuberculosi pulmonare." *Riv. di clin. med.* 30:1124–1149, Oct. 31, 1929.

Sprigge, S.; Moriand, E. eds. "Dietary treatment of tuberculosis." *The Lancet.* 217(2):404, Aug. 24, 1929.

Sprigge, S.; Morland, E. eds. "Dietary principles in tuberculosis." *The Lancet.* 217(2):617, Sep. 21, 1929.

Sprigge, S.; Morland, E. eds. "The Gerson diet for tuberculosis." *The Lancet.* 218(l):1415, Jun. 28, 1930.

Sprigge, S.; Moriand, E. eds. "Dietetic therapeutics of tuberculosis of the skin." *The Lancet.* 219(2):311, 1930.

Sprigge, S.; Moriand, E. eds. "Dietetic treatment of tuberculosis of the skin." *The Lancet.* 220(l):610, Mar. 14, 1931.

Sprigge, S.; Moriand, E. eds. "The Gerson diet for dermatoses." *The Lancet.* 220(l):1201, May 30, 1931.

Sprigge, S.; Morland, E. eds. "The Gerson diet." *The Lancet.* 220(l):1366–1367, Jun. 20, 1931.

Sprigge, S.; Morland, E. eds. "The Gerson diet." *The Lancet.* 222(l):629, Mar. 19, 1932.

Sprigge, S.; Morland, E. eds. "The diet of Gerson." *The Lancet.* 222(l):708, Mar. 26, 1932.

Starcke, H. "Erfahrung mit der salzlosen Diät nach Gerson und Herrmannsdorfer bei Kindern und Jungendlichen." *Beitr. z. Klin. d. Tuberk.* 74:61–88, 1930.

Stein, H. "Erfahrung mit Diätkuren bei der Lungentuberkulose." *Ztschr. f. Tuberk.* 58:426–431, 1930.

Strauss, H. "Dietary treatment in pulmonary tuberculosis." *Med. Klin.* 25:1383, Sep. 6, 1929.

Strauss, H. "Diät als Heilfaktor." *Med. Welt.* 4 (6):171–175, Feb. 8, 1930.

Stub-Christensen. "Dietetics and tuberculosis, with especial regard to calcium metabolism and to significance of vitamins." *Hospitalsitdende, Copenhagen.* 74:157, Feb. 5, 1931.

Stumpf, R. "Case of lupus vulgaris treated by Roentgen therapy and Gerson diet." *Irish J. Med. Sci.* 254–257, Jun. 1930.

Stumpke, G.; Mohrmann, B.H.U. "Dietary therapy of lupus and other skin diseases." *Med. Klin.* 27:235, Feb. 13, 1931.

Sylla, A.; Schone, G. "Zur Ernährungsbehandlung der Lungentuberkulose nach Sauerbruch-Herrmannsdorfer-Gerson (S.H.G.)." *Beitr. z. Klin. d. Tuberk.* 78:678–696, 1931.

Symposium. "Die Bedeutung der von Sauerbruch, Herrmannsdorfer und Gerson angegebenen Diät bei der Behandlung der Tuberkulose." *Veröffentl. a.d. Geb. d. Med.-Verwalt.* 32:541–632, 1930.

Szold, E. "Treatment of tuberculosis of the urinary tract with the Sauerbruch-Herrmannsdorfer-Gerson diet." *Orvosi hetil.* 75:1130–1132, Nov. 21, 1931.

Tesdal, M. "Die Diät von Gerson-Herrmannsdorfer-Sauerbruch und deren Einwirkung auf den Stoffwechsel." *Ztschr. f. klin. Med.* 121:184–193, 1932.

Tesdal, M. "Effect of Gerson-Herrmannsdorfer-Sauerbruch diet on metabolism in tuberculosis." *Norsk. mag. f. laegevidensk.* 93:1073–1082, Oct. 1932.

Timpano, P. "La dietoterapia e la radiumterapia del lupus vulgaris." *Rinasc. med.* 10:184–185, Apr. 15, 1933.

Traub, E.F. "A Case for diagnosis (tuberculosis)." *Arch. Dermat. Syph.* 30:592–593, 1934.

Unverricht. "The influence of an unsalted diet upon the gastric secretion, and the clinical use of such diet." *Deutsche med. Wchnschr.* Aug. 4, 1933.

Urbach, E. *Skin Diseases and Nutrition, including the Dermatoses of Children.* Trans. F.R. Schmidt. Vienna: Wilhelm Maudrich, 1932.

Urbach, E. 1946. *Skin Diseases, Nutrition, and Metabolism.* New York: Grune and Stratton, 1946.

Varela, B.; Recarte, P.; Esculies, J. "Sauerbasengleich und ionisiertes Kalzium im Blute der Tuberkulösen und ihre Veränderungen bei Mineral Diättherapie nach Sauerbruch-Herrmannsdorfer-Gerson." *Ztschr. f. Tuberk.* 57:380–390, 1930.

Valagussa, F. "La cura dietetica della tuberculosi medianti il metodo Gerson-Herrmannsdorfer-Sauerbruch." *Bull. e. atti d. r. Acad. med. di Roma.* 56:15–24, Jan. 1930.

Van Kampen, F. "De Gerson-Therapie." *Nederlands Tijdschrift voor Integrale Geneeskunde.* 8:53–57, 1985.

Van Kampen, F. "De Theorie van de Gersonbehandeling." *Nederlands Tijdschrift voor Integrale Geneeskunde.* 10:199–204, 1985.

Vaucher, E.; Grunwald, E. "Le Traitement diététique de la Tuberculose Pulmonaire, Revue critique sur les travaux de G-S-H." *Paris méd.* 1:25–30, Jan. 4, 1930.

Volk, R. "Therapie des Lupus vulgaris und die Gerson-Diät." *Wien. Klin. Wchnschr.* 43:1461–1466, Nov. 27, 1930.

Volk, R. "Zur Diättherapie von Hautkrankheiten." *Dermat. Wchnschr.* 91:1869–1873, Dec. 20, 1931.

Volk, R. "La dieta sin sal según Sauerbruch-Herrmannsdorfer-Gerson en la tuberculosis extrapulmonar." *Rev. mex. de. tuberc.* 2:5–23, Jan.–Feb. 1940.

Watson, C. "Gerson diet for tuberculosis." *The Lancet.* 218(2):161, Jul. 19, 1930.

Watson, C. "Gerson treatment of tuberculosis." *Brit. Med. J.* 2:284–285, Aug. 23, 1930.

Watson, C. "Diet and nutrition with special reference to the Sauerbruch-Herrmannsdorfer-Gerson diet." *Med. Press.* 130:207–209, Sep. 10, 1930.

Watson, C. "The 'vital' factor in diet: a theory of the nature of vitamins." *Edinburgh Med. J.* 38:91–104, Jan.–Dec. 1931.

Watson, C. "The 'vital' factor in diet." *Nature.* 128:154, Jul. 25, 1931.

Watson, C. "The Gerson regime in pulmonary tuberculosis: with a note on the radiological findings by Dr. J.S. Fulton." *Trans. Med.-Chir. Soc. Edinburgh.* pp. 6–20, Nov. 1932.

Weisl, N. von. "Einiges über die praktische Durchführung der Gerson-Diät." *Fortschr. d. Med.* 53:185–188, Mar. 11, 1935.

White, C.J. "Lupus vulgaris (treated by Gerson diet). Lupus erythematosus?" *Archiv. Dermat. Syph.* 24:323–324, 1931.

White, C.J. "Tuberculosis of the skin." *Illinois Med. J.* 6:1215–1218, Jul.–Dec. 1931.

Wichmann, P. "Über die Beeinflussung der Hauttuberkulose durch die Diät nach Gerson." *Beitr. z. Klin. d. Tuberk.* 66:464, 1928.

Wichmann, P. "Ergebnisse der Diätbehandlung der Hauttuberkulose." *Klin. Wchnschr.* 8:2366–2368, Dec. 17, 1929.

Wichmann, P. "Reply to Gerson." *Klin. Wchnschr.* 9:694, Apr. 12, 1930.

Wichmann, P. "Verschlimmerung von Haut- und Schleimhauttuberkulose durch Gerson-Diät." *Beitr. a. Klin. d. Tuberk.* 73:825–828, 1930.

Wichmann, P. "Ergebnisse der Gerson-Sauerbruch-Herrmannsdorfer-Diät-Behandlung bei Haut- und Schleimhauttuberkulose." *Beitr. a. Klin. d. Tuberk.* 75:100–103, 1930.

Wise, O. "Erfahrungen mit der 'Diätbehandlung nach Gerson-Herrmannsdorfer-Sauerbruch' bei verschiedenen Tuberkulose Formen des Kindesalters." *Ztschr. f. Kinderh.* 51:119–126, May 1931.

Wohlfarth. "Erfahrungen mit HGS-Diät bei Lungentuberkulose." *Ztschr. f. ärtzl. Fortbild.* 29:559–563, Sep. 15, 1932.

Wolff-Eisner, A. "Die Gerson Sauerbruch Tuberkulose Diät im Urteil der Fachkritik." *Beitr. z. Klin. d. Tuberk.* 73:829–834, 1930.

Zelinka, J. "Gerson-Herrmannsdorfer-Sauerbruch diet in therapy of osseous tuberculosis." *Casop. lék. cesk.* 71:357, Mar. 18, 1932.

Ziegler, O. "Die Gründe der Ablehnung der salzlosen Diät durch die Tuberkuloseheilanstalten." *Deutsche med. Wchnschr.* 57:11–13, Jan. 2, 1931.

INDEX